D1483320

Shining a Light on Stuttering:

How One Man Used Comedy to Turn his

Impairment into Applause

Dale F. Williams, Ph.D.

Jaik Campbell, M.Sc. by Research

Published by The Brainary® Australia and The Brainary® LLC United States of America.
Registered Office: 45 Pakington Street Geelong West 3218 Victoria Australia
www.thebrainary.com info@thebrainary.com
First published by The Brainary® April 18, 2016

ISBN: **978-0-9873476-2-6 (pbk)**
ISBN: **978-0-9873476-3-3 (e-Book)**

Title copyright: Shining a Light on Stuttering: How One Man Used Comedy to Turn his Impairment into Applause ©2016
Authors: Dale F. Williams, Ph.D. & Jaik Campbell, M.Sc.
Illustrations: Alberto Verdejo, 2016 www.sikk.cl

This publication is a textbook developed for students studying the field of Speech-Language Pathology and in particular the speech disorder known as stuttering. This textbook is not a substitute for professional advice and treatment, and should not be used as a substitute.

British Library Cataloguing in Publication Data
Title copyright: Shining a Light on Stuttering: How One Man Used Comedy to Turn his Impairment into Applause©2016
Authors: Dale F. Williams, Ph.D. & Jaik Campbell, M.Sc.
Illustrations: Alberto Verdejo, 2016 www.sikk.cl

ISBN:978-0-9873476-2-6 (pbk)
ISBN: 978-0-9873476-3-3 (e-Book)

National Library of Australia Cataloguing-in-Publication entry
Title: Shining a Light on Stuttering: How One Man Used Comedy to Turn his Impairment into Applause
Authors: Authors: Dale F. Williams, Ph.D. & Jaik Campbell, M.Sc.
Illustrations: Alberto Verdejo, 2016 www.sikk.cl

ISBN: **978-0-9873476-2-6 (pbk)**
ISBN: **978-0-9873476-3-3 (e-Book)**

Target Audience: Tertiary Students

Subjects: Stuttering, Speech disorders, Speech-language pathology

Praise for Shining a Light on Stuttering

The message from Jaik Campbell that stuttering and stand-up can be mutually beneficial is powerful and positive, and an encouragement and inspiration to stutterers and non-stutterers alike.

Michael Palin, Comedian, Actor and Writer

Jaik Campbell and Dale Williams offer a unique textbook on stuttering based on the collaboration of an autobiographer and an educator. Jaik's life story of stuttering and development to successful comedian is inspiring to the reader. As our human interest in the challenges he faces grows with each new chapter, so does the desire to understand the whys and hows of stuttering and what it takes to overcome it. Here, Dale's extensive knowledge, research, and clinical experience provides understanding and wisdom as he discusses Jaik's narrative. His chapter discussion questions are the best I've seen – thought provoking, relevant, and practical. This text is appropriate for students, practicing clinicians, family members, and people who stutter no matter where they are on their own journey.

Diane Constantino, Clinical Associate Professor and Director of the Fluency Center at Boston University
Chair, American Board of Fluency and Fluency Disorders 2010-2014

Jaik Campbell is not a typical stutterer, and that's part of the value of this book. There's no such thing as a "typical" stutterer because stuttering is a highly individual disorder: intensely personal for those of us who stutter and a complex puzzle for clinicians. Campbell's personal story, interspersed with Dale Williams' professional perspective, should be required reading for speech-language pathologists and will resonate with people who stutter.

Although Campbell's story is unique, the impact of stuttering on his life is something every person who stutters will recognize. Those who are struggling with stuttering can learn from his personal journey of coming to terms with himself and taking risks with his speech.

Campbell's narrative will give clinicians insight into the experience of people who stutter, while Williams' chapters provide a solid background of research findings and clinical expertise.

James A. McClure, Author, Advisory board member, National Stuttering Association

---

This book provides insight into the mind of a person who stutters while providing those readers a wonderful education about stuttering. The authors show their open-mindedness, along with their own humility, by presenting information about stuttering without pushing the reader. Instead, the link between Jaik's journey with stuttering and what the field of stuttering has found is presented seamlessly in a manner that encourages the reader to keep their eyes glued to the pages.

Scott Palasik, Assistant Professor and Director of the Mindfulness Behaviors ACT and Social Cognition Stuttering Lab, University of Akron

---

The organization of the book is indeed novel. Jaik writes very well, with a welcome and appropriate sense of humor. In other words, the medium he is using is a good match for his message. Both fit with each other. He is showing the personal side of stuttering and conveying to an audience the human aspect of the disorder.

David A. Shapiro, Robert Lee Madison Distinguished Professor, Western Carolina University. Author of Stuttering Intervention: A Collaborative Journey to Fluency Freedom

---

Dr. Williams does an excellent job bridging the personal and the scientific in his book *Shining a Light on Stuttering: How one man used comedy to turn his impairment into applause.* Many times books about stuttering written by professionals in academia leave out the real experiences of people who stutter. Juxtaposing the story of Jaik Campbell alongside research is a brilliant way to make the research come to life. The book seems ideal for the classes that discuss stuttering for this reason. I don't think a non-PWS could have done this good of a job with the integration of all aspects of stuttering.

Nina G, Comedian, Disability Advocate, Author, and Educator

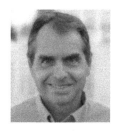

Dale F. Williams, Ph.D., CCC-SLP, BCS-F is a Professor of Communication Sciences and Disorders at Florida Atlantic University, where he also serves as Director of the Fluency Clinic. In addition, he is a consultant for Language Learning Intervention and Professional Speech Services.

He completed his bachelor's degree at Alma College, his master's at the University of Oklahoma Health Science Center, and his doctorate at Southern Illinois University. A Board Certified Specialist in Fluency since 1999, Dr. Williams served as Chair of the Specialty Board on Fluency Disorders for three years.

His publications are primarily in the area of fluency disorders and include the books *Stuttering Recovery: Personal and Empirical Perspectives* and *Communication Sciences and Disorders: An Introduction to the Professions* (Psychology Press).

A person who stutters, Dr. Williams coordinated the stuttering support group that has met on the FAU campus since 1996. He lives in Boynton Beach with his wife Misty, sons Brennan and Blaine, daughters Cayley and Caysey, and a wide variety of pets.

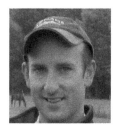

Jaik Campbell (BSc, MSc by Research) is a British stand-up comedian, writer and was an Edinburgh Fringe Festival regular between 2001 and 2008.

He completed his bachelor's degree in geography at Bristol University and his master's at Edinburgh University, but following various unfulfilling office jobs he decided to follow his dream of becoming a stand-up comedian.

After a few years on the London comedy circuit, he performed stand-up at prestigious venues such as The Comedy Store, Banana Cabaret and Headliners, appeared on BBC and ITV television, and reached the finals of several UK comedy competitions. He also campaigns for maintaining UK speech and language therapy services, early intervention for children and is a strong supporter of the British Stammering Association. He now lives and works in rural Suffolk, in the east of England, with his partner Jennifer, his two young children, Angus and Emma, a cat and ten chickens.

To speech-language pathologists and comedians everywhere. May your skills and dedication be supported by those who most benefit from them.

Acknowledgments

If we acknowledge people chronologically, we should begin with Sir Tim Berners-Lee, the inventor of the World Wide Web. Without Sir Tim's efforts, it is unlikely that a British comedian, an American professor, an Australian publisher, and a Chilean artist would have ever found one another.

Back in 2007 or so, the professor had an idea: base a stuttering book on one interesting subject. Over the ensuing years, however, he and five different graduate assistants (GAs) at Florida Atlantic University were unable to find a high profile individual who stuttered and was willing to take part. Then in January of 2012, a GA sent the following note, "I emailed a British stand-up comedian who stutters named Jaik Campbell and he said he would be interested in your project. Would he work for what you are looking for?" So if we keep the list sequential, we should next thank Jamie Heidenreich, the graduate assistant in question.

After that would be Hugh Kingsley, Managing Director of The Brainary, who responded enthusiastically to our unusual proposal and, over time, offered guidance, wisdom, and insight into the process, as well as patience with our many questions. In addition to Hugh, we would like to thank everyone at The Brainary for the help they provided.

Before we get off the topic of GAs, those who followed Jamie deserve mention for the many hours of research and summarizing they cheerfully completed. Their names are Krystal Garzon, Danielle Battaglia, Connelly Thompson, and Krystal Archibald.

Although mentioned once, we want to specifically thank Alberto Verdejo for the wonderful artwork. And author Jim McClure for his help with the title.

In addition to the formal reviewers cited on and within the book covers, we greatly appreciate the constructive comments and editorial suggestions we received from Joe Klein, Judith Maginnis Kuster, Paul Brocklehurst, and Phil Zimmerman.

We wish to also acknowledge our families for keeping us grounded during the years of writing, reading, and editing, and for putting up with some grumpiness during the darker days of this project. Alphabetically, they include Angus Campbell, Blaine Williams, Brennan Williams, Cayley Williams, Caysey Williams, Emma Campbell, Jenn Humphreys, and Misty Williams.

Our extended families also provided kind support over the years. Thanks in particular to Jaik's parents, Caroline and Christopher, whose energy and drive is astonishing, and to Dale's—Christel and Dale L.—who will place a copy of this book on their coffee table for all to see.

And finally, we acknowledge all those who stutter. May your world give you the patience, understanding, and respect that you all deserve.

Notes to Readers:

The odd-numbered chapters are a first-person account of the life of stand-up comedian Jaik Campbell. The even ones, as well as the Questions for Discussion at the end of every chapter, were written by Dale Williams. Because of this unique organization, stuttering topics do not follow any conventional order but, rather, are addressed as Jaik raises them. The Questions were designed to provoke thought in readers and inspire conversation among clients, support group attendees, and students.

It is our hope that Jaik's story brings you knowledge about stuttering while at the same time placing a human face on (and inspiring research about) this difficult disorder.

Table of Contents

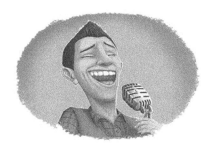

Chapter 1: Stand-Up Britain

Until the day my first child was born, I viewed Friday 18th October 2002 as the scariest, riskiest, and craziest day of my life. I was backstage with six other acts, all, like me, finalists in *Stand-Up Britain*, television's hunt for the best stand-up comedian in the United Kingdom.

All seven of us shared a variety of concerns common to stand-up: hecklers, running short of good material, forgetting lines, and, of course, rejection from the audience. Along with these worries, however, I had an additional one: I could get horribly stuck on a word.

You see, I have a stutter.

When I was younger, to stutter in front of anyone was very embarrassing. Now I was likely to do so in front of an entire nation. The speech therapy I received in my 20's had stressed the benefits of desensitization to listener reactions. Good thing, because I was about to experience the most desensitizing moment of my life!

When it was my turn—*to go on national TV!*--I remember standing behind a screen at the edge of the stage, waiting for MC Ed Byrne to introduce me. Once he did, I would perform my three minutes in front of a live audience, as well as 2 or 3 million television viewers.

I took some solace in knowing that I had a reasonably funny script, with material tried and tested in about 150 comedy club gigs. And I had survived an initial heat in front of network TV judges, and then a second one before a live audience, which was later televised and judged by a public telephone vote. On top of all that, we'd had a rehearsal earlier that day, which had gone well.

Still, I understood the stakes involved. Stand-up comedy requires laughter (and lots of it) and the rehearsal had been without an audience. What if the crowd gave me the same reaction—silence—that the empty studio had?

About a week before the event, I had contacted my friend Michael Knighton, who ran a comedy course I had attended two years prior. Michael told me that it was important to look as though I were enjoying myself on stage. He also told me to repeatedly visualise the gig going well, because having an optimistic visual approach often leads to positive outcomes. I thought about this advice during the days leading up to the final.

The day of the show was both exciting and tense. I had to arrive at the studio 11 hours before airtime. That's a great deal of time to spend with competitors. Despite the usual comradery that exists among comedians, conversation prior to this event was a bit strained. It was probably fortunate that the time was filled with rehearsal, hair and costume checks, and a comforting chicken and chip meal in the Granada Studios canteen. It was whilst I was eating that I first focused on what I would be doing that night and nearly became sick thinking about it. It's one thing waiting to perform in a comedy club, but quite another anticipating three minutes on live TV with all your family and friends watching, as well as competing for a £7000 prize.

Ninety minutes or so before the show, I remember drinking some lager and thinking it would either make me fall asleep or help my performance. Half an hour later, things started getting manic. Runners were making sure we were all ready and producers were giving last-minute instructions—mostly telling us not to swear excessively (even spelling out which words were most offensive). Then there were final hair and make-up checks. The show was about to start and the atmosphere became electric, with a hyped up studio audience and seven acts nervously waiting in the wings, desperately rehearsing their lines.

I knew I had to walk on stage confidently, without the appearance of anxiety. The lager helped with that. But I also had to tell the jokes. I had performed my routine so often in London comedy clubs that I was confident about remembering the lines. That, of course, was only half the battle. I also had to get the words out of my mouth. As usual, I had written a script full of words I could say fluently. I know this is a form of avoiding stuttering (i.e., basically the opposite of desensitization), but old habits die hard.

Although I worried about stuttering during my stand-up acts, it was, strangely, never as much of an issue then as during normal conversation. Even today, words that are typically difficult for me to say come out easier when I do comedy. Maybe performing allows me to escape from my internal image of a person who stammers. Or maybe I feel less exposed than when I have to choose words on the fly. That is, I don't have to think as much when the words are scripted, which reduces my risk of stuttering due to the mental indecisiveness[1]. When the material is right, in fact, I almost forget that I am about to walk out in front of a group of strangers and try and make them laugh. I know I'm funny and the audience will soon know it too.

Show Time

In all honesty, when I walked on stage for the televised *Stand-Up Britain* final, I was thinking not so much "I know I'm funny and the audience will soon know it too" but, rather, "This had better work!" Fortunately, the opening joke—*I went to my hairdresser and asked, "What have you got for my hair?" He said, "Extreme sympathy"*—received a good laugh from the audience. Many comedians say the first laugh is the most important one, as you then can judge how energetic and responsive the audience will be to the rest of the performance. With that in mind, I relaxed a bit.

Less than a minute into the set, the first stutter appeared, a tense repetition that happened right on the punch line. This was followed a few seconds later by a prolonged /w/ (also on the most important word of the joke). I was prepared for this, having written some stuttering material. My hope was that the audience would accept this new feature, stay relaxed, and not be turned off by it. I didn't want people to think that I was stuttering due to nerves or that I was faking it for a cheap laugh. "I've got a slight stutter," I said. Not a great start, especially when you've only got three minutes on live TV!"

Fortunately, the audience liked that line. Then I told them good night, "not because I am about to leave, but because I'm going to run out of time at the end so I had better say that now." This joke also got a big laugh.

1   Here and throughout the book, Jaik speculates about various issues related to stuttering. How his individual conclusions compare to general research findings will be addressed in the even numbered chapters. (Footnote by Dale Williams.)

I was pleasantly surprised how positively the audience reacted to the mention of my stutter. Given how I routinely avoid words that might trigger it, I found myself in the unique position of being open about my stutter at a time I had hoped to hide it.

Based on the applause at the completion of my routine, I did pretty well that night. I didn't win, but I believe I came across as someone who was relaxed, funny, and enjoying his three minutes of live TV. I also believe that I showed the viewers at home that someone with a stutter can perform well in the final of a national stand-up comedy competition!

After the Show

It took me quite a long time to mentally get over the *Stand-Up Britain* final. I'm not exactly sure why, but I think one reason was the stress of performing on national television. Even without a stutter, that sort of pressure can be quite immense, especially for someone with no formal drama or TV training. Along with the stress of the event, however, was the self-scrutiny once it was completed. I tend to over-analyse, but it dawned on me afterwards that, had my act gone badly, I would have embarrassed not only myself but also many who knew me. Truth be told, while I did get laughs, I was not as accomplished a stand-up comedian then as I am now. I was later annoyed with myself for not having funnier gags (something I am still trying to rectify over a decade later).

My long-term aims following this experience were to have a totally brilliant routine that would work on TV and to keep talking about stuttering, as I think the public still has much to learn and accept about it.

If nothing else, I would like people to realize that the "stutterer[2] stereotype"[2] (i.e., that people who stutter are passive, shy, and basically afraid of life) is wrong. We are just normal people who have slight problems talking.

Looking back, I'm almost pleased I didn't win that *Stand-Up Britain* final. For one thing, I learn more from flawed gigs. At the brilliant routines, comedians entertain and everyone loves them. But the lesser performance forces self-reflection, wondering why people did not find it hilarious. From mediocre gigs, comedians discover what needs to improve.

Just as important, however, the final put me on the road to desensitization and greater acceptance of my stuttering. At last I was being open about it. At school, university, and work, I had gone to great lengths to cover it up. Now people pay to hear me talk about it.

That may be the biggest reward of all.

---

2   Most professionals in the field prefer person-first language, i.e. *people who stutter* and not *stutterer*. Likewise, this text will typically (but not exclusively) use person-first designations. Most exceptions will be for the terms *stutterer stereotype* and *non-stutterer*, as these remain commonplace within the stuttering literature. (Footnote by Dale Williams.)

Questions for Discussion

What is your version of *Stand-Up Britain*, that is, the "scariest, risk-iest, and craziest" situation you have been in? What were you feel-ing? If you stutter, how did that impact the situation? If you do not, how would having a stutter have changed it?

How do you rate public speaking in terms of anxiety? Explain your rating.

For people who stutter, their speech is rarely a joking matter. Why did Jaik's jokes about his disorder get laughs?

Jaik stated the he learns "more from flawed gigs" than successful ones. Can you think of a skill that you obtained via much failure? Is there an application of this idea to treatment of people who stutter?

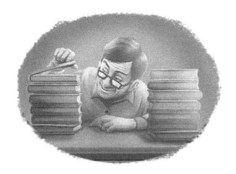

Chapter 2: Introducing Stuttering

Jaik introduces the topic of stuttering with two key phrases, "horribly stuck on a word" and "very embarrassing." Although there is no uniform definition of stuttering, nearly all include speaking disruptions in the forms of prolonged or repeated speech units and/or tense hesitations (e.g., Logan, 2014; Prasse & Kikano, 2008)—the "horribly stuck" part. For people who stutter, however, the disorder is far more than breakdowns of speech. As we will see, it is also filled with anxiety[1] and emotions, including, yes, embarrassment (to name but a few additional components).

The traits that normally define stuttering are:

- *Part-word repetitions*

  o Sound repetitions (buh-buh-buh-ball)

_____

1   Stuttering is frequently associated with anxiety (e.g., Manning & Beck, 2013; Murray & Edwards, 1994), yet the term is often left undefined in the stuttering literature. When attempts at definition are made, they are inconsistent (see Craig, 2014, for discussion). Throughout the book, we will use Barlow's (2000) definition of anxiety as a chronic, unpleasant state of inner turmoil, uneasiness, and apprehension

- Syllable repetitions (may-may-may-may-maybe)

- *Prolongations* (mmmmmine)

- *Tense hesitations* (My name is…Jaik)

Typically, these disfluencies are associated with above average duration[2] and tension. That is, with stuttering, there tends to be noticeable struggle to produce some speech sounds.

A question that often arises during explanations of stuttering is: Don't these disfluencies happen to everybody? The answer, of course, is yes. However, they can still be used to define the disorder because of fundamental differences in how and when they occur.

- The stuttering disfluencies defined above are observed almost ten times as often with children who stutter than with those who do not (Ambrose & Yairi, 1999; Logan & LaSalle, 1999; Yairi, 1997).

- Stuttering disfluencies make up about three-quarters of the total disfluency of children diagnosed as stuttering; for non-stuttering children, the majority of breakdowns are interjections ("um," "ah," "you know," "like") and revisions ("Let's—we are all going") (Yairi, 1997).

- The repetitions of non-stuttering speakers typically include 1-2 iterations—most often one, based on the average of 1.13 found by Yairi and Ambrose (2005). Sounds or sylla-

---

2   Research (e.g., Throneburg & Yairi, 2001) has typically found mean stuttering-like disfluency durations under 1.0 seconds, although individual breakdowns can last 20 seconds or longer.

bles are usually repeated 2 to 5 times in children identified as stuttering (Van Riper, 1982).

- The iterations of stuttering children are produced more quickly than those of their non-stuttering peers (Throneberg & Yairi, 1994).

It is important to remember that there are numerous exceptions to these data. For example, it is not a given that the core disfluencies of repetitions, prolongations, and hesitations will be the primary speech characteristics of all people diagnosed with stuttering (Einarsdóttir & Ingham, 2005). Moreover, they are not even required for a speech sample to be judged as stuttered. To this point, Hegde and Hartman (1979) found that excessive single-unit repetitions or interjections are identified as stuttering by common listeners. Taking these findings into account, it appears that attempts to define stuttering by its primary characteristics may not completely capture what listeners reflexively identify as stuttered speech when they hear it.

In addition to the core disfluencies, most definitions (e.g., Prasse & Kikano, 2008; World Health Organization, 2010) make mention of *secondary* (or *associated*) *behaviors*, which consist of actions designed to avoid or escape stuttering. Jaik mentioned his use of these behaviors (specifically, substituting easier words for those difficult to say) and they will be addressed in greater detail later in this chapter. I mention them now to make the point that the visible portion of stuttering is actually quite small relative to the entire disorder. Nearly everyone who stutters has heard the iceberg analogy (Sheehan, 1997) characterizing stuttering as an impairment that exists primarily below the surface. There is certainly truth to that idea. Think about it: Who has the bigger problem—Jaik, who gets stuck repeatedly while performing successful comedy routines, or the person who stutters far less often, yet avoids life aspirations that involve speaking?

Along with the stuttering disfluencies and behaviors secondary to them, there are characteristics that are often associated with the disorder. Examples include *word repetitions* and *phrase repetitions.* That is to say, words and phrases are repeated more often by people who stutter than those who do not (Ambrose & Yairi, 1999; La-Salle & Conture, 1995), yet these speech discontinuities are rarely used to define stuttering. Although one syllable words can be viewed as another type of syllable repetition, repetitions of multiple syllables (be they words or phrases) are more difficult to explain. The reasons they are not typically listed as defining behaviors are that:

> 1) Although they occur more frequently in the speech of those who stutter, their overall frequency is nevertheless so small that their impact on speech is considered negligible (Yairi, 1997),
>
> 2) Listeners tend not to identify these disfluencies as stuttering (Williams & Kent, 1958; Zebrowski & Conture, 1989), and
>
> 3) They are sometimes used as secondary behaviors. To wit, if Jaik feared stuttering on his name (a common occurrence with people who stutter), he might utilize voluntary phrase repetitions to "launch" himself past the feared word: "My name is, my name is, my name is, my name is Jaik." In such an instance, the problem word—*Jaik*—is the only one *not* repeated, yet it is the source of the disfluency.

Some stuttering trends are based on oral reading. For example, *adaptation* is the tendency for stuttering to decrease across successive readings of the same passage (Max & Baldwin, 2010). The average decrease in frequency of words stuttered is about 50% over five readings, after which the frequency more or less plateaus (Johnson et al., 1967). *Consistency* is the tendency for an individual to stutter on the same words on successive readings of the same passage (Johnson & Knott, 1937). Average consistency ranges from 40 to over 70% (Bloodstein, 1960; Neelley & Timmons, 1967), although for a given individual it can be anywhere from 0 to 100%.

Can adaptation and consistency coexist? Asked differently, how can a speaker stutter less while stuttering on the same words? In short, although the number of disfluencies decreases, those that remain tend to be words stuttered in a previous reading.

Although stuttering is likely to decrease over repeated readings, there are other circumstances under which it occurs even less often, sometimes not at all. Most commonly referred to as *fluency enhancing conditions*, they include situations such as choral reading, speaking under masking noise, singing, and talking to infants and animals, among others (Bloodstein, 1950; Ingham et al., 2012; Williams, 2006). Why they work is unknown, although theories abound that attempt to explain at least some of these conditions. For example, many of them force a change in speech by increasing phonatory durations and decreasing rate, features that allow for more right hemisphere processing than is typical with everyday speech (Andrews et al., 1982; Moore, 1990). Speaking may also be simplified when rhythm is imposed or interpersonal aspects of communication are lessened (Zocchi et al., 1990). Other research has focused on auditory feedback, given how many fluency enhancing conditions involve how speakers hear their own voices. More specifically, there is speculation that faulty feedback systems are tied to the source of stuttering (Shapiro, 2011). Thus, any condition that disallows or changes this flawed monitoring system—e.g., delayed auditory feedback, frequency altered feedback, masking noise—will reduce stuttering. It should also be noted, however, that some of these conditions also force speakers into a slower, more prolonged speech pattern (Stager & Ludlow, 1993), which, as noted above, is fluency-enhancing.

Another oft-cited tendency of people who stutter is the *apparent production of the schwa vowel*. For example, the syllable repetition initiating the word "ball" is more likely to sound like "buh-buh-buh-ball" than the actual consonant-vowel combination contained in the word ("baw-baw-baw-ball") (Montgomery & Cooke, 1976; Stark-weather, 1987). Although no uniform explanation exists for this phenomenon, it is possible that the restricted articulator movements result in a vowel of brief duration (perhaps an incomplete vowel production) which is perceived as a schwa.

No discussion of stuttering trends would be complete without mention of *word weights*, or, more specifically, the tendencies in adults for disfluencies to occur more often on consonants than vowels (Brown & Moren, 1942), content words than function words[3] (Howell, Au-Yeung, & Sackin, 1999), longer words than those shorter (Wingate, 1967), early words in an utterance (Logan & LaSalle, 1999), words used less frequently (Soderberg, 1967), words that convey much of the information of an utterance (Soderberg, 1967), and words involving relatively high linguistic stress (Wingate, 1988). The term word weight connotes that the heavier a word is (i.e., the more weight attached to it) the more likely it is to be stuttered. Of course, there is much overlap across these weights (e.g., content

---

3   Interestingly, children are more likely to stutter on function than content words (Howell, Au-Yeung, & Sackin, 1999), as well as words that are relatively low frequency (Anderson, 2007), early within an utterance (Richels et al., 2010), and lengthy (Zackheim & Conture, 2003).

words tend to be longer than function words; function words occur with relative high frequency), but they nonetheless indicate that stuttering is not completely random.

Finally, there is the notion that people who stutter experience a loss of control upon initiation of stuttering-like disfluencies (Perkins, Kent, & Curlee, 1991). That is, these breakdowns are differentiated from the non-stuttering variety (e.g., interjections, broken words) by the speaker's overall command of speech. Although non-stutterers can also be disfluent in overtly uncontrolled ways, this is still an interesting distinction. The moment of stuttering can feel as if continued speech is unmanageable, an experience not characteristic of everyday disfluencies.

To this point, we have reviewed general similarities that exist across people who stutter. It is important to realize, however, that stuttering is, by and large, an individualized disorder. The specific speech breakdowns, fears, avoidance behaviors, and tendencies all vary from person to person. Robert Quesal, a Board Certified Specialist in Fluency, put it this way: "The one thing stutterers have in common is that they are all different" (Quesal, R. personal correspondence). Stated another way, the only universal trait found among all people who stutter is stuttering.

Clearly, we still have a long way to go in our understanding of this mysterious disorder.

Subgroups

The variability across the stuttering population has led many theorists to speculate on the possibility of subgroups. For example, Cullinan and Springer (1980) found that children who stuttered presented significantly slower voice initiation and termination times than nonstuttering peers; however, when the authors divided the experimental sample into children who only stuttered and those with additional speech and/or language problems, it was found that only the "stuttering-plus" group differed significantly from the normal-speaking children in phonation times. That is, the two stuttering groups were dissimilar in terms of the measures of interest.

Differences within stuttering samples have also been identified based on the primary type of disfluency (Schwartz & Conture, 1988), the anatomical loci of disfluency (Borden, 1990), and whether or not there is a family history of stuttering (Janssen, Kraaimaat, & Brutten, 1990; Poulos & Webster, 1991). In addition to these groupings, subjects who stutter have been separated on the basis of severity. This follows from findings of physiologic and durational differences between samples differing in severity (Borden, 1983; Borden, Baer, & Kenney, 1985; Watson & Alfonso, 1987). Differences in gender, age, intelligence, motivation, and other personal characteristics have also been examined (Bloodstein, 1981; Culatta & Goldberg, 1995; Kent, 1983; Yairi, Ambrose, Paden, & Throneburg, 1996).

While it seems possible that different subgroups of people who stutter might respond to different therapy approaches (Yairi, 1990), at this stage that remains a question in need of more research.

The Stutterer Stereotype

Despite the individualized nature of the disorder, the idea of a stuttering comic would strike most people as strange. As Jaik notes, it flies in the face of the "stutterer stereotype," the notion that people who stutter are passive, nervous, shy, quiet, and withdrawn, among other comparable traits (Allard & Williams, 2008; Crowe Hall,

1991; Doody, Kalinowski, Armson, & Stuart, 1993; Healey, 2010; Lass et al., 1991; MacKinnon, Hall, & MacIntyre, 2007; Turnbaugh, Guitar, & Hoffman, 1979; Woods & Williams, 1976). People who stutter have been stereotyped in this manner by the general public (Craig et al., 2003; Schlagheck, Gabel, & Hughes, 2009; Silverman & Paynter, 1990), employers (Hurst & Cooper, 1983a; Logan & O'Connor, 2012), vocational rehabilitation counselors (Hurst & Cooper, 1983b), teachers (Abdalla & St. Louis, 2012; Arnold, Li, & Goltl, 2015; Hearne et al., 2008; Yeakle & Cooper, 1986), school administrators (Lass et al., 1994; Kiser et al., 1994), college professors (Dorsey & Guenther, 2000), college students (St. Louis, et al., 2014), nurses (Silverman & Bongey, 1997), pediatricians (Yairi & Carrico, 1992), and even speech-language pathologists (Cooper & Cooper, 1985; Woods & Williams, 1976; Yairi & Williams, 1970). Although there is little evidence that this stereotype is true (see Bloodstein & Bernstein Ratner, 2008 for a review of this research), its existence is reason enough for many people to be astonished by a stuttering individual telling jokes on stage.

As the "stutterer stereotype" will color much of Jaik's story, it is a concept worth exploring here. Different researchers have speculated on the existence of this sort of classification. Some of the hypotheses put forth include:

- Listeners react to the tension and anxiety of the stuttering moment and generalize that the speaker is always tense and anxious (Healey, 2010; Woods & Williams, 1976).

- The common perception of stuttering speakers is a function of their poor eye contact, though the authors of this conjecture (Thatchell, Van den Berg, & Lerman, 1983) offered no evidence to back the contention that the eye contact of people who stutter is abnormally bad.

- All people experience anxiety and tend to withdraw when they are disfluent. Thus, people overtly and abnormally disfluent will be viewed as perpetually anxious and withdrawn (MacKinnon, Hall, & MacIntyre, 2007; White & Collins, 1984).

In addition to such speculation, some researchers (Alm & Risberg, 2007; Bleek et al, 2011, 2012) have reported above normal neuroticism scores in some people who stutter. Neuroticism is associated with moodiness, emotional instability, anxiety, and intense emotional and physiological reactivity to stress (Bleek et al, 2012; Gunthert, Cohen, & Armeli, 1999). The existence of such traits would surely encourage belief in the aforementioned stereotype.

Perhaps the best place to go when attempting to figure out the stutterer stereotype is the research on attitudes toward speech (see chapter 8). From early childhood, people who stutter present negative speech-related attitudes in comparison to non-stutterers (Clark et al., 2012; DeNil & Brutten, 1987). Given their past experiences with speech, it makes sense that stuttering individuals are, overall, more likely to avoid speaking situations. From this conclusion, it is an easy (and often incorrect) overgeneralization to assume that similar traits exist in non-speech situations.

A separate issue from how this stereotype is set is how it (and stereotypes in general) are maintained. Theories abound regarding this question as well:

- Because we humans interpret data in ways that make us comfortable (i.e., see what we want to see) (Williams & Diaz, 2006), we remember the introverted individuals who stutter and ignore the outspoken ones (or call them the "exceptions that prove the rule," whatever that means). It is similar to why people watching a political debate are likely to report that their favored candidate won.

- White and Collins (1984) wrote of a self-fulfilling prophecy whereby people who stutter are induced to behave in a manner consistent with the listener's beliefs about them. For example, a speech-language pathologist who believes a new stuttering client is likely to be shy might purposely limit the client's speaking opportunities (on the assumption that he or she will not talk much anyway). Thus, the perception of shyness will be reinforced.

- Media portrayals could also play a part. In general, such depictions can influence beliefs about groups (Mackie et al, 1996), including effectively changing negative perceptions (Zhang & Tan, 2011). More specific to stuttering, Shapiro (2011) argued that the common stutterer stereotype is pervasive in arts and literature. More recent portrayals (e.g., *The King's Speech*) have been fairer, but do not occur with great frequency.

- The stereotype associated with stuttering is particularly susceptible to maintenance when passivity, nervousness, and the like are considered socially unacceptable traits (e.g., most Western cultures), in part because denigrating other groups is often used to enhance one's view of self (Williams & Diaz, 2006). Many who consider themselves bold extroverts, for example, need to assert the comparative undesirability of passive introverts in order to boost their own self-perceptions.

The effects of this stereotype can be both personal and societal. Social interactions are changed when one has to work past oth-

31

ers' misperceptions. Academic and professional opportunities are limited when an individual is perceived as passive, anxious, and/or nervous (Gabel et al., 2004; Logan & O'Connor, 2012; Rice & Kroll, 1994), although it is unclear how often this occurs with people who stutter (Gabel, Hughes, & Daniels, 2008; McAllister, Collier, & Shepstone, 2012). It is also worth noting that, over time, individuals may modify their self-concepts to match the perceptions held by others (Jones, 2004; McCrosky et al., 1977; Schlagheck, Gabel, & Hughes, 2009). In the case of people who stutter, this can result in a negative self-concept and failure to pursue their life goals (Bricker-Katz, Lincoln, & Cumming, 2013).

It is important for people who stutter, speech-language pathologists, and others to help the public expand its limited perception of this disorder. Means of controlling the stutterer stereotype include education about and exposure to individuals who stutter. That is, the more one learns about a group of people, the better his or her sense of the group's complexity and variability. Similarly, meeting individuals who stutter provides the best evidence of their heterogeneity. Through such processes, it is hoped that others can understand that actions such as social isolation or professional limitations are not justified (Worchel & Rothgerber, 1997). Readers are referred to Williams and Diaz (2006) for a detailed discussion of these concepts.

Onset of Stuttering

Those well-versed in this disorder may well be surprised by Jaik's story for reasons other than a false stereotype. As noted earlier in this chapter, the negative communicative experiences of people who stutter lead many of them to fear and thus avoid difficult speaking situations. That is, while not naturally anxious or passive, they might still shy away from communication circumstances associated with negative consequences. By way of example, the stuttering boxer will be just as apt as his opponent to aggressively throw punches, but not to be interviewed after the fight. The stuttering teacher might be a strict disciplinarian in class, but appear passive elsewhere. The stuttering comedian will take the stage on national television, yet be afraid of single words. This speech-associated wariness has much to do with how stuttering develops.

Stuttering typically begins during preschool years (Mansson, 2007; Reilly et al., 2013; Yairi & Ambrose, 2005), frequently before age 3 (Ambrose & Yairi, 1999; Yairi & Ambrose, 1992). Although it usually develops gradually over the course of many weeks (Williams, 2006; Yairi & Ambrose, 2005), it can arrive suddenly, even within a single day (Yairi & Ambrose, 1992; 2005). Less clear is whether the abrupt occurrences are in response to distressing emotional events. Parents often report such incidents close to onset (Yairi, 2005), though establishing cause and effect is difficult.

The notion of traumatic onset is prevalent enough that speech-language pathologists sometimes have to address it within clinical settings. Parents speculate whether disruptive events, such as moving or changing babysitters, are the causes of their child's stuttering. More serious situations, such as divorce or abusive parents, have been suggested by the clients themselves. My brother told me that he was taught in school that stuttering arises *only* in response to a disturbing childhood event (in a *World History* course, of all places).

Given that the cause is unknown, notable life experiences cannot be ruled out as contributing factors. However, there is simply no way of knowing whether stuttering onset in a given individual would have occurred anyway.

When it does begin, parental concern ebbs and flows along with the child's disfluencies. This brings us to a common developmental myth, that stuttering results from overanxious parents worrying about normal speech breakdowns. This misconception almost surely derives from early learning theories of stuttering, many of which seem to blame listeners for convincing children to change the way they speak in order to avoid imperfections (see chapter 14 for a more detailed explanation of such theories). It is not difficult to see what a large role parents could play in such a process. In truth, parents (and indeed listeners in general) are good at differentiating normal and abnormal speech disfluencies. In my clinical experience, when parents suspect stuttering, their fears are usually tangible. In fact, I can only remember one instance when this was not the case. With that child, there was a strong family history of stuttering (including the child's mother and older brother), so the high level of concern was understandable.

Spontaneous Recovery

In time, the stuttering flows outnumber the ebbs and the parents seek guidance. What they are often told is that stuttering is normal and will likely go away on its own if it is not brought to the child's attention. This is unfortunate advice, given that 1) stuttering is a communicative disorder and therefore is, by definition, not part of normal development, 2) the likelihood of spontaneous recovery (i.e., remission without intervention) is capricious at best (and certainly not a phenomenon on which to base a guarantee), and 3) denying stuttering can be a tough habit to break.

Within the field, published research is sometimes used to support the contention of high spontaneous recovery. At those times, the phrasing is this: three-fourths of children who stutter eventually outgrow it. It is a statistic that can both supported and misused.

This oft-quoted recovery rate originated from the results of massive longitudinal and retrospective studies published around a half century ago (Andrews & Harris, 1964; Cooper, Parris, & Wells, 1974; Sheehan & Martyn, 1970). Mountains of data were obtained on various aspects of human development, including stuttering. Researchers found a five percent incidence (that is, five percent of the individuals investigated stuttered at some point in their lives) and an overall population prevalence (or percent presenting the condition at a given point in time) of one percent. Therefore, the reasoning went, four of five recovered from (i.e., outgrew) the disorder.

When some of the early research was reanalyzed, it became apparent that, whatever it reflected, it was not true spontaneous recovery from stuttering (Martin & Lindamood, 1986). Subjects had self-reported stuttering, relying on their own memories or those of their parents. Definitions of stuttering varied. People reported as recovered continued to present mild stuttering. Nonstuttering adults had received therapy as children. In other words, some of the *spontaneously recovered* may not have presented the condition in the first place. Others had not actually recovered. Finally, there were those for whom recovery was anything but spontaneous.

A later study depicted spontaneous recovery as the exception rather than the rule (Ramig. 1993). Because the subjects of that study were older children (aged 4 years, 9 months to 8 years, 6 months), and thus past the point of likely recovery, many experts did not embrace this depiction. But it did emphasize the importance of age as a variable in this process (or, perhaps more accurately, time since onset). That is, samples of younger children showed greater recovery than those comprised of older children. It seems that once stuttering is established, it is less likely to go away. This affirms research suggesting that when remission happens, it will probably occur quickly (within a year) (Andrews & Harris, 1964; Yairi et al.,

1996). However, such a rapid recovery is more a likelihood than a certainty; remission can still occur in adolescence (Andrews & Harris, 1964) and, in rare cases, even adulthood (Finn, 2005; Quarrington, 1977).

More recent research in this area (e.g., Yairi & Ambrose, 1992, 2005) suggests that the 80% figure is not far off. All things considered then, one can make a case for high spontaneous recovery and, in turn, for waiting to see if the stuttering disappears. And indeed some (e.g., Yairi & Curlee, 1995) have questioned whether early intervention is necessary, or even ethical, for a disorder that is likely to resolve itself, particularly given the lack of strong treatment efficacy data.

It is important, however, not to carry this idea too far. For one thing, research on brain plasticity (see chapter 6) can be interpreted to suggest that preschool therapy may well alter disordered neural patterns for the better, increasing the chance of normal fluency development. Furthermore, as noted, the time of likely spontaneous recovery is relatively short. By the time parents observe their child's disordered speech, discuss it, watch it get better and worse, ask their friends about it, then wait for the kid's next physical to ask the pediatrician, the period of probable recovery may have passed. Viewed from a different perspective, a "wait and see" approach might work with a 3 year-old who has been stuttering a month or two, but would be less likely to succeed with a 5 year-old who is two years post onset.

But what if we ignore all that? For the sake of argument, let's say that *all* preschool children who stutter have an 80% chance of recovery. *Now* is it a good idea to tell parents to ignore it? Does an 80% spontaneous recovery rate amount to strong odds that a given child won't be the unlucky one in five who continues to stutter? Stated another way, should parents decline early intervention based on a 20% likelihood of stuttering? My experience tells me that most consider that to be too high a risk to take, a conclusion I completely understand. I can firmly state that I would choose to treat the stuttering with my own children. After all, if I know there is "only" a 20% chance that my home will be flooded by an oncoming storm, I'm still moving my family out of the house.

Further complicating the issue is the paucity of data telling us which children are likely to recover and which ones are not. Research in this area has revealed some trends but little for speech-language pathologists or worried parents to bank on.

Probably the factor that appears most tied to recovery is gender. Researchers (Ambrose & Yairi, 1999; Yairi, 1981; Yairi & Ambrose, 1992) found close to a 1:1 sex ratio for stuttering for children aged around 2 years. This is a stark contrast to the population male-to-female ratio of about 4:1 (Craig, et al., 2002) and suggests that little girls recover more often than their male peers. Given the protective effects of the female hormone estradiol (Tuong, Traystman, & Hurn, 1998), it is tempting to state that these findings indicate a neurological component to stuttering onset. In truth, however, gender differences in neurological recovery of any sort are complex and not precise enough to draw such a firm conclusion (see Wilson, 2013).

In addition to including many females, the population of children who recover present fewer relatives who stuttered (Yairi & Ambrose, 2005; Yairi et al., 1996). Given that it has long been known that stuttering runs in families (see chapter 14 for a more detailed treatment of this topic), it would appear that there is a hereditary component not only to the occurrence of stuttering, but also to its persistence.

Speech production differences have also been found between children who did and did not recover (Logan, 2014). With respect to the stuttering itself, for example, preschool children who show considerable reductions in frequency post-onset are more likely to recover than are those who present no or slight reductions (Ambrose & Yairi, 1999; Throneburg & Yairi, 2001). In addition, children whose stuttering persisted presented greater variability for other production measures, including fundamental frequency, timing of voice onset, vowel duration, and articulation rate (Brosch, Häge, & Johansenn, 2002). These data may be indicative of less stable speech production systems.

Language differences were uncovered as well. Given that stuttering develops at a time of great language acquisition, hypothesizing a connection is understandable. The association between the two, however, is unclear. Most children for whom stuttering persists present normal language (Watkins & Yairi, 1997). As a whole, however, this population presents delayed phonological development (Paden, Ambrose, & Yairi, 2002) and greater variability of both development and proficiency of expressive language (Watkins & Yairi, 1997) compared to those who recovered.

Development

Of course, the parents don't know all of the research on spontaneous recovery. In many cases, they only know what they are told by those outside the field of speech-language pathology and will thus attempt to wait out their child's stuttering without comment.

Initially, such an arrangement seems to work out fine. The parent monitors and the child stutters without concern. There soon comes a time, however, when awareness increases and the child becomes distressed about the speech breaks (Bloodstein & Bernstein Ratner, 2008; DeNil & Brutten, 1987). The parents experience guilt, wondering whether they 1) are the cause or 2) should be the solution (Wright, 2002). If they respond to their child at all, it is generally with unhelpful advice such as "take your time" or "think about what you want to say before you talk." Such reactions may only serve to increase the speech-related anxiety.

In such instances, the child is unlikely to talk about stuttering because of the associated shame. The parents will not force the issue due to their ongoing guilt (plus they might still be following the advice to ignore it). Thus, an obvious part of everyone's reality is largely disregarded. The child is in effect secluded, as the proverbial (and overused analogy of the) elephant in the room is not discussed (Rustin & Cook, 1995). It becomes the child's problem to solve, alone. And, as we will see with Jaik, it can continue as a lonely disorder for quite some time.

The child's initial solutions often involve the strategy discussed by Jaik: avoiding the stutter. Some common avoidance behaviors include:

- word substitutions (e.g., "Beggars can't be, well... pickers"),

- rephrasing utterances ("I need to go shopping for...let's go to the mall"),

- interjections ("My name is um, ah, um, you know..."),

- answering with "I don't know,"

- describing a concept rather than using a feared word ("It wasn't one but I don't think it was three either"), and

- purposely mispronouncing words to dodge a problem sound.

Sometimes, avoidance behaviors are more extreme, for example:

- ordering food based not on what one wants to eat, but on how easy it is to say,

- giving oneself a nickname,

- pretending to be sick (e.g., because it's book report day),

- feigning an accent,

- evading speech altogether, and,

- as we saw in chapter 1, rewriting a comedy script so it's void of feared words.

In addition to avoidance behaviors, there are, as noted earlier, maneuvers designed to escape a stutter in process. These strategies can be the result of the great muscle tension associated with stuttering, attempts to distract the speaker, or strategies to help propel the problem word. Some common examples include:

- eye blinks,

- throat clearing,

- foot taps,

- pitch change, and,

- as noted earlier in the chapter, the use of easy words or phrases to help launch the difficult ones.

Although these avoidance and escape maneuvers are known as secondary behaviors, because they would not exist without the primary stuttering behaviors of repetitions, prolongations, and hesitations, they are nevertheless a significant part of the stuttering experience (Blomgren, 2010; Bloodstein, 1981; Conture & Kelly, 1991; Logan, 2014). It is also important to note that the aforementioned lists are by no means exhaustive. In fact, I would venture to guess that every motor or verbal act humankind is capable of performing has been used as a secondary behavior by some stuttering individual at some point in time. The *Behavior Checklist* (Brutten & Vanryckeghem, 2006) lists 95 behaviors identified as secondary behaviors and even *that* is far from a complete list.

When we discuss therapy in chapter 6, it will become evident that secondary behaviors are repeatedly taken into account when trying to manage stuttering. For now, it is important to realize that their use is fraught with problems. For one, their effectiveness is temporary. The behaviors themselves, however—e.g., the foot tapping or throat clearing—are often maintained long term. In those instances, the secondary behaviors become unusual movements that accompany speech without helping it. A person struggling with a word may go through numerous motor actions that at one time effectively propelled him or her past stuttering, but are now just bad habits. This is one reason why the stuttering of school aged and older clients does not look like that associated with onset. That is, preschoolers often present disfluencies with minimal tension and escape maneuvers whereas the breakdowns of older clients are tense and chock full of extraneous movements. Although stuttering is not a learned behavior per se, much of what is visible with adults includes actions learned as a result of stuttering.

Another problem with secondary behaviors is that their temporary effectiveness serves as reinforcement for their use. Social penalties associated with stuttering are averted when no one can detect its presence. As is the case with any reinforcement, a particular behavior then increases in frequency. But because it is a secondary behavior, it eventually stops working and needs to be replaced by another (which initially works and is reinforced, etc.). Over time, this cycle can increase both stuttering fears and frequency. For example, the child (or adolescent or even adult) who substitutes words as a secondary behavior might use the term *tune* because it is easier to say than *song*. Because he or she associated stuttering with a new word, in time, this speaker will likely have difficulty with *tune*. Then he or she will have to resort to less typical synonyms, such as *melody* or *number*, until those too present difficulties. In essence, the individual has taken one problem word and turned it into many.

While the stuttering is becoming more layered, the family's unspoken covenant to disregard it strengthens. As a result, the child becomes very sensitive about the condition, discussing it with no one. The fears, anxiety, embarrassment, and humiliation all remain internalized. Not surprisingly, associated behaviors continue to increase. The muscle tension needed to escape stuttering intensifies and becomes more overt. Secondary behaviors are increasingly unwieldy, unusual, and frequent. As the individual ages, avoidance behaviors can significantly impact life, from refusing to socialize to turning down promotions because the new job would involve public speaking.

In some cases (including with Jaik, as subsequent chapters will show), secondary behaviors are used to deny the disorder, regardless of whether it is actually hidden.

Listeners might not recognize certain mannerisms as avoidance behaviors, yet they will still understand that something is amiss when a speaker says, for example, "My name is uh, um…well, um…"

Blissfully unaware of such listener reactions, some people who stutter carry these types of behaviors to unusual extremes, constantly monitoring and altering speech, doing whatever they can to avoid core stuttering behaviors. This is known as *covert* or *interiorized stuttering*. As the name suggests, it is a condition characterized by perpetual avoidance and a need to pass as a non-stutterer at all costs (Hood & Roach, 2001). And it is not only the disfluency that is interiorized. These individuals additionally attempt to hide the anticipation, stress, fear (of stuttering, of not conforming, and/or of the stuttering secret being discovered), guilt (about stuttering and/or about making listeners feel uncomfortable), shame (for being a person who stutters), and denial (of stuttering, of an inability to manage stuttering, and/or that anyone can detect the stuttering) (Douglass & Quarrington, 1952; Hood & Roach, 2001).

Because they desperately want to pass as fluent, covert stutterers may take pride in the notion that no one sees them stutter. Of course, one could easily argue that the aforementioned emotions (fear, shame, etc.) are worse than occasional speech breakdowns, as are the noted dangers of using so many secondary behaviors. On top of all that are missed activities and opportunities, and the cognitively exhausting effort required to constantly monitor and adjust speech. Although they do not stutter overtly very often, emotionally these individuals can be quite impaired.

So yes, stuttering is characterized by repetitions, hesitations, prolongations, and secondary behaviors. But it is also marked by loneliness, self-consciousness, embarrassment, and a host of other emotions.

It can be so consuming that it wears the person down to denial, or to a point where communication hardly seems worth the effort.

Addressing Speech-Associated Anxiety

So how did Jaik get up on stage? He mentions desensitization, often a major component of stuttering therapy (Blomgren, 2010; Williams, 2006). Certainly, to stutter openly, one would need to become desensitized to listener reactions as well as one's own negative reactions to stuttering (Van Riper, 1973). And one of the most effective desensitizers is disclosing the stutter (Guitar, 1998; Murphy, Yaruss, & Quesal, 2007), which Jaik did roughly a minute into the routine described in chapter 1.

Disclosure (or *advertising* the stutter), though rarely done with millions watching, serves a number of related purposes. It lets those who are listening know what they are hearing, thereby reducing potential confusion (and increasing the chances of an appropriate reaction). Perhaps that explains why listeners tend to react favorably to stuttering speakers who self-disclose (Collins & Blood, 1990; Schloss et al., 1987). Mentioning the stutter also makes it less tempting for the speaker to employ his avoidance behaviors and begin the harmful cycle referred to earlier. That is, when stuttering is out in open, there is no real reason to try to hide it.

The ways in which Jaik's other stage fright remedy—alcohol—affects stuttering are less clear. Although not advocated for stuttering (or much of anything else for that matter) or typically used by those who stutter (Iverach et al., 2010), alcohol does tend to suppress social inhibitions (Steele & Southwick, 1985). Informal clinical reports suggest that people who stutter respond to alcohol in a wide variety of ways—for some, severity increases, others improve, and a third group shows no change. It could be that there are individuals whose stuttering behaviors are closely tied to anxiety and thus disappear under the effects of inebriation, while others present more speech discoordination (so basically the alcohol further damages an already-damaged speech neurological system). Dr. Joseph Klein of Appalachian State University conjectured that speakers who maintain precise controls on their speech will experience an increase in stuttering, as this control will diminish while drinking (Klein, J. personal correspondence). Such speculation is certainly logical, but the truth is that nobody knows.

As Jaik noted, it is ironic that his moment of mass disclosure began with a script designed to help him avoid stuttering. Among those who stutter, unfortunately, avoidance is far more common than openness. Even Jaik admits that it took a while to reach a point where he had somewhat accepted his disorder (not to *like* it, which may never happen, but to accept that he would have to live with it). Jaik's story will present this journey.

Questions for Discussion

In this chapter, the question was posed: Who has the bigger problem—Jaik, who gets stuck repeatedly while performing successful comedy routines, or the person who stutters far less often, yet avoids life aspirations that involve speaking? What does the iceberg look like for each of these two examples?

List and explain a possible connection between secondary behaviors and fluency-enhancing conditions.

Which theory about fluency enhancing conditions best explains the phenomenon?

The prevalence of stuttering is quite low in the population of people with severe hearing impairments (Montgomery & Fitch, 1988). Could this finding be related to fluency enhancing conditions?

Can you explain the great number of trends—adaptation, fluency enhancement, word weights, etc.—in such an individualized disorder as stuttering?

Do nonstuttering speakers experience a loss of control upon normal speech discontinuities (e.g., interjections, single unit repetitions)? How would you differentiate this feeling from the loss of control experienced by people who stutter?

Were you surprised by the idea of a stuttering comedian? Why or why not?

Do you or did you hold the stereotypical view of people who stutter (i.e., shy, introverted, passive, etc.)? Why or why not?

As defined in the chapter, would you consider neuroticism a cause or result of stuttering? Why?

Do relatively high neuroticism scores in some people who stutter suggest that the stutterer stereotype has some basis in fact?

Different theories have been proposed regarding how the stutterer stereotype is maintained. Apply one of these theories to a different stereotype.

Can you think of examples of how the media influenced perceptions of a group (good or bad)?

Do most people you know describe themselves as extroverts or introverts? Are they accurate? Explain.

Describe an example from your own life in which exposure to individuals of a particular group gave you a better sense of that group's complexity and variability.

Why do you think stuttering begins? Has your view changed?

If you were diagnosed with a disease for which researchers claimed an 80% spontaneous remission rate, would you seek medical help? Why or why not?

Why do you think some parents employ a "wait and see" approach to their child's stuttering?

Would you advocate early intervention for a preschool child starting to stutter? Why or why not?

Is it possible to make stuttering development a less lonely experience for the children suffering from the disorder?

Which of the following topics is most in need of additional research—preschool development, subgroups and how to treat them, or fluency-enhancing conditions? Why?

In addition to the strategies listed, can you think of other ways to avoid a feared word?

Think about a trait or instance that causes you shame. How difficult would it be to disclose it to listeners?

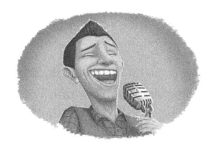

Chapter 3: Early Memories of Stuttering

I was brought up on a small farm in rural England. Most referred to my village as Darsham, but I always used the full title—*the village of Darsham*—because I could say it without stuttering. The family farmhouse was over 300 years old with oak beams and four fireplaces, and I lived there until I was 18.

According to my mother, I spoke well from an early age and articulated a wide vocabulary. Despite these skills, my brother Guy (more than four years older) did much of the talking for me throughout my early childhood. If I wanted to ride my tricycle, Guy would ask my mother. If I needed to get out of the bath, he would call out that I was finished. Sharing a room for more than four years, we became close and I spent hours following Guy's interests: Toy "Action Men," BMX bicycles, pop music, football, TV, and films. Some days we amused ourselves by recording silly radio shows on his cassette recorder.

Confident and out-going (and fluent), Guy was a positive influence on me. My mother was as well. Always supportive and kind, she often joked that she only passed art and cookery O-levels at school, knowing they would be her specialities in life. As was typical of her generation, she was content to stay home while the man went to work every day.

My stuttering was probably caused by a mixture of reasons, largely connected to my father in terms of both nature and nurture. That is, he stuttered (as did *his* father), so genetics played a part. It is also possible that I copied his hesitations and stuttering. The sheer intensity with which he addressed everyday situations probably didn't help either. (By the way, although neither of my siblings stutter, some of my cousins on my mother's side also have speech impediments. Playing *Trivial Pursuit* in our family is certainly not trivial!)

My father — always father or Christopher; he hated "dad" or "daddy"— has been a big influence on my life. He was born in London in 1938 to a woman impregnated by her physician. The doctor was, quite inconveniently, married to someone else at the time. Kept in the dark by all who knew him early in life, my father didn't discover the man's identity until after the doctor had died.

A year after his birth, the UK entered World War II. My father was privately evacuated to live with a family in Buckinghamshire, leaving his mother in London. This was undoubtedly a traumatic experience for a toddler. They were not reunited until after the war.

My father remained an only child, raised in a single-parent home. Growing up without a father of his own had serious repercussions for him. From what I know, he was an insecure and angry child, which likely exacerbated his speech difficulty. I have been critical of my father over the years, but I have also learnt how navigating childhood fatherless can result in lasting psychological damage, manifested in overt frustration, anger, and depression. These emotions can, in turn, lead to verbal outbursts, difficulties interacting and socialising with peers, and even physical violence (particularly in males)[1]. My father suffered all of that and more. Predictably, then, he had a tough childhood, displaying unruly behaviour at home and in school. After the turmoil and stress of the war, he surely craved guidance and support, needs which a single mother would have had difficulty fully providing. Unfortunately, he did not have access to professional counselling services. He met my mother in the sixties and she became his support system. She would openly say that she sometimes felt she was put on this Earth to look after her husband.

They married in 1968, an event that went less than smoothly. A few weeks before the wedding, my father told his bride-to-be that he no longer wanted to get married. She told *him* that it was too late to back out. He relented and even sang for her on their wedding day. Unfortunately, she missed the song he sang, which led to an argument. Thus began the marriage; this was the first of many, many rows between the two of them, some of which resulted in my father leaving home for a few nights.

He began his career in the late 1960's as a cattle feed advisor/debt collector. He was sacked from this job when he was 27 for the sin of belonging to a rock group. In 1980, he and a business partner (with whom he still works) decided to run their own feed company, calling it *Protein Feeds Ltd.* This was probably a good decision, as my father hated being managed by anyone or any expectations that he respect authority, traits possibly related to his development in a single-parent household. Even so, I believe that his decisions to work in agriculture and to start his own company were primarily based on his stutter. Agriculture is ideal for someone with a stutter,

---

1   Although conventional wisdom is that two-parent households result in happier and healthier children than do those without fathers, research does not always support this notion (e.g., see DePaulo, 2009). (Footnote by Dale Williams.)

as animals and fields tend not to answer back. And being one's own boss eliminates the need to communicate effectively with a hierarchy of managers on the way up the corporate ladder.

It is no secret that starting a business can be a tough, stressful, and time-consuming process, especially in a rural county such as Suffolk, which is paved more with mud than gold. I was born on 31st December 1973 and by the time I became aware of my father's company, it was still in its early development. His business partner was a man 20 years younger and my father spent long hours training him. This was the start of another complicated relationship in my father's life, one marked by periods of disrespectful behaviour (from both men) and struggles for control that continue to this day. Few people they employed lasted, most ending their stays in turmoil and screaming walk-outs. In my father's eyes, his business partner was a highly practical genius, very capable and incredibly hard working. Unfortunately, his own sons appeared impractical and lazy by comparison. He regularly reminded me that I had never experienced a hard day's work.

Oddly enough, my own feelings toward his partner are overwhelmingly positive. I am glad that he absorbed so much negativity over the years because it alleviated some of the abuse that my mother would have had to endure and it allowed my father to remain employed.

My father wasn't particularly interested in family, so my mother did the majority of the child care, housework, and cooking. On top of that, she started her own antique restoration business. She and her male business partner attracted many customers, which was good for the family finances, but also required many late nights of stripping furniture. (After a few years, my father decided that her partner had to move on, and so that business wound down.)

Around the same time that the family businesses were being established, we were getting ready to relocate to Brakes Lane Farm, in Darsham. Unfortunately, much of the farmhouse required reconstruction and renovation before we could move in, a process that literally lasted for years. This, of course, only added to the family's stress and financial strain. Adding unneeded fuel to that fire, my maternal grandmother moved into our house during this period. Over time, considerable discord developed between her and my father. When I was about 6 years-old, he kicked her out of the house, which I remember finding fairly traumatic.

In the years that followed, my father's mood further deteriorated. Maybe it was linked to the stress of working with a man much younger than him, or perhaps he missed his rock band days. He always seemed jealous of any type of performer he saw on television. As an apparent solution to this envy, in 1981 he opened *Barnabees Restaurant* in Westleton, Suffolk. My father would act as the resident "host" for diners, serving wine to people (even if they weren't drinking wine) and making them laugh. In other words, he was again an entertainer. Some people loved this, others resented having their privacy constantly interrupted, but my father usually made sure that *he* had a very good night.

In actuality, *Barnabees* was a converted house owned by my mother's side of the family and, like everything else during those years, became a stress magnet. Its location in a tiny village made it difficult for potential customers to find, helping to generate a history consisting largely of arguments, late working nights, walk outs, firings, and more than a few tears.

In all of his endeavours, my father spoke very loudly. The combination of volume and brazenness made people think he was either super-confident or slightly crazy. Perhaps that helped him at work, where he spent most of his time. As demanding as he was with those he employed, however, the perfection required at home was even worse (to me, anyway). He demanded that children be quiet and still at meal times. Despite his own stutter, my father found it quite hard to accept mine. As such, he showed very little patience when conversing with me.

Ironically, because I was worried that he would get angry if I stuttered, I tensed up and probably stuttered more whenever I spoke to him. This situation still exists today.

When I asked my father questions, I got long, complex, and critical lectures in return. The few times I received advice, it consisted of "it's a tricky world" and "try to always be independent." More often, he either did not pay attention to what I said or he misinterpreted and twisted my words, then held his version of my statement against me for years to come. He seized any golden opportunity to lay blame. I once threw a coffee mug on the floor in front of him when I became frustrated during one of his long and critical monologues. For years thereafter, every time he spoke of my faults he mentioned the thrown cup.

My father thrived on arguments, displaying a complete disdain for conflicting opinions. The result was that the rest of the family said very little, for fear of the consequences. My sister (10 years younger and, like Guy, normally fluent) lived with my parents well into her 20s and claims she has never had a proper conversation with my father. And my mother told me that she was afraid to leave him, for fears about what might happen to their property or children.

As noted, I was certainly not spared his argumentative side. Always critical (even if I was doing something right), my father undermined and disagreed with whatever I said, a pattern which played havoc with my self-esteem. There is a balance between teaching a son how to be self-reliant and maintaining his confidence levels. My communication strategies were to either excuse myself from the conversation or to "go with the flow," that is, to find ways to be agreeable even though I believed him to be wrong. Letting my father vent his emotions was easier than battling against them. Defiance not only took energy, it also set off his controlling behaviour. At the end of the day, he could make me pretend to be something I wasn't, but he couldn't change who I actually was.

Eventually I developed a third strategy: get a witness. When he wanted to speak to me, I suggested someone else, such as my mother, be present. The increased audience size made it more difficult for him to be as abusive. As with all bullies, he found controlling a crowd to be relatively problematic.

Thinking back, his communication style may have been caused by his own frustrations about his stutter, combined with a lack of empathy. Whatever the reasons, speaking at home always seemed to be quite pressurized and it was difficult competing with my father and brother. Life was fast moving and crowded, populated by my parents, their work colleagues, my siblings, family friends, and people at the numerous social events and parties that we attended or hosted. I remember too that we were always late for everything, which only added to the stress. In my teens, I began to deal with it via alcohol. But that's a subject for another chapter.

The only times I remember my father looking happy were at the social events. After a few glasses of red wine, he would talk constantly or dance with someone else's wife or start singing (sometimes after first grabbing the microphone away from the band). Some people wondered whether he had multiple personalities, as he could be happy one moment and then totally argumentative and negative the next. Although he would never have taken any medication for these mood swings, my mother kept him on a diet designed to reduce them. I dread to think where he would have been without her love and emotional support.

It is telling that my father displayed more pleasure during social occasions than he did with family. Such events were his rewards for hard work. He laboured diligently to provide financially, at the cost of being away from his family. Still, the importance of economic success and hard work were lessons he never neglected to impart. He wanted to make me into more than someone who goes to school and then spends the next 40 years working toward the day he receives a handshake and a gold watch. My father believed that to be one's own man in a capitalistic society, one must "learn to attack because someone is always attacking you." It is a lesson that he knew all too well, given the rigours and challenges he faced in the commercial world. Maybe he just wanted to prepare me for that life. I was an opportunity to right his wrongs if he could only make certain I avoided the mistakes that he had made. As a result, he seemed to take my shortcomings as his own personal failures.

Even now in his seventies, my father doesn't let me finish a sentence. But today it is less frightening than a tiresome reminder of childhood. I do not believe that he intends (or has ever intended) to be unkind. In fact, at times he is the most charming and charismatic man I have ever known. But he presents a strange hostility about life, one not easy to isolate. I recently asked him whether having children has given him any happiness and he responded that he married my mother because she wanted a business partner; he therefore felt the marriage would not last. Of course, that was not the most positive response for a son to hear! I believe that children were a burden to him in terms of both economics and responsibility, just another bother in the series of hassles that define life. Add to that the stress of the dog-eat-dog business world and his certainty that he could have been a rock star and a bitterness resulted that was both overt and layered.

Life at School

Although I remember stuttering a little around the ages of six or seven years, my first vivid speech memory was at the Abbey, a private pre-main school in Woodbridge, at the age of eight. I had to register to sit my entrance exams and the lady at the registration desk asked me my name. I remember standing there beside my mother, unable to say it.

Clearly, my academic career did not get off to a flying start.

Once enrolled at the Abbey, things did not get any easier. During my first week, I was dismissed from the classroom at the start of a lesson. I assumed I had done something wrong. Out in the hallway alone, I stuck my ear to the door and heard the teacher telling the class, "Now everyone, Jaik has a slight problem. He can't speak very well. So I want no one to be unkind to him and just to be nice and respect him." I was then called back in to the stares of my classmates. In many ways, I have never felt quite normal since.

I went through stages of working very hard at the Abbey, which may well have been an attempt to prove that I wasn't some stuttering idiot. Other times, however, I was disruptive and attention seeking, enough so that I was told to sit outside the classroom. These instances had less to do with stuttering than with my overall make-up. In various forms, attention-seeking behaviours continued all the way through University and beyond.

All in all, life at school was okay. The stutter never really held me up too much, although I remember an instance when I was nine and sitting on a fence waiting to join a football game. Eventually, one of the players came over.

"Hi. What's your name?" he asked.

I tried to speak, but nothing came out.

"What, have you forgotten your name?"

Thinking quickly, I answered, "Well, yes, sorry. Let me check what it is." I looked at the back of my shirt and said "Yes, sorry, it's Jaik. That's it. Silly me."

Playing rugby could also be a little embarrassing. I was a hooker in the first team, which required me to call out the secret code name of the player to whom I would throw the ball. After a few blocks on words and barely stifled laughter from the opposing team, our captain decided that using sign language might be a quicker option.

Despite the awkward instances, however, I was rarely teased about my speech. I attended schools in Suffolk, where children were generally brought up to be tolerant of differences. Years later at Bristol University, such tolerance continued. My cousin has a similar speech impediment and went to a state school, where he was routinely bullied. I am thankful I did not attend schools where survival depended on blending in.

Even with the lack of teasing, however, stuttering did present barriers to my education. For one, I was loath to participate in classroom discussions. I also couldn't say my name very easily, which made morning register a stressful and embarrassing time.

All I wanted to do was hand in a note that said, "I'm sorry, but Jaik is in today."

When I was 15 years old, I attended the school's Friday activity drama group. Immediately (albeit quietly), I was asked to leave. I was placed into a plane model making class instead. Interestingly, I was later able to get on stage for the school musical because I could sing without stuttering.

The Abbey and Woodbridge were fee paying, private schools and, although I am grateful to have attended them, life there at times did seem like an endless barrage of classroom contests, exams, sports, music lessons, and extra school courses. The constant competition required one to be disciplined, hardworking, and confident. I was thankful that I had learned how to be the first two, but the lack of confidence often served to increase my stress level.

I was also frustrated that I couldn't talk as well as my peers. As a teenager, most of my friends were praying to get a girlfriend. I just wanted to say my name. It was a bit like unrequited love: depressing, humiliating, worrying, and emotionally traumatic. I remember secretly wanting to be like James Bond (as did most boys at the time), but not because of the cars or the gadgets or the girls. My desire rested on a workplace where I could call people by just one letter such as "Q" or "M." Perfect!

I dealt with my frustrations by working hard, playing sports aggressively, and, despite the aforementioned attention-seeking behaviours, being reasonably self-disciplined. The latter had less to do with willpower than lack of distractions. Watching TV in the evening, for example, was out because of my father's aforementioned envy of celebrities. He also disliked having my friends to our house and I had difficulty speaking to them on the phone. As a result of these factors, I spent a lot of time studying in the solitude of my bedroom or riding my BMX bike, Both activities were ways I could have space away from being criticised.

Parental disregard of school furthered my feelings of isolation. My father never really paid any attention to my results or school reports, as the business always had to come first. He thought that school events such as rugby matches, speech days, and parent evenings were a waste of his time. On one occasion he even asked me to say that he had malaria—a disease with an approximately 0% prevalence rate in the UK—when he wanted to avoid going to speech day.

The time spent studying paid off with good grades in difficult courses and even a national General Certificate of Secondary Education history course work prize. Despite this award, and over the objections of teachers, I decided not to do history A-level, a decision that plagued me for years. But I felt that I wasn't really that good at history. Also, it is customary for history students to study English when obtaining an arts degree at university, and I wasn't particularly interested in English Literature. I didn't have the patience to read long fictional novels and wasn't particularly adept at understanding poems. On top of all that, the bourgeoning comedian in me thought it would be amusing to forego history A-level when my teachers, friends, and family were all expecting me to sign on.

In addition to personal reasons for avoiding the arts, there were also outside pressures. For one, there was a big push at school for students to pursue science based A-levels, as it was felt that the best jobs required them. As a result, many of my friends enrolled in applied sciences and I followed suit, even though I knew chemistry and biology were going to be struggles. My thinking was that science courses were a surer path into a quality university. There was also some pressure from my father to eventually work for his cattle feed business, for which biology, chemistry, and geography would be more useful than English literature or history. In the end, my decision was probably the right one, as subsequent science writing projects helped me get into Bristol University (luckily for me, their admissions procedures did not include interviews).

All in all, my memories of school are positive. I was generally near the top of the class and my teachers were understanding of my difference. I learned how to get along with people and made good friends. In retrospect, however, it is clear that stuttering impacted these years to a large degree. I learned early on that I could express myself better in writing than I could by speaking, and so wrote numerous stories for school and even for fun. Later on in life, the restraint placed on my capacity for expression by my stammer only served to concentrate and intensify my desire for words, writing, and later, stand-up comedy. I sometimes dreamed of a kind of utopia where I did not stutter and did something really creatively impressive, allowing me to live in a retreat-like existence, a bit like Ian Fleming took refuge in Jamaica to write his highly acclaimed *James Bond* books. In fact, during my summer holiday at the age of 16, I built a full sized log cabin, complete with fire place and chimney, about ten metres from my parent's house. This was part retreat and part symbol of leaving my parents' control. The cabin still stands today, over two decades later.

Life on Vacation

Stress was not limited to home life or school. It trickled into vacations too. In fact, going on holiday as an adult these days and watching families playing happily by the pool or calmly having a quiet meal together seems strange to me. My family never did anything peacefully.

Our holidays could be summed up in three words: *crazy*, *rushed*, and *traumatic*.

My first recollection of a vacation was at the age of six, when we flew to South Africa to stay with some friends in Durban. Going to the Kruger National Park, getting out of the car, and nearly being killed by charging elephants are events that still haunt my memory, as is the time moments before when the ranger told us not to exit our vehicle under any circumstances. Then there were the Sudwala Caves, where my father caused a scene by being loud and rude to a group of German tourists. I didn't know it at the time, but this trip was the beginning of a deleterious pattern.

The following year we spent a taxing vacation in Europe. The plan was to drive a *Comma* (a motorised home) around Italy and France. At the time, parents had to register children on their adult passports, but mine had neglected to do so. As a result, every time we crossed a border, I had to hide in a cupboard. Adding to the stress, the Comma's engine wasn't powerful enough for our weight, so getting up hills or going through mountain underpasses was always a nightmare. One evening we stopped the Comma alongside a mountain road in Italy and my father, for motives long forgotten, decided to pick up an iron girder. He was unsuccessful, dropping the girder on his foot. This resulted in perhaps the worst blood curdling scream I have ever heard. My father ran into the Comma with a nail hanging off his toe.

My mother bandaged his wound, but he still spent the next few days hobbling around on crutches, a circumstance that further worsened his already-foul mood.

When I was 11 and we went to Paxos, Greece, my father spent the entire trip arguing with the tour rep, criticizing the villa, finding fault with the beaches, complaining about the mosquitoes, and basically disparaging anything in sight. At the end of the trip, for reasons known only to him, he started a fight with the tour rep's boyfriend. Even worse, we were on a boat at the time, so there was no escape from the combatants.

At the age of 15, I travelled around Spain, Portugal, and France with my parents and five-year-old sister. During that trip, our car was broken into, money was stolen, we lost our hotel room keys, and, for various reasons, we met several local police officers. Needless to say, my father was unpleasant throughout.

Perhaps the most memorable vacation of all was in 1994 when my father came to Los Angeles to join the rest of the family on what, until then, was a good trip. Shortly after he arrived, my brother and I accidentally locked the keys in the hire car. A normal father would have been mildly annoyed. Mine went absolutely berserk. Things got worse from there. As parking is difficult in LA, my father would leave the car next to fire hydrants or in illegal spaces, leading to tickets he subsequently refused to pay. Instead, he drove to LA police stations to lodge unsuccessful complaints. My brother was a student at the University of Southern California at the time and he ended up paying the fines after the rest of the family had returned to England.

In Palm Springs, someone told us where Bob Hope lived, so my father drove us to the estate. At the entrance gate, he used his most posh English accent to tell the guard, "The Smythe family has arrived and we are personal guests of Bob Hope."

The guard simply said, "Do not get out of the car, Sir."

Of course, the next thing my father did was to get out of the car, exclaiming in the same posh accent, "I'll have you know, good man, we've driven 4000 miles to be here, and Bob is expecting us!"

At that, the guard reached for his gun and repeated, "Do not get out of the car, Sir."

Luckily, my father slowly returned to the driver's seat and we drove away, my mother and me speechless and white as sheets.

Life at University

Given the soul-searching that went into my higher education subject decision, it was with some relief that I enrolled in Bristol University at the age of 18. University life included activities such as indoor go carting, drinking, and more rugby. Oh, and some studying. Looking back, I should have joined more clubs, such as the Drama Society or the Revue Team, but I guess my stutter lowered my confidence to do so. Or maybe I was just being lazy and self-conscious.

I didn't have a "gap year" before university, as I knew some of that time would have been spent at my parents' house, something I wanted to avoid. I could have travelled instead, but earning the necessary money would have been difficult, given the types of jobs that were available where I was living (such as unskilled catering). In addition to those factors, stuttering played a part in my decision. Working or traveling would have involved talking and my speech at the time was not good. All things considered, it was far better to get to Bristol, get my degree, and then worry about applying for jobs.

During my second year at university, most Saturdays were spent in speech therapy, which took up quite a bit of time and energy (this therapy will be elaborated in chapter 5). Unfortunately, the treatment did little to help my day-to-day existence. In the long term, however, these sessions did give me the confidence to tackle my stutter, and thus were probably more productive than the likely alternatives: being on a rugby pitch or watching TV with my housemates.

Unless I was aided by alcohol, I did not display a great deal of self-assurance at university. Half of me thought, "Wow, this is great. I'll meet new people. Possibly get a girlfriend. Brilliant." The other half was more: "Right. I'm locking my door, and never going outside again until I'm educated." I had such little confidence that if I walked into a room full of people I didn't know, I felt as though I would suddenly forget how to walk properly. Finding a girlfriend at university was similar to banging my head against a brick wall, only more painful. People say that the most difficult parts of university life are always being broke and dealing with tough course work. For me, the hardest thing was coming to terms with the fact that the pretty posh blond girl will never go out with me.

But I ventured on, for various reasons:

- I knew how annoyed my father would be if I had wasted this opportunity and not passed.

- I understood how competitive life would be once I left university, especially with a stutter. Leaving without a degree would have made it that much tougher.

- I had come from a competitive group of generally over-privileged kids at Woodbridge School and it was important to me that I matched or surpassed them.

- I was also competing with my university friends, most of whom were going to become lawyers, accountants, doctors, and other professions often associated with success.

- I thought a degree would help my self-confidence and perhaps even help me to overcome my stutter.

- I realised early on that with a bit of hard work, university life was manageable for me. There was really no excuse for not obtaining the degree.

- I needed to achieve financial independence as quickly as I could. I hoped the sooner I escaped from under the shadow of my father, the sooner he would recognize my declaration of independence and stop his controlling behaviours. It didn't actually work out that way, but that was my thinking at the time.

Life After University

Because I couldn't stay at home after leaving university, due to the complicated relationship I had with my father, I moved to London instead. This meant that I had to find some kind of employment in order to pay the rent.

Early jobs included data input, soil map digitising, crime mapping, and geographic information system (GIS) technician. The trouble was that it took me a long time to learn the necessary life skills to actually survive a normal Monday to Friday, 9 to 5 working week. I was often late for work, hung-over on Mondays, prone to answer back authority, and generally unfulfilled.

I also had some social anxiety which made meeting new colleagues, attending work meetings, or simply saying "hello" to someone in the corridor quite difficult.

Then there was the ever present spectre of family. It would begin when my mother would phone me up and ask me to come back to Suffolk for a weekend. I obeyed and soon found myself bombarded with negativity from my father about how I was wasting my time at whatever job I was doing. This pattern was followed so often that one boss actually pleaded with me not to visit my parents.

"I can always see when you've been with your father over a weekend, as you are more irritable on Monday morning," he explained.

I was more independent and paying my own way, but some things hadn't changed.

Conclusions

In a way, my experiences with my father were valuable life lessons. In comparison to dealing with him, getting along with anyone else was easier. Even performing stand-up comedy was not that consciously stressful, maybe because I had been conditioned to stress from a young age. In fact, I almost craved stress, like a drug. It is true that no careers officer ever said, "So Jaik. You're quite shy, show no confidence, and have a terrible speech impediment. Have you considered being a stand-up comedian?" But I was actually quite well suited for it, as charming a large audience was genuinely easier than having a one-on-one chat with my father.

In addition to their help with stand-up comedy, my experiences growing up made me more patient, compassionate, and determined. They gave me an inner strength which I have used in many aspects of my life. Maybe that was my father's intent all along. Or maybe it's this cloud's silver lining. Now that I have children of my own, it is something I think about. Any father has a responsibility toward his child. Should he bring that child up to be a kind and caring individual who will one day become a responsible and comfortable citizen? Or should the parent teach that there is more to life than that and the possibilities are in fact limitless with a willingness to push the boundaries? Maybe it is a father's responsibility to teach a child that comfort zones are to be expanded, in which case my father did a pretty good job. That said, these days I take relaxed vacations. Furthermore, I would like my children to see me gain respect from people by being kind and straightforward, rather than loud and rude.

A problem with so much stress (in addition to the arguments, injured toes, hiding in cupboards, armed guards, etc.) is that it may well have increased my stuttering. It certainly didn't help.

Related to the disfluent speech—by cause, effect, or both—was my lack of confidence. I just wasn't very assertive or decisive. In fact, when I was 15 or 16, a friend of mine used to tease me, not because of my stutter, but, rather, my indecisiveness. Indecision has always been part of my life: Do I do these A-levels? Do I do that degree? Do I do that job? Do I ask her out on a date? Do I stay in London? Do I go travelling? Do I eat that? Should I buy that? The list is endless, every decision a wrestling match between options. But what drove me crazy about this was the regret that often followed decisions I had made. Because I did not know what I wanted in the first place, I always wondered if the alternative was better.

I don't know whether I was born indecisive or had too much confidence eroded from me. Part of me feels that I should have been stronger. I believe that many of my life decisions were designed to make my father happy. It also seems, however, that the lack of self-assurance and self-worth that goes with having a controlling father tends to make decisiveness more difficult. My father ran the family with anger and manipulation, and I was afraid to voice an opinion. His decisions were the right ones solely on the basis of intimidation.

When I didn't agree with them, I would rethink my opinion, looking for ways to accommodate his (being a middle child, this accommodation comes quite naturally). As I was always "wrong" in these instances (because his verdict was the one that stood), I began to question my ability to make good decisions.

I thought decisions would be easier to make when I was out on my own, a time for which I could hardly wait. Looking back, I may well have wasted too much of my childhood wanting to be an adult. I saw academic success as a ticket out of the control I experienced at home, so I worked hard at school—maybe *too* hard. Although I am happier being out on my own, it is also true that childhood years are precious and we do not get them back.

Mine just would have been simpler without the stress.

Questions for Discussion

Are there any keys to the cause and/or precipitating factors in his story of growing up stuttering?

Neither of Jaik's siblings stutter, despite growing up in the same environment. How do you explain that?

Growing up, Jaik "tensed up and probably stuttered more" whenever he spoke to his father, a situation that continued into adulthood. Why would he still have trouble talking to him today?

Jaik provides a lot of background information about his father. How might that be related to his stuttering?

Young Jaik was dismissed from class so that the teacher could inform the other students about his stuttering. Was that an appropriate way to handle the situation? Why or why not?

Why do you think Jaik remembers being asked his name when he was 9 years-old?

Was it good for the school's drama teacher to steer Jaik toward an activity that required less speech?

In Jaik's ideal world, everyone's name would be one letter. Do you believe, as he claimed, that would have made speech easier?

Were you surprised to find out that Jaik was not the class clown? Why or why not?

Jaik thought a university degree would help his self-confidence and perhaps even his stutter. Are these realistic outcomes? Explain your answer.

Jaik stated that "charming a large audience was genuinely easier than having a one-on-one chat" with his father. What does that say about situational fears?

Do you feel that the stress of Jaik's childhood increased his stuttering severity? Why or why not?

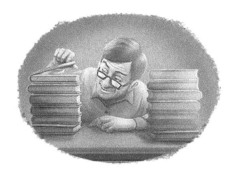

Chapter 4: Parents, Stress, and Confidence

Jaik's story of growing up with a stutter was dominated by the themes of family, stress, and self-confidence. Even those topics, however, were overshadowed by one dynamic: Jaik's relationship with his father.

What first needs to be pointed out is that Jaik's experience is not typical. Parents of children who stutter are like any other parents. That is to say, they differ in terms of belief systems, methods of discipline, and every other way imaginable. One must be careful not to read Jaik's story and assume that stuttering is caused by argumentative fathers. Nor, as suggested elsewhere in that chapter, does it result from imitating stuttering parents. In fact, the stuttering disfluency of children is generally quite different from adult patterns.

Having said all of that, however, it is also true that no single cause has been found. Many (e.g., Smith & Kelly, 1997; Wall & Myers, 1995), see stuttering as arising from a biological susceptibility paired with environmental agents. That is, a complex interaction of multiple factors—genetic, linguistic, neuromotor, cognitive, emotional, environmental, and others (Smith & Kelly, 1997; Starkweather, 1990)—is responsible (these factors will be discussed throughout the text, particularly in chapter 14). Thus, Jaik's speculation on nature vs. nurture is accurate in the sense that both play a part. In truth, however, the two are not easily separated. They interact in numerous ways. For example, prospective stressors may be environmental but which ones an individual identifies as taxing and how he or she reacts to them could well be organic (or, more likely, a combination of organic and cultural). Applied to stuttering, children are exposed to potentially stressful events on a constant basis; parsing out which ones contribute to the onset of the disorder would be difficult at best. And even if it could be determined that a child's stuttering began right after his father booted his grandmother out of the house (or any other significant event), not even that would place the blame squarely on dad's shoulders. If the child was that predisposed, it is almost a certainty that if the event in question (in this case, the eviction) had not brought it out, something else would have.

Parents

As for the role of parents, that is also complex. There is no evidence that parents cause stuttering, but that is not to say that their behaviors have no influence post-onset. Environmental recommendations to parents of children beginning to stutter routinely include advice such as relaxing their own speech and communicating with their child in a turn-taking milieu (e.g., Williams & Williams, 2000), acknowledgments that family influences are very real. If parental behaviors increase the chances of recovery, one can argue that opposing behaviors decrease it.

Once the stuttering has developed, the faster that parents accept it, the better life will be for the disfluent child. Unfortunately for everyone involved, the road to acceptance is not without obstacles. Getting in the way are worry, frustration, anger, and/or a host of other conflicting and often simultaneous emotions. Most prominent among these feelings is that of *guilt*.

Parenthood in general is characterized by insecurity (Starkweather, 2000). After all, there is no manual to instruct parents how to nurture a helpless being seemingly chock full of potential. What happens, then, when their child displays an abnormal behavior such as stuttering? Very likely, the first signs of parental confusion and guilt will arise (Buscaglia, 1975; Crowe, 1997; Kendall, 2000; Wright, 2002). Something beyond their understanding—breaks of speech that do not sound normal—is happening and they simply do not know what to do. Confusion, however, does not feel like an adequate response when the subject is one's own child. Parents feel an imperative to do the right thing (Kendall, 2000), but the combination of insecurity and confusion makes it difficult to trust their own instincts. Parents will consult friends, neighbors, family members, textbooks, the Internet, and anyone or anything else that might possess some insight into stuttering. Unfortunately, the large amount of information they get is likely to be 1) questionable, 2) contradictory, and 3) overwhelming (Plexico & Burrus, 2012). As noted in chapter 2, many misunderstandings surround this disorder. Upon such misunderstandings lie some really bad pieces of advice (e.g., "Just wait it out," "Don't let him get away with talking that way"). When such advice does not work, parents worry that they made poor choices—followed bad recommendations, didn't follow good ones correctly, or both. Each subsequent point of confusion—dealing with insensitive listeners, wondering how to talk to their child, and finding the right speech-language pathologist, to name just a few—that is not handled perfectly generates more guilt (Wright, 2002).

Because of alleged poor parenting, parents feel that their child will have difficulty communicating, get teased by peers (or rugby opponents), be excluded at school, and generally face a lifetime of challenges.

Parents may also feel responsible for the disorder itself (Sen & Yurtsever, 2007). With any childhood variance, parents wonder whether they should have done something differently during pregnancy (Kendall, 2000) or the child's formative years (Crowe, 1997). Learning theories of stuttering certainly do not help, particularly when all parents know about them are quotes such as "stuttering begins not in the mouth of the child, but in the ear of the parent" (Johnson, as cited in Williams, 1992). Such theories are elaborated in chapter 14, but the point here is that parents buy into the idea that their anxiety and misguided corrective measures caused their child to speak unnaturally. There is no real evidence supporting this position (e.g., see Alm, 2014), but they are unlikely to know that.

Even when parents do not blame themselves, emotions can still run high. Anger can surface, directed at professionals for lacking information or guarantees (Wright, 2002), or life in general. And given the unlimited potential they see in their children, defects cause some parents to actually grieve the loss of the perfect child (Boström, Broberg, & Hwang, 2010; Crowe, 1997; Kendall, 2000; Webster & Ward, 1993; Wright, 2002). An early stage of the grieving process is denial (Sen & Yurtsever, 2007), which can be manifested as denying either concern about the disorder or the disorder itself. Of course, even though denial is part of the grieving process, it cannot go on indefinitely. When it continues too long, the child does not receive the needed intervention (Wright, 2002), a potential source of even more parental guilt.

In some instances, grieving leads to depression (Resch, Elliott, & Benz, 2012). This is an emotion characterized by submission and retreat (Crowe, 1997; Wright, 2002). As with confusion, parents are quite willing to accept whatever others tell them. Thus, more guilt can arise if and when yet more bad recommendations are followed.

Outside forces affect parents of stuttering children in more ways than dubious advice. People can ask questions in ways that sound (to the parents, at least) accusatory (e.g., "Why does he talk that way?"). Professionals refer to the parents as neurotic, unrealistic, and/or overprotective, as if these are ingrained traits and not parts of the acceptance process (Buscaglia, 1975). If the parents view their neurotic behaviors, unrealistic thoughts, or overprotectiveness as precipitating factors in their child's stuttering, guilt again rears its ugly head.

Given that parental guilt can be based on perceived responsibility for both causing a condition with no known cause, and not curing a condition with no known cure, it is clearly unfounded. With proper education about stuttering, parents can generally understand this point, at least on an intellectual basis. Emotionally, however, true acceptance does not come easily.

As difficult as they already are, the negative emotions can be magnified for the parent who stutters. Although nobody can control genetics, parents nevertheless feel guilty about passing along an unwanted trait. Each disfluency can serve as a reminder of this perceived failing. Is guilt the reason that Jaik's father disliked his son's stuttering so much? Years later, it is difficult to say with any certainty. It is worth noting, however, that most people who stutter demonstrate great tolerance with others suffering from the same disability. In fact, Jaik reported that his experiences growing up made him more patient and compassionate, as he knows what it is like to be on the other side of impatience and callousness. Presumably Jaik's father has been on the receiving end of negative listener reactions himself. So how to explain his antagonism? No clear answer emerges.

While Jaik's father may or may not have blamed himself for his son's stuttering, he clearly had a lot on his mind. He needed to support a wife and three children, choosing to do so via his own business. And that, he apparently felt, required a "dog eat dog" mentality that might have been difficult to leave at the office. Unfortunately, the aforementioned parental ideals—relaxed speech, turn-taking, and other behaviors that will be elaborated in chapter 6—would have been absent from Jaik's developmental years.

Some of the other claims pertaining to Jaik's father are interesting to examine. Did he choose a relatively isolated lifestyle because he stutters? Again, there is no way of knowing, but such decisions are not unheard of. I personally know adults who have turned down promotions and worked isolated jobs because stuttering made the alternatives too difficult. Then again, there are people who stutter who become stand-up comedians (and others who pursue rock stardom). (As a side note, it is interesting how Jaik was steered away from drama. As will be discussed in chapters 11 and 12, outside forces can serve to keep people who stutter from situations that might make listeners uncomfortable. Jaik then noted that he was able to perform in a musical without stuttering. This report is not particularly surprising. Singing is a strong fluency enhancing condition.)

Jaik also speculated that his father spoke loudly as a way to compensate for the stutter, meaning, I suppose, that he wanted to appear harsh and in control (or basically the opposite of the stutterer stereotype). As with the insulated vocation, he would not have been the first to try this tactic. On the other hand, that could have been a secondary behavior designed to mask the stuttering.

In many ways, it is a shame that Jaik could not discuss stuttering with his father. Unresolved issues with parents can interfere with the recovery process (Starkweather, 2000). Parental disapproval (real or imagined) can be a major obstacle keeping a person from fully accepting his or her own stuttering. In Jaik's case, he appears convinced that having a meaningful conversation with his father is unrealistic. Unfortunately, desensitization to parental reactions is likely to be difficult for him as well.

Other Factors

Jaik's relationship with his brother is interesting in light of research and clinical reports regarding siblings. That they were very close is consistent with qualitative data on stuttering-nonstuttering sibling relationships (Beilby, Byrnes, & Young, 2012). Normally fluent siblings sometimes experience increased responsibility and power in such relationships (Beilby, Byrnes, & Young, 2012). It is unclear which (if either) was the case for Guy when he spoke for Jaik. Perhaps some light is shed on this question by Jaik's later statement that he was unable to verbally compete with his older brother; communication dominance is a common way of exerting power over a stuttering sibling.

Another recurring theme in chapter 3 was stress, mostly in the forms of paternal demands and family financial constraints. Overall, Jaik believes that he was born into an environment that increased the probability that stuttering would not merely be a transient developmental event. The difficulty of identifying environmental stressors in the development of stuttering was addressed earlier in this text but, in a way, it is much like confidence, another trait Jaik linked to fluency. Do stress and lack of confidence increase stuttering? More often, they are reactions to the disorder, responses that should be monitored (e.g., Yaruss, 2010). Although the stress within the Campbell household didn't help Jaik's speech development, it is also certain that it didn't turn a normally fluent child into a stuttering one.

At school, Jaik worked hard to show that stuttering is not detrimental to academic potential. Although decreased intelligence is not part of the stutterer stereotype (see chapter 2), it is not unusual for stuttering clients to report being treated as if their brainpower is lacking. And it has been reported that children who stutter score about five IQ points lower than those who do not (Andrews & Harris, 1964; Berry 1938; Okasha et al., 1974). However, it must be pointed out that stuttering-like disfluency has a greater prevalence among the intellectually disabled in comparison to the general population (Bloodstein, 1995; Delfoor, Van Borsel, and Curfs, 2000; Hanson et al., 1986; Kleppe et al., 1990; Schlandger and Gottsleben, 1957). Thus, the population difference in IQ has basically no application to an individual stuttering person. In fact, other research studies found higher non-verbal cognition scores for stuttering preschoolers when compared to their non-stuttering peers (Reilly et al., 2013) and that college students who stutter are more intelligent than their peers, a finding that could reflect numbers of each population who pursue a college education more so than actual intelligence (Hulit, 2006). In truth, there is no real evidence demonstrating that people who stutter are any more or less intelligent than people who do not.

Jaik reports that stuttering did not affect his academic performance to any great extent and doesn't blame his failures on it. Still, like most people who stutter (see Daniels, Gabel, & Hughes, 2012), he faced many challenges at school, both overt and covert. He did not participate verbally, a common aversion for people who stutter

(Daniels, Gabel, & Hughes, 2012), due likely to past history with speech difficulty. He also struggled to say his own name, another difficulty often associated with stuttering (Marland, 2013).

In part because of his stutter, Jaik did not spend as much time with friends as he would have liked. This report is also consistent with the research. Although adolescents tend not to take stuttering into account when choosing friends (Blood et. al, 2003; Evans et al., 2008), the stuttering speaker's embarrassment can get in the way (Hearne et al., 2008). Jaik was not the first person who stutters to hold himself back socially.

Teasing and Bullying

Although Jaik faced some intimidation at home, he was rarely teased at school. In this regard, he was fortunate. Based on retro-spective survey data, Hugh-Jones and Smith (1999) concluded that nearly 9 of 10 grade-school children who stutter experienced bul-lying. What's more, stuttering adolescents are almost three times as likely to be bullied as are teens in general (Blood et al., 2011). These data are not particularly surprising, given that stuttering is associated with traits such as insecurity, nervousness, and pas-sivity (Blood & Blood, 2004). Essentially, the stutterer stereotype makes these children appear to be easy targets for bullies.

Bullying is an issue justifiably gaining much media attention in re-cent years. It is clearly not a phenomena limited to childhood. And even when it is, the effects can be long-term. It can lead to loneli-ness, depression, violence, social isolation, poor academic perfor-mance, loss of self-confidence and self-esteem, and even health problems such as weight loss or substance abuse (Blood et al., 2011; Centers for Disease Control and Prevention, 2010; Dake, Price, & Telljohann, 2003; Murphy & Quesal, 2002; Roth & Beal,

1999; Starkweather & Givens-Ackerman, 1997). It is also not, as some might argue, just part of growing up. In fact, widespread anti-bullying programs (e.g. Utterly Global, 2015) exist on the basis that it not only can be stopped, but that it must be.

Resources designed for people who are bullied on the basis of their stuttering stress empowerment by educating these individuals that the stuttering is not their fault and, thus, they don't deserve to be mocked for it (Murphy, 2000). They also learn that they are not alone; many people are teased and bullied about a variety of differences (Lew, 2000) and they should not consider themselves weak because of it. In addition, understanding that bullies do what they do for reasons of insecurity (that is, they need self-validation or attention) and ignorance (Lew, 2000; Wong, Cheng, & Chen, 2013) makes the teasing less abstract, more controllable.

Williams (2006) outlined six strategies for dealing with a bully. Some of them are used more than others (see Blood et al., 2010). As the reader will see below, all have their pros and cons.

1. *Avoid the bully.* That is, the individual hides from the tormentor or stays in crowds.

Pro:

- Bullies rarely pick on groups.

Cons:

- This strategy is difficult to employ for someone who is socially isolated. Groups will be hard to form, mostly because others fear being teased themselves if they socialize with an outcast.

- Avoiding a persistent bully may require costly sacrifices (Roth & Beal, 1999). Missing school or work, for example, is a high price to pay to hide from teasing.

2. *Ignore the bullying.* With this approach, the one being teased does not respond to it.

Pro:

- Because the bully is not getting the desired reinforcement (attention or a self-validating reaction), he or she might stop (Lew, 2000; Murphy, 2000).

Con:

- While this may work, it will undoubtedly take some time. Meanwhile, the severity of the teasing may increase (Roth & Beal, 1999).

3. *Confront the bully.* The targeted individual can stand up to his or her tormentor verbally or even physically (see Dugan, 1998; Lew, 2000; Murphy, 2000; Roth & Beal, 1999).

Pros:

- It could "teach the bully a lesson" or lead him or her to find a less challenging target.

- A forceful reply (Dugan, 1998; Lew, 2000; Roth & Beal, 1999) such as "Yeah, I stutter. So what?" or asking the bully to stop teasing fits with common clinical advice that people who stutter present themselves with assurance and confidence.

Cons:

- Assuming that the bully prefers victims of comparatively small stature and/or who are unable to talk back quickly, expecting that victim to mount a successful physical or verbal challenge may be unrealistic. Perhaps because of these reasons, children who stutter rarely defend themselves (Roth & Beal, 1999).

- Progressing a victim to the point of confrontation often requires a lengthy process of desensitization. Those who are not desensitized will obviously have a tough time projecting the necessary assurance and confidence to successfully discourage a bully (Roth & Beal, 1999).

4. *Using humor against a bully.* This has been advocated for decades (Lew, 2000; Manning, 2001; Starkweather & Givens-Ackerman, 1997).

Pro:

- This tactic could disarm a bully without a physical confrontation.

Cons:

- The person responding with a statement such as "If you're going to stutter, do it right. Let me show you," is relying on verbal skills, which is the source of the bullying problem to begin with.

- Expecting someone to have the presence of mind to create and implement a witticism in the face of danger may not be realistic.

5. *Education*. This strategy can involve explaining stuttering, bullying, or both, either in general terms or those traits specific to the individual (Lew, 2000; Murphy, 2000).

Pros:

- Education can effectively combat the ignorance on which much of teasing is based.

- It may offer the opportunity to educate the entire class or workplace not only about bullying, but also about stuttering.

- Bullies can get some idea of how it feels to be on the other side of teasing.

Cons:

- Educating others requires much confidence, a feature that might not be present while the individual is suffering bullying.

- Even if others are doing the teaching, the person who stutters could feel shame and/or embarrassment if not desensitized properly.

- If the bully's goals are self-validation and attention, he or she is not likely to be interested in learning about stuttering.

- Learning about stuttering may only provide the bully with additional material to mock the stuttering child.

6. *Getting help.* The person being teased can tell someone what is happening (Blood, 2014; Lew, 2000; Murphy, 2000; Roth & Beal, 1999; Starkweather & Givens-Ackerman, 1997).

Pros:

- The victim is decreasing his or her social isolation by forming a helpful alliance.

- If an anti-bullying program is in place, help should come quickly.

Cons:

- The "helper" might turn out to be anything but helpful. Those in supervisory positions do not always understand the potential danger of bullying and take inappropriate (or no) action (Plexico & Burrus, 2012; Roth & Beal, 1999).

- There may be a fear of retaliation, that the bullying will become more severe if trouble is caused for the perpetrator (Lee, 2003) (not to mention the risk of *actual* retaliation).

This is a primary reason why bullying often goes unreported. Victims understand the value of reporting it, often stating that they will do so if and when it occurs, yet do not.

- Some feel that getting help shows weakness, an admission that they cannot solve their own problems. Interestingly, clients will admit asking for help with other problems all the time. A student who cannot figure out a math problem, for example, has no qualms about bringing it to someone who is good at math. Yet within the realm of teasing, they have been conditioned to behave differently. All too often, unfortunately, the bullies get to set the rules.

Questions for Discussion

Do you believe a root cause for stuttering will ever be found? Why or why not?

Variations of the word *guilt* appear ten times in the section on *Parents*. Why do you think it was stressed so much?

A parent tells you that he or she caused a child's stuttering. How do you respond?

List in importance the factors that you believe caused or perpetuated Jaik's stuttering.

What do you think is the best way to handle teasing/bullying? Why?

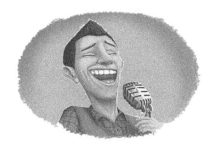

Chapter 5: Speech Behaviours and Therapy

Based on my parents' recollections, between about four to six years of age, my speech was characterized by slight repetitions and pro-longations of sounds, syllables, and words. There were no anxieties or avoidance behaviours related to these disfluencies. After the age of seven, the breakdowns were uncontrollable, so I started using fillers and starters, such as *er, um, I mean, so, but*, and *well*. These extra syllables allowed me to take a kind of "run up" before saying a feared word. For example, if someone asked me what my name was, I'd say, "Yes, well it's um, it's er, I mean, it's normally, Jaik Campbell."

They'd then say, "Well, what is it the rest of the time?"

And I would reply, "Um, Samantha."

Although these behaviours hid the stuttering (arguably), I know they still came across as strange. In the movies, when someone asks James Bond for his name, he is always very confident and sure of himself. He doesn't say, "Err, m-my name.

Well, um, well, it's B- B- B- B- ha ha ha ha, er er er er er, B- B- Bol-locks, J- J-J- James – Bollocks. Sh- Sh- Sh- Shaken, with a speech impediment."

My stuttering was not too noticeable until I started "blocking" at age 9 or 10. Blocking occurred when my lips came together with too much force to form a plosive normally. That is, rather than part-ing my lips gently, rapidly, and easily, I was unable to release the contact between them. A great deal of tension and inner frustration built up, resulting in a prolonged initiation of whatever word I was saying. In severe cases, I was stuck on the blocked sound for 5-10 seconds, which affected my breathing (because I was holding my breath during the block). So the more I stuttered, the worse my breathing got and the worse my breathing got, the more I stuttered. As a result of this downward spiral, head, neck, and chest muscle tension increased and talking became quite an exhausting process.

My solution was to come up with more tricks to speak fluently. If I was stuck on the first sound of "Jaik," I would make novel move-ments of the lips and tongue—and perhaps actions involving my hands, arms, and legs too—just to get the word out. Sometimes I resorted to slapping the side of my leg to propel the word, but I found I couldn't really get away with that in a normal conversation.

Such behaviours were accompanied by a lack of eye contact with the listener, which were either a result of embarrassment at not being able to produce the word, a way of helping me better concen-trate on speaking, or both. Later, I developed a carefully controlled swapping of my words, so that I never quite said all that I wanted to say. This made speaking a fairly frustrating experience. For ex-ample, I'd go into a newsagent to buy some tissues, and say "Hello, do you have anything I can blow my nose on?" rather than saying the word *tissues*.

As a teenager with a stutter, I remember putting off telephone calls to friends, and avoiding lengthy class discussions, auditions for school plays, and even routine speaking situations. I gradually developed an overall fear and avoidance of certain letters, words, and people, especially those in authority.

An accompanying inner frustration, embarrassment, and shame developed that slowly filtered more and more into my life.

At university, more secondary behaviours developed, including facial grimacing, which was really embarrassing. Someone would ask, "What's your name?" and I'd just make a weird facial grimace.

"That's a strange name," would be the response.

"Yes," I'd answer. "It's Greek for complete moron."

Other secondary behaviours included covering my mouth with my hand, blushing, tension, clenching my fist, refusing to speak in tutorials, and using vocal techniques such as changing my speech rate, utilizing a monotone, or even feigning an accent. Speaking became a complicated process.

As an adult, I avoided certain social situations, such as answering the telephone, making presentations, asking for bus fares, speaking to work colleagues, or regularly meeting up with friends. I also used to switch direction mid–sentence when I was speaking, which made me appear indecisive, unsure of myself, and unassertive.

Childhood Therapy

I went to a speech therapy course in Suffolk when I was 8 years-old. I can't remember that much about it (and I didn't save any of the notes I was given at the time), but I do recall something called "easy speech" that made me sound like a robot on weak battery power.

Easy speech involved beginning speech a little slower, with less tension and loudness. Once I had achieved fluent speech at the word level, the length and complexity of responses was gradually increased.

Self-monitoring was also taught, and well as practising certain "plosive" letters such as p's" and b's.

I used to tell a joke about the unnaturalness of the speech techniques I learned in therapy:

> I can speak to you tonight because I had speech therapy lessons when I was younger. They taught me something called easy speech clicking which makes you speak very slowly, whilst clicking your fingers.
>
> However, I realised this didn't work very well after a series of unsuccessful interviews.
>
> I would go into the interview and say, "Hhhh- Hello, my name is Jaik Campbell. I applied for the post as your communications administrations assistant."

On one occasion they said, "Well, that's fine. What's your telephone manner like?"

I said, "It's verrrrry good. Just as long as I can use easy speech clicking."

They said, "Maybe you should consider getting a part in West Side Story" (whilst clicking fingers).

I said, "Thank you very much" (whilst clicking fingers).

(OK, the clicking fingers part was made up.)

The real problem was that at age eight there were many other things going on in my life. It was an academically competitive year, so my time was taken up with homework and trying to keep up with my peers. Sitting down for as little as ten minutes a day to practise speaking was very difficult to fit in. Even my parents didn't bother to encourage such practice, and so I simply wasn't worried about it. I was not being teased that much at school and so the impetus to actually put the time in to get rid of my stammer was reduced.

In addition to formal therapy, I also remember when I was about 11, my form mistress advised me to record myself speaking on tape and then play back my words. This task was designed to improve my speech. As with the easy speech, I generally neglected the advice.

Adult Therapy

When I was 20 and in my second year at university, I gradually became aware that my stutter was becoming more noticeable. So I visited the university general practitioner who referred me to a speech therapist. For most of the next three months, I attended block modification group therapy with eight other adult males.

Block Modification Therapy

The course introductory letter stated, "Speech and language therapy can only guide you with how best to help yourself, so during the course, you need to put it as a high priority in your life." Consistent with that message, therapy lasted full days (9.30 am to 4.30 pm), a large time commitment, especially as some of the days were Fridays. In truth, completing my degree and attending this course was a bit of a strain, but I really needed to improve my speech. My mother also really encouraged me to continue with it.

The course demanded emotional and mental energy and also the completion of quite a bit of homework. In addition, we were asked to practice new techniques in our "real lives." The goals were to develop more positive attitudes toward communication and to control and monitor speaking rate and breathing. The result was speech that was slightly slower and less physically tense.

The course was based on the writings of Charles Van Riper, a renowned speech therapist who became internationally known as a pioneer in the development of speech pathology, and who stammered himself. It consisted of a series of building blocks, each forming the basis for the next. We learned what we did and how we felt (e.g., anxious) when we stuttered, the idea being that this would help us change our attitudes and feelings and make the experience of stammering less negative. We also worked on breaking habits and modifying our core stuttering behaviours. The aim was to change the tense disfluencies to an easier, more fluent style of stammering.

I managed to attend nearly all of the eight day sessions, despite missing the odd lecture/geography practical (fortunately, university officials were OK with this). Not surprisingly, the sessions were quite intensive. One of the techniques I remember best was called pausing. Pausing was described as "a deliberate delay after a stammered word to remove the communicative profit from stammering." We had to train ourselves to stop and wait after each instance of stammering. The purpose of pausing was to reduce the time pressure and resume control of speech by taking a breath or two and relaxing the tense areas of the speech mechanism (namely the muscles of respiration, voicing, and/or articulation). The pause was also a way to acknowledge that a stammer had occurred instead of rewarding ourselves (i.e., the "communicative profit") by running away from it or trying to deny that it had actually happened, something of which I was definitely guilty.

Another session involved pausing mid-sentence, then identifying areas of the face and body that were too tense. From there we went to voluntary stuttering in a range of activities such as reading aloud and making phone calls. We ventured out in public in pairs and observed listener reactions to voluntary stammering.

This course allowed me to make changes in my speech and how I contended with listeners. More specifically, I was able to:

- Place phone calls in which I mentioned that I stammered,

- Tell more new people about my speech impediment,

- Discuss my stutter with my girlfriend,

- Try out a few voluntary stammers with friends,

- Use fewer of the "ums" and "ers" designed to hide stuttering,

- Utilize more pauses after bad blocks, and

- Modify my stammer by sliding into the vowel sound, such as "S-----u-----n" or "P----en-----cil".

Like most people in their 20's, I wanted to be a confident, fluent-speaking, self-assured, and decisive individual who was able to handle a job interview, go on dates, and get on with his life in a positive and constructive manner. However, block modification therapy made me realise that my stutter wasn't going to disappear following a few hours of speech therapy. Addressing it was going to take a long time and require a great deal of hard work and self-discipline.

Unfortunately, due to school/work/university commitments, I probably didn't devote enough practice time to reduce it significantly.

Actually, I *never* practiced voluntary stuttering with anyone except friends, as I was far too scared, self-conscious, and embarrassed of actually purposefully stammering with strangers. Other desensitisation activities, such as telling friends at university that I had a stammer, were also too difficult for me. Even the recommended physiological relaxation or block modification techniques were rarely practised. One reason was that I feared silence, as it reminded me of having a stammer in the first place. Thus, to purposefully add a forced gap in a sentence went against my instincts. Also, the pause needed to be at least three seconds to have the desired impact, which is a long time in conversational speech.

Overall, I was pleased that I took part in the block modification course, as it helped me to regard my stutter in a more positive way, as well as providing me with the tools to adapt the way I stuttered. Despite my lack of follow-through, the course forced me to push my comfort zones and practise speaking in more varied situations. This practise, in turn, probably led to me to conclude that standing up in front of audiences could help my speech. Comedy also offered a way of telling people that I had a stutter, thus decreasing my sensitivity about it.

Given my schedule and residual fears, however, it was not easy to continue using the techniques once the course ended. I was doing on average three gigs a week, in addition to numerous comedy competitions (including the path to the *Stand-Up Britain* final). My energy went into learning my lines rather than practicing the techniques I learnt in the course.

For someone whose schedule allows, this course is perfect way to start the recovery process, as it equips clients with all of the necessary tools for immediate and long-term results.

It has taken me ten years to refine and repractice the techniques, and to truly understand their importance to my life.

Wembley Therapy

Several years after completing my university studies, I became a Crime Mapping Officer for Brent Council in North West London. When my contract expired, I had to reapply for a new Geographical Information System (GIS) Analyst post at Brent Council. The application process involved a three person panel interview and a ten minute presentation. The day was a stuttering disaster and I was duly dismissed.

I was 25 years old and out of work.

A series of failed interviews followed, but they did result in a referral to a speech and language therapist at the Wembley Centre for Health and Care. At the time I was quite annoyed that I had to see a speech therapist, but in hindsight it was the best thing I could have done. I had not only just lost a job, but also a girlfriend. I was a stuttering wreck; the sheer act of breathing was often difficult, the ability to relax impossible.

The Wembley course entailed four 2-hour sessions spread out over two months. It began with breathing drills "to be practiced at least once a day for ten minutes." I was then taught voice exercises performed while lying down—breathing in for a count of four and then phonating slowly and evenly for another 4-count. I was told to focus on relaxation, posture, and establishing a correct breathing pattern. Relaxation exercises included tightening my toes by curling them under the soles of my feet, holding them taut, and then letting them go; and turning my feet upwards toward my knees to tense my ankles, then relaxing them to enjoy the feeling of ease.

Perhaps helped by the speech therapy sessions, I finally had a successful job interview. The interviewer told me that the stutter wasn't an issue, mainly because the job involved fairly little speaking. However, my new post as "GIS Technician" did become one of many distractions in my life at the time. As a result, I don't think I practised the therapy techniques enough to notice any real effects.

More Block Modification Therapy

The technician job lasted two years, after which I needed to find work again. Whilst in Edinburgh in August 2001, I saw my former MSc supervisor who suggested that I make sorting out my stutter a top priority, as he felt it would affect any profession I decided to enter. Based on that advice, I started a new series of block modification sessions at the City Lit, in London. Going on the course also gave me an excuse to be out of the house in the evenings, which was a welcome diversion at the time.

Term 1 involved attending weekly 2-hour sessions. During this time, I was also doing a great deal of stand-up performances, but I still made it to every session. In fact, they helped my confidence and comedic timing on stage.

Again, the aims of the therapy were to help me become less sensitive about stuttering and to reduce the tension of the actual stammers. As with the Bristol course, it was group therapy, which was normally subdivided into smaller groups for parts of each session. Apparently group sessions are better than individual sessions as clients gain mutual support as well as experience communicating in life-like situations. Stammerers often feel isolated because they believe no one else stammers in quite the same way they do. Through participation in the group stammering course, I learnt that most of us had faced similar challenges and had similar thoughts relating to our speech, both of which were useful.

One of their aims was to make us become our own therapists, which seemed like a useful concept. We were told that the more regularly we attended, the more likely we were to benefit from the therapy. We were also encouraged to complete daily home assignments because "a reasonable amount of therapy each day is better than cramming a lot in the night before." Finally, greater progress was anticipated if we could involve some of our workmates, friends, or family in the desensitisation process.

As a group, we agreed:

a) To participate as much as possible in group activities, (a - c)

b) To be open with each other (with sensitivity), and

c) To be punctual as far as possible.

Some of the highlights from this course include the following:

- We were introduced to the idea that many problems are made easier by treating them "as a series of small, interrelated steps, called a hierarchy."

- I came to realise that the severity of my stammer had increased over time as my school, university, and work environments became more stressful.

- The situations in which I feared I would stutter closely correlated those in which I actually did. These included making calls and answering the phone, speaking in groups, asking for directions, requesting items in a shop, buying train tickets, introducing myself to others, and job interviews.

- Identification exercises showed me that I blocked on particular plosive letters such as p and b. These created tension on my lips at the front of my mouth.

- I realised that my breathing needed to be more relaxed when I spoke.

- Telling people that I had a stammer increased my self-confidence.

- Watching too much TV tended to clutter up my mind and increase my blocking.

- It was important to focus on my speaking, rather than being too sensitive to the people/events going on around me.

Like at Bristol, this therapy was based on the Van Riper (1973) approach. The actual modification of stuttering involved three steps: pausing after a word (called "cancellation"), in-block modification, and finally, pre-block correction. The aims of this part of the course were to teach us strategies for the modification of a blocked word, thereby learning how to stutter more fluently.

Cancellation or "post-block modification" involved taking action after stuttering. It was step 1 because it is apparently easier to work on a block after, rather than before, it happens. My notes related to the relevant steps read as follows.

1) *Complete the problem word, pause for about three seconds and then continue. (numbered)*

2) *Use the pause to calm down and to pantomime the way you have just stuttered, i.e. suddenly recreate what you did when you stuttered. Though pantomiming is done silently, you should actually execute the actions rather than just thinking about them.*

3) *Also pantomime the new way you intend to say the word, slowly moving from sound to sound.*

4) *Repeat the stuttered word aloud, but in a modified version. The aim is not to produce the word fluently, but to say it slower, more deliberately, and with complete conscious control.*

Apparently cancellation is not designed to increase fluency, but, rather, to set up a model for easy stuttering. In other words, mastering cancellation is a step toward speech control.

At the time, post-block modification was difficult for me to practice in real-life situations, and it wasn't something I felt I was likely to use outside the classroom. If I were meeting a new person, I just couldn't bring myself to pause three seconds after each stammer. I felt that was worse than stammering. In hindsight, I was letting my stutter control me rather than controlling it.

In-block modification was a bit more functional. During a moment of stuttering, we were asked to deliberately prolong what we were doing. While holding on to the stuttered sound, we mentally searched the sequence of movements that would take us through the rest of the word. The important point was to "stutter forward", rather than stopping and starting again. From the tense stuttering position, we tried to work toward a more appropriate way to make the sound. This could involve, for example, repositioning our mouths, unscrewing our faces, and then gradually easing the sound out. All our attention and monitoring needed to be directed at how we were producing the word, feeling our way through the sounds successively.

Once we got the hang of finishing stuttered words more smoothly, we could try to grab hold of the stutter earlier and earlier. We tried to change the moment of stuttering into a slow, forward-moving release as soon as possible after recognising that we were stuttering. In other words, we tried to apply the modification technique progressively sooner in time.

In order to achieve in-block modifications successfully, various conditions were necessary. We had to:

1. Be able to recognise moments of stuttering,

2. Be prepared to work on them,

3. Avoid panic at the recognition of stuttering, and

4. Remember that it was possible to assume control over stuttering by focusing on what our mouths were doing, rather than how we felt about stuttering.

Sometimes I blocked on a word and virtually no sound escaped. In these instances, I needed a way to transition from the tense and silent block to "easy vocalisation." The recommended bridge was the use of "vocal fry" or "creaky voice." In time, I alternated creaky voice with my natural voice to move slowly into the next word. For example, if I had a silent block of the word "Daniel", I used progressively less creaky voice (shown underlined), such as D d d Daniel, and then D d d d Daniel, followed by D d d Daniel.

One benefit of techniques such as this was the knowledge that it if I got into a stammering situation, I could do something about it. This, as any stammerer will tell you, is more than half the battle. Such awareness made me more relaxed and meant that I was less likely to stammer in the first place. The new cycle of fluency replaced a previous vicious circle of "I'm going to stammer. I'm nervous, therefore I stammer. I can't do anything about it, so I get more nervous and stammer more." Now my thought process was more "if I do stammer, so what?" It sounds simple but it's easier said than done, and requires much practice!

The final level of modification, pre-block correction, was designed to correct the block on the approach to the word. We did this by pausing just before we said the feared word. During the pause we then planned an easy way of saying it. With practice, the procedure was very quick and accurate. However, in learning this technique, there were many stages which need to be tackled slowly and carefully:

1. Pause before the difficult word,

2. Relax the throat and mouth muscles,

3. Recall the way in which the word is normally stuttered,

4. Plan the corrections needed to eliminate the hard stutter (e.g., tongue position at the front of the mouth/less tension in the jaw), and

5. Prolong the word aloud, keeping the sound flowing.

Apparently, it was vitally important that the pause was not used as a postponement device. Instead, it was designed to prepare and rehearse the new plan of action. As soon as possible, I was to move slowly into the problem word.

In order to become proficient in our use of this technique, we were told to practise it as much as possible, on both feared and non-feared words. As we became more accustomed to using pre-block corrections, we could gradually eliminate the pause. We found that we could prepare to say the word smoothly from the moment we anticipated stuttering, even while talking. If we practiced it sufficiently, it could become an automatic response to the anticipation of stuttering.

Effective Communication in the Workplace for People who Stammer

Soon after completing the second Block Modification course, I attended a 3-day course (from 10 am to 4 pm each day) designed to explore the issues of stammering and the workplace. Topics included stress management, dealing with authority relationships, and effective listening. I was also encouraged to mention my stammer more. In addition, we looked at our rights at work, noting that we were entitled to 1) be treated with respect and dignity and 2) express our feelings and opinions.

A major focus of the course was telephone fears, for which we learned some do's and don'ts:

- Do not put calls off.

- Develop tolerance for silences/pauses on the phone.

- Answer the call in our own time, instead of rushing.

- Be aware of areas of physical tension during speech and to try to allow these areas to relax.

Overall it was a detailed and useful course, which again I perhaps should have read over again in the ten years since!

My Story Course

Later that same year I attended a group course called "My Story." The ten 2-hour sessions focused on the psychological and personal issues related to stammering. It allowed us to reflect on our personal life stories, defined as our past, present, and future hopes, fears, dreams, aspirations, losses, and gains related to being someone who stammers. By creating a story about ourselves as people, we could make sense of confusing experiences from the past. We explored the idea of the "personal myth" representing our identity and how our "selves" are created through narrative and within a social context.

This time I put quite a bit of effort into the homework exercises, because I found the course to be interesting and because I wanted to gather some new material for my stand-up routine. Initially, the homework involved listing eight critical incidents from the past, focusing on the impact those events had on my life story and what they said about who I was or am as a person. This was a useful process as it made me think about my key changing points over the years.

The eight key life events were:

1. *Peak experience: A high point in your life story; the most wonderful moment in your life.*

One of the events I listed was my first holiday abroad on my own in Gran Canaria. This occurred about 18 months prior to this course and lasted a week. I hired a car and spent the time feeling very free, confident, and independent. There was also the day I found out I graduated with honours from Bristol University. Both incidents made me feel more sure of myself as a person, and I realised I could do things on my own and not feel self-conscious. Anything that can improve confidence and make it stay is a wonderful moment!

2. *Nadir experience: A low point in your life story; the worst moment in your life.*

I was at Heathrow Airport, saying goodbye to my long-time girlfriend, knowing that I would probably never see her again. She was going home, never to return to London. Three weeks later, this low point sunk even further: She wrote to me saying that she had been cheating on me for six months. This experience took me a while to get over and made me quite tough, isolated, and self-reliant. For a time afterwards, I became negative about life and relationships, which probably helped put me on course toward stand-up comedy.

3. *Turning point: An episode which led to a significant change in your understanding of yourself. It may be that you did not realise it was a turning point when it happened. What is important is that now, in retrospect, you see it as a turning point or at least as symbolising a significant change in your life.*

I identified two episodes that led to the reclusive and solitary Jaik Campbell of the *My Story* course:

- I ended a relationship (prior to the cheater) to focus on my third year university exams, reconsidered, but unfortunately wasn't able to restart it.

- Trying to come to terms with the repercussions of my father pulling a knife on one of my friends at my twenty-first birthday party took a lot of soul searching.

4. *Earliest memory: One of the earliest memories you have of an event that is complete with setting, scene, characters, feelings and thoughts. It does not have to seem like an especially important memory.*

I remember my first girlfriend from primary school, at the age of 6 or 7. I realised that I was too young to be having a girlfriend, but enjoyed spending time with her. I remember feelings of happiness, excitement, embarrassment, and stress! This "relationship" ended when we changed schools, but we kept in touch during our teens (although she wasn't quite so keen on me then).

5. *An important childhood memory: Any memory from your childhood, positive or negative, that stands out today.*

I noted two memories, both of which were related in chapter 3:

- I recall going to the Abbey entrance exam and not even being able to say my name upon arrival and then later being told to stand outside while the teacher told the class that they were to be kind toward the new stuttering child. I realised that I wasn't exactly the same as everyone else and made sure I worked harder to compensate. This event led to me being a very studious person. In fact, I was top of the class in my first year at the Abbey.

- I also have a vivid memory of travelling with my family to Europe and my father hitting his toe on a massive iron bar. It was about that time that my stutter began and I feel that the stress of this trip was a possible catalyst for my speech difficulties.

6. *An important adolescent memory: Any memory from your teenage years that stands out today. Again, it can be either positive or negative.*

My late teens were fairly memorable:

- At aged 17, I failed my first driving test. No surprise, my father got very stressed out by it and told me off. He thought that the examiner and driving instructor were in collaboration with each other to make more money!

- That same year at the sixth form school ball, I became drunk on red wine and ended up sleeping in my car, a circumstance caused by frustration, depression, and exhaustion, all related to my inability to make any real connection with a girl I quite liked.

- Also at 17 (it was a busy year), I crashed the car and my father went absolutely crazy when he found out. (I had stupidly left opened the drawer in which the insurance forms were kept, in my attempt to sort out the mess myself.) My father then phoned up the owner of the car I crashed into and had a massive argument with him before driving me up there to meet him. As we were driving away, I was still buckling the car door, as my father was in a rush and had forgotten to close it!

- At 18, I went off to University and met lots of new people. I did not speak very confidently and became fairly depressed when I realised I had little or no self-confidence. I felt I would never find a girlfriend or maintain a proper conversation with anybody.

7. *An important adult memory: A memory, positive or negative, that stands out from age 21 onwards.*

- After a year and a half without a girlfriend, I met an attractive woman who amazed me by actually agreeing to go out. What followed was a very exciting time, one which made me feel very grown up, confident, and independent from my parents, all positive steps. Also my stammer seemed less of a problem during this time for some reason.

- Numerous failed job interviews qualified as bad adult moments, in particular being told twice that I could have the job only if I lost my stutter.

8. *Other important memory: One other particular event from your past that stands out. It may be from long ago or recent times. It may be positive or negative.*

Instead of a specific memory, I went with a stream of consciousness for this item. I broke up with my girlfriend, had second thoughts, then went to her house and realised that the relationship was completely over. I later saw her around with a new boyfriend and became very depressed about this. I drove up to Edinburgh University to do an MSc as a way of coming to terms with the loss. Whilst up In Edinburgh, I lived and studied with some very interesting people from many different cultures. I also saw a few comedy shows at the Edinburgh Festival and recognized that I wanted to be part of that too. Realising that self-fulfilment was more important than being in a relationship at that stage, the experience helped make me into a very self-reliant person (while still a bit angry over my break-up mistake).

Significant people. The final exercise dealing with the past was to list significant people in our life stories. This began with identification of individuals who had major impacts on us. We were asked to reflect on the kinds of relationships we had with them and the impressions they made on our lives. At the age of 28, my list consisted of the following:

1. My father – Although, as noted, this was not an easy relationship, his impact cannot be denied. It can be described as severe, tough, and hard, especially in my 20's. He also has a stutter and for various deep psychological reasons was a narcissist and maverick control freak, perpetually frustrated, unhappy, and loud.

2. My mother – This was a good relationship, filled with friendship and support. She always tried to make me practical, able to earn money, but, overall, she has been very understanding, supportive, and kind to me over the years.

3. My MSc supervisor (Professor Peter Furley) – I would term Prof. Furley "useful support." He improved my self-discipline and confidence in my academic abilities by being quite strict with me, which I probably needed at the time. He also forced me to focus on my speech difficulties and advised me to get help to cure it.

4. A previous girlfriend – The woman I left at Heathrow helped me believe in myself, which facilitated self-confidence. In

addition, spending time with her always cheered me up to the point that I felt I could do whatever I wanted to do. Unfortunately, she also did whatever *she* wanted to do, marrying another and making me feel quite hurt and angry. But I forgive her. I couldn't be there for her enough and we weren't 100% compatible, so it probably wouldn't have lasted anyway.

We also had to identify any particular heroines or heroes that we had in our lives and tell why we chose them. I listed:

1. Rowan Atkinson

2. John Cleese

3. Bruce Willis

4. Daniel Kitson

I selected these people because I believed I understood their goals: exerting a bit of creative influence in society, being admired, and having fulfilling and meaningful careers. Talented and self-disciplined, they are people who are focused and believe in themselves. They did what they did (i.e. acting, comedy) driven by a need to perform for an audience.

I think it's important to enjoy one's occupation, given that so much of life is spent working. The people I chose seem to enjoy what they do while still having an influence on mankind and making money.

Rowan Atkinson, Bruce Willis, and Daniel Kitson all had stammers when they were younger, and it is interesting that they have all excelled at performing. Perhaps their stammers made them overcompensate in other areas of their lives or gave them the sensitivity and pathos needed to be likeable, humble, and endearing actors/performers at an internationally acclaimed level. The public likes celebrities who have overcome the odds rather than being handed something on a plate.

Stresses and Problems. Moving on to our everyday present lives, we were instructed to think about two causes of significant stress or major conflict/challenge that needed to be addressed. Specifically, the assignment was to write a brief history of each stressor and a plan for dealing with it in the future. I found this to be a useful process. All of us have challenges in our lives, but we don't actually take the time to sit down and systematically attempt to resolve them. Instead we bury ourselves in work or watch television, in the hope that they will go away, which, of course, they never do.

Ten years ago, I identified the following stresses and problems:

1) Nature of stress, problem, conflict, problem, or challenge

I had to decide whether or not to continue at comedy/acting or go back to Suffolk to get more involved with my father's cattle feed business. (This is slightly amazing that a decade ago I had the same problem that I have now. This one still hasn't been 100% resolved yet!)

2) Source of concern

I'm worried that if I don't start getting more involved back home soon, I will never do it. On the other hand, comedy/acting is my dream, albeit one that might never happen. It's a bit of a lottery with a lot of negative aspects to it.

113

3) Brief history of its development

I believe that my father always assumed that I would get more involved with his business. After all, my geography degrees and work experience are relevant to that type of work. But I also always wanted to do stand-up comedy and to act. Due to being brought up by self-employed parents, I work better on my own, without a manager and in a fairly unrestrictive time/day structure.

4) Plan for dealing with it

If I go home, the comedy/acting will be very difficult to do, as I will be expected to work very hard on the animal feed business/farm (i.e. 9 am - 6 pm every day). Although London is not too bad, I am getting a little sick of it.

(Note: Five years after writing the above paragraph, I left London and moved back to Suffolk. It subsequently turned out my father and I couldn't really work with each other. The amount of criticism he could fit into a work day was too much for me. On the plus side, I took comfort in the fact that he criticised everyone, so it was not just me!)

1. Nature of stress, problem, conflict, problem, or challenge that must be addressed soon

I wanted to see my ex-girlfriend one last time. We were together for 14 months, but now living in different cities.

2. Source of concern

She was not only distant at the time, but I was worried that she would soon be even further away, as in was going back to her home country, half a world away.

3. *Brief history of its development*

We had become friends, until she found a new chap, fell in love, and married just a few months after we broke up.

4. *Plan for dealing with it*

I needed to go and see her. I knew that probably wouldn't help things very much, but she was difficult to forget.

As a result of writing this exercise, I organised stand-up gigs at comedy clubs in the big city nearest her village. I hired a car and drove 160 miles to see her, just hoping that she'd be there. Luckily she was. I slept in the car that night in order to see her the next day. I was successful, as she granted me a whole hour of her precious time.

It was worth it.

1. *Nature of stress, problem, conflict, problem, or challenge that must be addressed soon*

Living with my current roommates is destroying our friendships.

2. *Source of concern*

I'm woken up every morning at 6.30 am by one of them getting ready for work. Their conversations and general way of acting are stressing me out. I don't really get on with them very well these days. The situation makes stand-up comedy more tiring than it should be. Still, I perform as often as possible because I can't stand being in the flat in the evenings.

3. Brief history of its development

We've been living in the same flat together for two years and it's no longer any fun. In fact, it's very depressing and tiring.

4. Plan for dealing with it

I have various options:

- Move out and live on my own (but that's too expensive, as I'm not earning any money at the moment).

- Earn more money (but it's difficult to get a place for one as the average rent for a single bedroom flat is quite high).

- Go back to Suffolk, work hard, then return (which would involve working for my father).

- Stay in the flat with the landlady, whist my roommates move out (which is what eventually happened; it was a messy situation that totally ruined my friendship with both roommates).

Future Script – Where is your story going? Having explored my past and present, I was then asked to think about the future. I was to describe my overall plan or dream and how it enabled me "to be creative in the future and to make a contribution to others."

I identified three dreams:

Dream 1) To be a famous stand-up comedian/actor. This one had many sub-goals:

- get more paid gigs,

- write more entertaining and educational material,

- have my own successful 1-man comedy show at the Edinburgh Fringe,

- do more TV work and become an acclaimed television personality,

- comedy acting on TV or in a film, and

- have my own chat show in 5 to 10 years' time (ironic for someone who can't really chat).

Being a comedian is creative and makes a contribution to others by providing entertainment and laughter, ideally in an educational and positive way. In my case, comedy could possibly be used to increase public awareness about stuttering.

Dream 2) To earn a PhD. First of all, this dream can assist with achieving dream 1 by providing money, skills, and education. It would be stressful, but more useful to society than doing stand-up comedy. It also requires less alcohol. At the time, I thought that a PhD was only really necessary for a career in academia, but in the years since I've realised that doing a PhD is recognised by employers across a wide range of sectors as a sign that a candidate can creatively combine subject-specific knowledge and a distinctive skill set to their organisations. As such, contributions can be made to education (teaching, administrative and professional roles), public sector positions, research and development, publishing, or general entrepreneurial activities, to name just a few areas.

Dream 3) To help my father's cattle feed business. This opportunity would provide an income and help continue the business. Also, business-related work has an element of creativity attached to it, although obviously not as much as writing and performing comedy. And providing dairy feed to farmers contributes to the milk and beef industries in the UK. On the other hand, I would have to learn all about the cattle feed industry which would take time to interest me.

Eventual outcome. Because of the high cost of living in London, and the fact I wasn't suited for the place, I eventually moved back to Suffolk whilst still returning to London for stand-up gigs. In addition to the aforementioned criticism from my father, various arguments ensued. I spent much of my days doing menial tasks, such as painting and sweeping. Also, a series of barn conversions involved me helping builders, rather than learning about the cattle feed business. Once the barns were completed, I was put in charge of their management, which was a good opportunity but involved a great deal of time doing cleaning and maintenance.

Stuttering in Society. The final part of the course was to think about the messages we have received about stammering over the years. To this I wrote:

> *Overall, I think the media and films haven't had a positive influence on stammering over the years. For example, in the film "A Fish Called Wanda," Michael Palin plays a stammerer who seemed like a clumsy half-wit, sex starved and having chips up his nose. I don't think this helped the plight of stammerers.*

Also the film "Die Hard with a Vengeance", starring Bruce Willis, the main antagonist in the film, played by Jeremy Irons, had a stammer and he was made to seem a little psychotic.

In "Smoky and the Bandit" (starring Burt Reynolds and Sally Field), Mel Tillis (the country music star who stutters) did a cameo appearance as a stuttering amusement park employee, and when he stuttered badly, he was made to look like an idiot by the main characters.

Since that time, the Oscar winning movie *The Kings Speech* has given the public better insight into the trials and tribulations of dealing with a stammer (not to mention showing that it can inflict even someone as important George VI, who was King of Great Britain from 1937 until 1952). I also felt certain that comedians helped put stammering in a more positive light. For example, Patrick Campbell was an Irish journalist, humourist, and television personality in the 1960s, who suffered from a stammer, but nevertheless delighted television audiences with his wit, most notably as a regular team captain on the long-running show *Call My Bluff*. Some of his funniest short stories described stammering incidents. Patrick turned his stammer to his advantage and I found this to be quite inspirational.

I also read about Frankie Howerd, an English comedian and comic actor whose career spanned six decades. Frankie was neither a slick professional stand-up nor a rapid joke machine, but audiences loved the way his stammering delivery side-tracked and fluffed straight-forward punch lines. He made a career out of being a mixed-up, pretentious, pompous man who sent-up his own act and the performances around him. As a side note, Frankie Howerd also had quite a depressive personality, to which I could relate!

119

We were also asked how the media's overall portrayal of stammering affected who we are. In my case, having a stutter made me want to act and perform more. I'm not sure why—maybe as a way to practice speaking or to prove that even with a stammer I can be successful at talking. I didn't want my stammer to stop me from doing things I wanted to do. Perhaps that is why I tended to put my professional goals in front of everything else.

Well, almost everything else.

The *My Story* course taught me that I tended to make decisions to please my parents rather than myself. Such are the problems of growing up with a narcissistic father. Family business activities always came first. They still do today.

Questions for Discussion

Jaik employed secondary behaviors to hide his stuttering when saying his name. How well do you believe that, "Yes, well it's um, it's er, I mean, it's normally, Jaik Campbell" fooled his listeners?

Why do you think people who stutter often have difficulty saying their own names?

Jaik writes:

> Someone would ask, "What's your name?" and I'd just make a weird facial grimace.
>
> "That's a strange name," would be the response.
>
> "Yes," I'd answer. "It's Greek for complete moron."

Why did he use a derogatory term when referring to himself in this situation?

When Jaik was 11, he was advised to record himself speaking and then listen to the recording. What was the purpose of that advice?

As a young adult, stuttering was important enough to Jaik to attend all-day therapy, but not to practice regularly. Can you explain this apparent discrepancy?

During Block Modification Therapy, Jaik realized that simply possessing strategies to modify stuttering resulted in fewer instances of stuttering. Why do you think this was so?

The *My Story* course involved describing life events in order to "make sense" of them and better understand one's self. How might this help with stuttering?

Jaik related a childhood memory of one of the family's stressful vacations, noting that it "was a possible catalyst" for his stuttering. What do you think he meant by that?

Take the *My Story* course (i.e., answer the same questions Jaik answered). What did you learn about yourself?

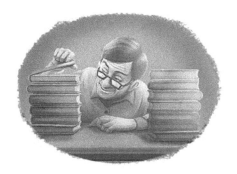

Chapter 6: Assessment and Management

Jaik's description of his therapy journeys began with a description of his early stuttering. Reportedly, it consisted of both repetitions and prolongations which, all in all, is fairly typical. Although repetitions are the more common feature (Onslow & O'Brian, 2013), prolongations are not exactly rare at onset.

Later, Jaik began to "block," a designation usually used, as it is by Jaik, to refer to tense hesitations of speech. Caution is urged with this term, however, as it is employed by others to mean *any* type of disfluency. For that reason, this text has used (and the even numbered chapters will continue to use) the word *hesitations* to denote silent fixations that disallow the initiation of sounds.

While we're dealing with vocabulary, there are a couple of other items that need attention. The term *stammering*, though not widely utilized in the United States, is used interchangeably with *stuttering* in other English speaking countries (Logan, 2014), including those of the UK. For American readers, then, Jaik uses the word stammering to mean stuttering.

Assessment

Jaik's description of his stuttering—repetitions, prolongations, hesitations, secondary behaviors—almost perfectly fits the definition laid out in chapter 2. Even so, these characteristics alone would not be enough to diagnose it. For one thing, there are other fluency disorders that can look a lot like stuttering, yet respond much differently to treatment (see Table 1). Misdiagnosis can result in recommendations that are ineffective and a waste of the client's time and money.

Table 1: Disorders of Fluency Other Than Developmental Stuttering

Type/Name of Disorder of Disfluency	Primary Characteristics	Treatment Strategies
Neurogenic Disfluency • Acquired, i.e., not developmental but resulting from a neurological insult of some sort (lesion or disease) • Damage can be widespread or limited. • Among other conditions, disfluency has been associated with the following: 1. Basal Ganglia Lesions 2. Right Hemisphere Lesion 3. Left Hemisphere Lesion 4. Diffuse CNS damage 5. Cerebellar Lesions	Neurogenic disfluency is not a unitary disorder. Characteristics and responses to treatment can vary with site and severity of damage. More frequent characteristics include: • Part-word, word, and phrase repetitions • Prolongations • Onset often within one month of neurological event • Fluency less likely to vary based on word position or type (i.e., content vs. function) • Often no secondary behaviors are observed • Anxiety can accompany disfluency • Typical fluency enhancing conditions do not always help these individuals	• Research has shown that enhancement or modification treatment methods used for developmental stuttering can be applied to neurogenic stuttering. • Electromyographic biofeedback • Delayed auditory feedback • White noise masking auditory feedback • Transcutaneous nerve stimulator • Medications

Table 1 Continued

Type/Name of Disorder of Disfluency	Primary Characteristics	Treatment Strategies
Cluttering • Low incidence disorder • Official etiology is idiopathic • May be tied to basal ganglia dysfunction • Can co-exist with stuttering	Some of the most commonly reported characteristics include: • Rapid, irregular rate of speech • Expressive language deficits • Language formulation disorders • Difficulties with narrative cohesion • Poor social skills • Misarticulations • Tendency to repeat phrases or words • Lack of awareness of speech differences • Reading deficits • Short attention span • Sloppy handwriting • Atypical placement of pauses • Excessive talking • Typically preschool onset • Affects males more often than females	Treatment often focuses on: • Awareness • Rate control • Language deficit areas • Self-monitoring • Production of word endings • Loudness control
Disfluencies associated with Intellectual Disability	• Primarily part word repetitions that increase in frequency as speech becomes more excitable. • Repetitions can occur in final word positions • Low levels of concern and amount of secondary behaviors • Disfluency increases when word length increases and with less familiar words • Severity tends to increase with degree of intellectual disability • Adaptation may be present • Low expectancy	• Fluency enhancement

Table 1 Continued

Type/Name of Disorder of Disfluency	Primary Characteristics	Treatment Strategies
Psychogenic Disfluency • Disfluency associated with psychological disorders • Client history likely to include sudden onset in response to a significant event	• Part word repetitions • Does not necessarily respond to fluency enhancing conditions • Situational variability • Periods of no disfluency • Frequency may increase as speech task level decreases • Extraneous movements unrelated to speech production	• Symptomatic therapy • Counseling • Delayed Auditory Feedback • May respond to treatment very rapidly and completely disappear
Palilalia Associated with basal ganglia dysfunction	• Repetitions of words, phrases, or sentences of at least 2 but often numerous iterations • Disfluencies may include utterance-final repetitions • Often no facial tension • Awareness of speech differences • Seen in individuals with Parkinson's, pseudobulbar palsy, schizophrenia, and Gilles de la Tourette syndrome, among other conditions	• Stuttering modification • Fluency enhancement • Speech devices such as pacing board • Electromyographic biofeedback • Delayed auditory feedback • White masking noise auditory feedback • Transcutaneous nerve stimulator • Medication
Disfluency associated with genetic syndromes • Reported syndromes include: • Down • Fragile X • Prader-Willi	• Part-word repetitions • Prolongations • Tension accompanying disfluencies • Cluttering-like behaviors (Down Syndrome) • Final sound repetitions (Down Syndrome) • Final sentence position disfluencies (Fragile X Syndrome)	• Fluency enhancement

Table 1 References: Azevedo et al., 2012; Boller et al., 1973; Bonfonti & Culatta, 1977; Borsel, Drummond, & de Britto Pereira, 2010; Chang et al., 2010; Chapman & Cooper, 1973; Cooper, 1986; Coppens-Hofman et al., 2013; Craig, 2010; Daly & Burnett, 1996; Duffy, 1995 Howell & Davis, 2011; Jokel et al., 2007; Krishnan & Tiwari, 2013; Langevin & Boberg, 1996; Lebrun & Borsel, 1990; Market et al., 1990; Myers et al., 2012; Otto & Yairi, 1974; Preuss, 1990; Scaler-Scott, 2011; Stansfield, Collier, & King, 2012; St. Louis et al., 2003; St. Louis & Myers, 1995; Theys, van Wieringen, & De Nil, 2008; Van Borsel, Drummond, & de Britto Pereira, 2010; van Zaalen-op't Hof, Wijnen, & De Jonckere, 2009; Ward, 2010; Ward & Scott, 2011; Ward et al., 2015; Williams & Wener, 1996.

When discussing diagnosis, it is also worth reiterating that stuttering-like disfluencies may be observed with nonstuttering individuals, although the frequency would likely be lower. This raises the question of how many disfluencies are required for stuttering. Some (e.g., Anderson & Felsenfeld, 2003) have offered three per 100 words as a rule of thumb, which is sensible in that few normally speaking children would produce that many. Of course, duration and tension need also be taken into account when diagnosing fluency disorders. A child may produce one prolongation in 100 words, but if it is one in which he struggles for ten seconds, he is not presenting normal fluency.

For frequency measures, percent of stuttering-like disfluencies can be reported in either words (as noted above) or syllables. The use of syllables (i.e., number of disfluencies divided by total number of syllables spoken) is recommended here simply because more than one stutter can occur within a single word. From a personal perspective, I also find syllables easier to count. They are all similar in duration, as opposed to words, which can vary greatly. Of course, such discussion might soon become outdated with the advent of electronic devices that can utilize speech processing technology to measure frequency, such as the *MyLynel* ® (Kale & Williams, 2014).

Although frequency of stuttering is not absolutely necessary for making a diagnosis, it is still important to record. For one thing, frequenmcy is often viewed as a primary component of severity[1] (see Riley, 2009), and can thus be helpful in situations in which the diagnostician is required to provide a severity rating. Using the same

---

1   Although severity is often based on stuttering frequency (Craig, 1998; Hancock & Craig, 1998), this limited view has been called into question (e.g., Manning, 2001). Other factors that have been associated with severity include disfluency duration, secondary behaviors, and the impact that stuttering has on one's life (Riley, 2009; Yaruss & Quesal, 2006).

premise, should frequency levels diminish over time, that may well be an indication that the client's stuttering issue is becoming less handicapping.

Unfortunately (given its potential importance), frequency counts are often unreliable (Cordes, 2000). Straightforward stuttering-like disfluencies that match contemporary definitions (e.g., instances of "p-p-p-potato" or "buh-buh-buh-buh-ball") are relatively simple to count. But what about single-unit repetitions that involve a lot of tension? Or multiple iterations that include interjections ("d-uh-d-dentist")? Or hesitations of some but not excessive tension that occur at clause boundaries? Examples such as these can make tallies more difficult and lessen the agreement across counters.

Given that core and secondary behaviors are insufficient to differentially diagnose stuttering, the question becomes what else is needed. Because there is no universal test (i.e., one for which a particular result indicates stuttering), diagnosticians are left to develop case profiles based upon what is known about the disorder. With stuttering, fortunately, we have learned much over the years. *Un*fortunately, despite decades of research, there remain some pieces of information that elude experts (the cause, for example; and the cure). To substantiate a diagnosis of stuttering with any degree of certainty then, numerous data are required.

In short, the more information that can be obtained, the better. Along with stuttering-like disfluencies and secondary behaviors, we can also determine—through testing, interview, and observation—whether any or all of the following features exist:

- Preschool age of onset,

- Episodic development,

128

- Family history of stuttering,

- Handedness[2],

- Adaptation,

- Negative speech-associated attitudes, and

- Reduced stuttering under fluency-enhancing conditions (such as whispering, singing, choral reading, or another easily testable condition).

For example, say a client presents part-word repetitions that began around the age of 3 and, in addition, displays avoidance of speaking situations, speech-related fears, and total fluency when speaking in unison. In such a scenario, much evidence has been accumulated that fits the general profile associated with stuttering.

Unfortunately, in the real world, the client's profile will more likely consist of some of these tendencies but not others. Thus, the speech-language pathologist (SLP) often has to determine whether the weight of the evidence indicates stuttering.

In addition to supporting the diagnosis, the SLP also needs to ascertain as much as possible about the individual client's stuttering and make appropriate recommendations (see Table 2). For these reasons, the fluency evaluation should yield additional information, such as:

---

2   Non-right handedness—i.e., individuals who are left-handed or ambidextrous—occurs more frequently among those who stutter than in the general population (Cavenagh et al., 2015; Starkweather, 1987).

- Consistency, which can help determine whether the stuttering is triggered by certain sounds (what Jaik terms "letters") or words, as opposed to being more situational.

- Speaking under different conditions. For example, does a child stutter more with a parent in the room? What about a sibling or a stranger? Does frequency change when going from conversation to reading? These types of observations can tell SLPs much about the individual's situational stuttering factors.

- Testing for concomitant disorders such as phonological or language deficits. Such additional conditions are common with stuttering (Bauman et al., 2012; Blood, et al., 2003; Ntourou, Conture, & Lipsey, 2011; Wolk, Edwards, & Conture, 1993) and can complicate therapy (LaSalle, 2014).

- Identification of communicative stressors. As Jaik noted, feared situations often closely correlate those in which stuttering occurs with great frequency. Life stressors—in Jaik's case, his father, roommates, love life, and others—certainly do not help. In fact, at least one of them (his father) appeared to be clearly detrimental to his speech.

Table 2. Selected evaluation tasks and information applied to the common 3-step diagnostic process (e.g., Williams, 2012).

Step 1: Find out if there's a problem.	Step 2: If so, find out about the problem.	Step 3: Recommendations (i.e., what to do about the problem)
Client's or significant other's description of the problem	Client's or significant other's description of the problem	Listener reactions
Onset description	Awareness of speech difference	Daily impacts of disorder
Family history	Frustrations related to speech	Awareness of speech difference
Handedness	Frequency of stuttering	Frustrations related to speech
Presence of secondary behaviors	Specific secondary behaviors	Specific secondary behaviors
Speech samples	Situational factors	Situational factors
Adaptation	Easy/difficult sounds or words	Easy/difficult sounds or words
Speech under fluency-enhancing conditions	Easy/difficult sounds or words	Previous therapy
Attitude scales	Speech samples	Speech samples
	Expectancy	Attitude scales
	Consistency	Concomitant disorders
	Attitude scales	
	Concomitant disorders	

Note: The reader might find it easier to think of the three columns as 1) data that help with making a diagnosis, 2) learning about the client's particular fluency disorder, and 3) the information that can benefit the treatment plan.

On this last point, it is worth mentioning that none of the primary generalized stressors were resolved with any real closure. Jaik's father was always looming as a potential employer. His roommates left under "messy" circumstances. Old girlfriends were revisited. One could make the argument that young adult Jaik was overthinking those aspects of life most important to him. As we will discuss, this is a trait that can complicate therapy.

With respect to speech characteristics, a common question is how long should a diagnostic speaking sample be. Logan and Haj-Tas (2007) recommend 300-syllable samples, which is reasonable and should provide the fluency data that the clinician is seeking (disfluency frequency, type, duration, word position, and secondary behaviors observed), as well as allow the tester to informally assess parameters of voice, resonance, speaking rate, intelligibility, and non-stuttering disfluencies. Clinicians must realize, however, that if a client does not produce that much language during an evaluation, all is not necessarily lost in terms of making a diagnosis. For example, three sound repetitions in 100 (or 50 or 20) syllables does not provide as much information as nine in 300 syllables would, but combined with history information and attitude scale scores may very well still allow the SLP to make a confident diagnosis.

Another frequent question regarding the samples is whether to record them for later scrutiny. Doing so will likely improve the precision of the analysis, particularly if the stuttering is severe or the client speaks rapidly. However, clinicians are advised that 1) some disfluencies appear as relatively quick moments of tension and these could be missed with an audio-only recording and 2) bad things can happen when recording—a paper covers the microphone, a battery dies—which could leave the clinician with no data at all if he or she were depending solely on a recording.

Sometimes stuttering-like disfluency information is very different for reading samples in comparison to conversation. A common reason for the dissimilarity is that many secondary behaviors (e.g., changing words, pretending to gather one's thoughts, circumlocution) are comparatively difficult to employ while reading an unchangeable passage aloud. Such a difference provides the SLP with some insight into the conversational usage of such behaviors.

Sample assessment plans for children and adults are included in appendix A of this chapter. Some explanation is incorporated, but it should be noted that these outlines are by no means comprehensive. Everything from history questions to evaluation tasks can vary.

Outside of the attitude scales, neither plan includes formal, norm-referenced tests for stuttering. Although this author rarely uses such instruments, this in no way suggests a lack of value. Probably the most commonly used stuttering test is the *Stuttering Severity Instrument* (Riley, 2009), which can not only compare the client to other people who stutter, it can provide the tester with a severity classification when one is required.

In both plans, the reader will see that the final entry consists of recommendations. It is important to note that the evaluation will not always lead to therapy. If the SLP feels that an adult's neurological impairment involves more than speech, for example, a referral may well be the appropriate course of action.

With a child, if stuttering-like disfluencies are not observed by the SLP, this will be discussed with the parents. Although therapy could still be an option in such an instance (based on parental concern), it is also possible that the child does not stutter. Recent clinical examples of this scenario include:

- Other disorders that looked like stuttering, including spasmodic dysphonia, cluttering, and linguistic pauses due to word-finding deficits.

- Normal disfluencies that are misdiagnosed as stuttering. As noted, this scenario is rare, given that listeners can generally identify the presence of abnormal fluency. (In fact, the only actual clinical example I have of this is the case noted in chapter 2 in which the basis of the concern was not only the client's speech breakdowns, but also the fact that his mother and brother both stuttered.)

Sometimes children present stuttering-like disfluencies but regular therapy visits are not recommended. Instead, the SLP advises parents how to alter the child's communicative environment to make the act of speaking easier (Williams & Williams, 2000). The specific alterations will be discussed in the section on preschool therapy. For these children, a probable additional recommendation is a re-evaluation after an interval of time that the SLP has determined is suitable for the environmental changes to have an effect.

With children, the controversial area of spontaneous recovery can impact recommendations as well. The question that may be considered is whether a young child should receive treatment if he or she is still within the window of likely spontaneous recovery and not distressed by speech disruptions. As alluded to in chapter 2, some (e.g., Yairi & Curlee, 1995) cite a lack of evidence necessitating direct therapy for such children. Others (e.g., Starkweather & Givens-Ackerman, 1997) urge early intervention on the basis of neuroplasticity, the ability of the central nervous system to adapt to changes (Ludlow et al., 2008). Pre-school years are a period of maximal neuroplasticity for speech and language acquisition (Mundkur, 2005). Chang (2011) argues that such plasticity makes young children more likely than older individuals to respond to treatment that shapes disordered neural growth patterns into those more normal. In other words, early therapy is seen to take advantage of this period of neuroplasticity to actually alter brain development for speech. The desired result, then, is lasting fluency.

Clearly, more research is needed to clarify the benefits of early intervention. At this point, my advice to SLPs is to spell all of this out to parents (i.e., the stuttering may be destined to go away on its own, in which case the time and money invested in therapy will be unnecessary; but there is still a 1 in 5 likelihood—at worst—that it will persist and become more ingrained before treatment begins). My experience is that most parents opt for immediate therapy.

When the rapy is recommended, it is the SLP's responsibility to explain it—in general terms. Two reasons for this are 1) the recommendations are what the clients, or the parents, have been waiting for (i.e., the whole reason they showed up for the evaluation): to find out how the problem can be helped, and 2) if the professional recommendation does not match the client's desires, this discrepancy needs to be addressed.

As a final note on diagnosis, it is important to note that it is not necessarily isolated to one evaluation session. The conclusions drawn from that first session (everything from the diagnostic classification to the recommended goals for therapy) may be adjusted over time, as new observations are made and additional information obtained. It is best to think of diagnosis as an ongoing, open-ended venture that may include later testing to revise therapy or monitor progress (Williams, 2012).

Treatment of Preschool Children

Jaik first entered therapy at age eight. My guess is that it would have been sooner today, given the increased emphasis on early intervention. The idea now is to eliminate stuttering before it becomes ingrained (Onslow & O'Brian, 2013). Intervention with preschool children can be quite effective (Manning, 2001), at least in comparison to adult therapy.

Eradicating stuttering can be accomplished with either indirect or direct treatment methods. When both are attempted, indirect precedes direct (Sidavi & Fabus, 2010; Walton & Wallace, 1998). Therefore, our discussion of preschool children will begin with indirect therapy.

Indirect Therapy

While there are various forms and definitions of indirect therapy (e.g., Hegde & Davis, 1999; Millard, Nicholas, & Cook, 2008; Roth & Worthington, 2001; Yaruss & Quesal, 2001), for the purposes of this discussion, we will consider it simply as the implementation of therapy without feedback. In essence, what this means is that intervention is based primarily on modeling and environmental changes. In most cases, parents are trained to 1) utilize a speech model that is fluency-enhancing (in the hope that the child picks up on it and begins using it) and 2) effect subtle changes in the child's day-to-day life that make the experience of communication easier (e.g., Boucand, Millard, & Packman, 2014). In some cases (e.g., Millard, Nicholas, & Cook, 2008), parent training is so extensive that it can be considered the basis of the treatment plan.

The speaking model conducive to fluency often involves decreasing both the loudness and the rate of speech. Sometimes the latter is controlled by slowing the movement of the articulators (Andrews et al., 2012; Trajkovski et al., 2009; 2011), but more often this is accomplished by adding pauses (Guitar & Conture, 2005; Williams & Williams, 2000). The resulting rate should still sound grossly normal; it is just on the slower end of the normal range. The intent is to let the child know that speech need not be rushed, but can instead be produced in a relaxed and deliberate manner.

This idea of making communication comfortable is also the basis of the environmental changes. Examples of such changes include the following:

- Allowing the child plenty of time to respond.

- Stressing turn taking in speech and other activities.

- Being a patient listener who responds in a calm, unemotional manner.

- Asking yes/no questions or at least those that can be answered with relatively few words.

- Asking only one question at a time.

- Encouraging slow and thoughtful answers.

- Paying attention to the content of the child's speech rather than to the presentation.

- Rephrasing disfluent utterances prior to responding to them as a means of showing the child that the content of the message is important and was received.

- Occasionally modeling a disfluency in order to demonstrate that speech need not be perfect in its presentation.

Making communication an easy and relaxed activity lowers the communicative demands placed on the disfluent child and, with it, the frequency of stuttering (Logan & LaSalle, 2003). It keeps him or her from rushing, encouraging instead the production of speech at a manageable pace. With this in mind, there are certain actions that parents should be instructed to avoid whenever possible, for example:

- Interrupting

- Finishing the child's sentences

- Instructing the child to slow down[3] or think before speaking

Such behaviors, no matter how well intentioned, rush the child, forcing him or her to speak in a manner that is difficult, given the relatively limited capacity of a preschool speech neuro-motor system. In other words, these actions make speech more challenging, exactly the opposite of what indirect therapy is designed to achieve.

---

3   Although it is true that many therapies include rate control goals (several are noted in this chapter), these are effective because the child has been taught *how* to slow down. In the absence of such instruction, the child will likely find this advice unspecific (and thus confusing), or punishing, given that it is often delivered in an unfavorable tone on a frequent basis.

It should be noted that indirect therapy is not necessarily administered only by the parents. More often, there are regularly scheduled sessions in which the speech-language pathologist provides a model and monitors how frequently the child uses the targeted fluency-enhancing speech (speech void of excessive loudness or rate), as well as how often he or she stutters. Given these objectives, the formal goals of indirect therapy may be variations of the following:

- The client will produce fluency-enhancing speech in 90% of syllables spoken in conversational speech.

- The client will produce stuttering-like disfluencies in less than 1% of conversational speech.

Short-term goals often follow the same themes, but at lower operational levels. For example, the SLP may initially record the frequency of relaxed speech and disfluency in one-word answers. When criterion is met at that level, the child will be asked to produce, say, prepositional phrases, then lists of attributes, and, finally, responses to open-ended questions (Sacco, 1992). Other SLPs may choose the more familiar operational treatment levels of word, phrase, sentence, and conversation.

In addition to speech goals, regular sessions may well include ongoing parent counseling. Parents come to therapy with a host of conflicting emotions. They need to understand that they are not at fault for their child's stuttering, and, more constructively, that they can engage in behaviors to further its demise. Parents should also know that the window of opportunity for eliminating stuttering does not stay open forever. Thus, their participation is essential from the start (Mewherter, 2012). Home assignments will be an immediate and ongoing part of therapy. Such assignments help with the transfer and generalization of easy, fluent speech by encouraging its use between sessions and expanding the environments in which it is produced. It is important that clinicians keep the initial assignments simple—for example, giving parents a specific time to model and asking them to provide an overall rating of target (i.e., fluency-enhancing) speech and amount of stuttering (e.g., 0=none, 1=a little, 2=some, 3= a lot). Generally, once the home plan is established, the SLP can begin assigning more complex tasks.

Asking the parents to rate stuttering may require first teaching them what disfluencies are and are not normal for their child's age. As noted, parents and other listeners are generally good at identifying the presence of stuttering. Defining it, however, is another matter. Add to that an additional problem: Once parents have determined that their child stutters, they may listen differently. Often, every little speech bump—be it an interjection, pause for word selection, or anything else preschoolers are prone to do—is judged to be stuttering. The hope is that instruction on proper identification will improve the accuracy of their ratings and limit potential overreaction to normal disfluencies.

Parents must know what to expect from therapy (and this is true for both indirect and direct treatment). Improvement is not guaranteed, nor is it linear. There will continue to be good and bad periods of speech. Hopefully, there is overall improvement (i.e., the good periods get better and more frequent), but parents should understand that recovery from stuttering behaviors is a gradual process. While improvement in fluency may occur in a relatively few sessions (McKeehan & Child, 1991; Jones et al., 2000), achieving and maintaining stutter-free speech often takes time. How much time varies with each child, but, in general, it is a process measured in months, not days or weeks.

Because the severity of the child's stuttering will continue to fluctuate, parents should stay the course (i.e., continue with the home plan) during periods of greater disfluency. Such periods do not necessarily mean that an indirect approach is destined to fail. Similarly, when fluency is high, this is not the time to stop the modeling and other changes, given the likelihood of a decline in the near future.

In addition to receiving instruction from the SLP, parents are often brought into treatment sessions. In this way, the clinician can observe them with their child and make any necessary recommendations pertaining to the speech model used. The SLP can also determine whether the child's speech or disfluency changes with parent interaction. If, for example, the child begins to speak faster when the parents enter the room, even if the parents' model is adequate, this is a sign that something about the parents' presence cues the child to rush. Such a scenario would need to be explored with the parents in order to determine what sorts of adjustments can help the child.

Many SLPs like to begin stuttering therapy with this sort of an indirect approach. Their justifications for using it generally focus on the child's language. That is, small children often do not have the metalinguistic skills necessary to understand instruction related to slowing or relaxing speech (McKeehan & Child, 1990). Also, indirect therapy feels like less of an imposition on speech development. What I mean is that speech and language are allowed to develop without the interference of instruction. Related to that idea, SLPs may worry that placing a focus on speech production could result in children making incorrect adjustments on their own.

Of course, the best reason for using any approach is its effectiveness. Although indirect therapy has not been the subject of extensive research, there is evidence that it has helped many preschool children reduce or eliminate stuttering (de Sonneville-Koedoot et al., 2015; Franken, Kielstra-Van der Schalk, & Boelens, 2005; Millard, Nicholas, & Cook, 2008; Millard, Edwards, & Cook, 2009).

Direct Therapy

Research also backs the use of direct therapies for preschool stuttering (e.g., Jones et al., 2000). Whereas the emphases of indirect therapy are modeling and environmental changes, direct therapies aim to shape fluent speech via teaching, reinforcement, and other feedback to the child. As noted, there are various reasons why SLPs often begin with an indirect approach when treating preschoolers. Greater effectiveness is not among them (de Sonneville-Koedoot et al., 2015; Franken, Kielstra-Van der Schalk, & Boelens, 2005; Frymark, Venediktov, & Wang, 2010). In addition, no evidence exists that using a direct approach right from the start will be somehow harmful to the child's speech or language development. With this in mind, the decisions about whether and when to use direct therapy will likely be based more on SLPs' personal preferences and clients' characteristics than reasons having to do with prognosis. In fact, some clinicians advocate starting with direct therapy with all preschoolers (e.g., Bothe et al., 2006), on the basis of efficacy data. And based on examination of the Lidcombe program, a direct method of treatment, such procedures may be more efficient as well; clinical results (Guitar et al., 2015; Jones et al., 2000) indicate a significant reduction in many preschoolers' stuttering in fewer than 20 sessions. Not all comparative research supports this conclusion, however (e.g., de Sonneville-Koedoot et al., 2015).

There are also client attributes that can point an SLP toward direct therapy:

- Age—as noted, the window of opportunity for eliminating stuttering does not stay open forever. If the child is an older preschooler, this window may be a narrow opening. In such an instance, aggressive treatment may appear to be a more sensible approach.

- Secondary behaviors—their presence indicates that awareness and concern about speech are high (thus nullifying the justifications for using an indirect approach) (Sidavi & Fabus, 2010).

- Previous therapy—perhaps an indirect approach was already attempted and the client did not respond to it.

Of course, there are also times when the clinician must change from the indirect to direct. But when? The easy answer is that a switch should be made when the indirect approach is clearly not going to work. But how does one know? Below are some specific indicators that it is time to alter the treatment plan.

- The child's parents cannot or will not make the necessary adjustments in speech or environment.

- Siblings engage in verbal competition with the child, making a relaxed communication environment all but impossible.

- Even after listening to it for weeks, the child does not respond to the relaxed speech model.

Clearly, the reasons and rationale for using direct therapy are varied. And the same can be said for the methods used. The main goal, however, is always the same: the reduction of stuttering-like disfluencies. Whatever the specific tasks used to achieve this goal, it is likely that the approach will include many of the aspects of indirect therapy outlined above. For example, parent participation and environmental changes will almost surely be components of the treatment plan. Unlike with indirect therapy, however, parents may be able to address their child's speech in more overt ways. This can take the form of rewarding fluent speech (e.g., Onslow, Packman, & Harrison, 2003) or reinforcing a fluency-enhancing speech model (McKeehan & Child, 1990; Walton, 2008).

One quick note on reinforcing fluency-enhancing speech: I have found that it helps to find a term for it that motivates the child. I have referred to the exact same speech model as easy speech, good talking, quiet voice, turtle talk, inside voice, and palace speech (with a little girl whose goal in life was to one day be a princess), among other terms.

Some SLPs prefer reinforcing easy speech over fluent speech. They do not like sending the message that stuttering is bad, thereby making the child think that his or her usual speech is unacceptable. Others take this idea a step further and teach easy disfluencies in order to show the client that 1) he or she can manipulate and, in time, fix speech and 2) disfluencies need not be a source of shame or embarrassment (Coleman, 2013; Walton, 2008). Although all of these reasons for focusing on easy speech are sensible, it should also be noted that programs in which fluent speech is reinforced, most notably Lidcombe (Onslow, Packman, & Harrison, 2003) have shown documented success (Goodhue et al., 2010; Guitar et al., 2015; Jones et al., 2000; 2008).

In addition to its reinforcement of fluency, the Lidcombe approach is notable for the structure of reinforcement used. In short, there are four ways of giving feedback, depending on what the child needs.

These include acknowledging the target speech ("That was your smooth speech"), praising it ("Wow! Your speech sounded great!"), requesting self-evaluation when utterances are fluent ("Was that your smooth speech?"), and requesting self-correction when it is not ("Can you say that with your smooth speech?") (Onslow, Packman, & Harrison, 2003). These sorts of feedback are initially given by parents in 10-15 minute periods every day (though once the child is accustomed to them, they can be given throughout the day). It is worth noting that any or all of them could also be used to reinforce a fluency-enhancing speech model (as opposed to fluent speech).

Just as with indirect therapy, home plans should be simple and realistic. Rating the amount of stuttering each day (Guitar & Tozier, 2002) and also the amount of fluency-enhancing speech used (if that is a treatment goal) should be achievable for most parents. Asking them to find times throughout the day to model relaxed speech (for example, story time) is also realistic. Requesting that they to do so 24 hours a day is not. In every household, there will be times when commotion is high, people are talking quickly, and the only communication possible is, "You can tell me later. We're already running late. Just get in the van!" Parents should know not to beat themselves up over these situations, but should understand that the greater number of relaxed communication situations they can create, the more opportunities there will be for their child to practice fluent speech.

While it is important not to overwhelm parents, it is also true that some will want to do more than they are asked. Particularly when progress is slow, parents feel helpless when their child is struggling and all they have been instructed to do is continue modeling and occasionally comment on instances of good speech (which may be few and far between). In such instances, I usually allow the parents to use some reminders throughout the day. I do this for two rea-

145

sons: 1) this practice can give the parents a feeling that they have more control over the situation and 2) realistically, many parents are so frustrated that they are going to say something to the child anyway; thus, I may as well determine what it is. Therefore, we not only discuss what sorts of reminders are likely to help get the child back on track (e.g., "Remember your good speech" is all right; "Slow down" is not), I also set severe limits on these reminders, often with instructions such as, "Use only two or three per day. Save them for when your child is really struggling. Remember, you only have a few to use. Use them wisely." If such limitations are set, the SLP needs to be sure to explain the reason why: When the child feels that he or she is being harped on, the reminders become counterproductive. That is, some children will resist excessive parental instruction, perhaps even resenting the mere mention of "good speech." And what if the child is struggling all day and the parents again feel helpless because they have used their limited reminders? In such cases, the parents can occasionally model instances of fast or loud speech themselves, then immediately call attention to it (e.g., "I didn't use my best speech there, did I?"). As this sort of indirect reminder is focused on the parent, it is unlikely to be received by the child as a reprimand.

Assuming that there is progress with preschool therapy, be it direct, indirect, or a combination of the two, the question becomes: When should the child be dismissed? The easy answer, of course, is to do so when long-term goals are reached. However, caution is urged here. For one thing, the job of the SLP is not only to teach skills, but to transfer them to different environments and assure that they are maintained. For another, relapse occurs with stuttering often enough to be considered an ongoing clinical issue (Shapiro, 2011). For these reasons, dismissal from therapy should not occur the moment speech goals are met. A better strategy is to end gradually, reducing the frequency of visits while monitoring progress. Increasing the time between sessions can assure both client and clinician that performance can be maintained without regular therapy.

A possible course of action is to ask a twice-a-week client to start attending therapy once a week. Then, frequency can be reduced to once every two weeks, then once a month. Should gains be maintained and the client discharged, follow-up telephone calls to parents are recommended as a way to help monitor the child's speech. Also, it should be understood that the therapist can and should be contacted in the event of relapse.

Treatment of Older Children and Adults

As is probably clear from what you have read of Jaik's story so far, stuttering (school-aged and beyond, anyway) involves more than occasional breaks of speech. There are also fears, frustrations, anxieties, and all the other metaphorical hecklers awaiting in the crowd. In the face of such barriers, it follows that treatment should address both the speech and non-speech components of stuttering. Exactly how this is accomplished—in terms of treatment activities, overcoming barriers to success, and other therapy objectives—will be different for school-aged children, adolescents, and adults. The fundamental principles, however, are largely the same across the three groups.

Unlike treatment with preschoolers, goal setting with older clients is a collaborative practice wherein the speech-language pathologist and client discuss what is appropriate, taking into account the client's needs, motivation, severity, and any other factors pertinent to therapy. Of course, the role of the SLP is larger when setting goals with a 6 year-old client than with an adult, but in both cases the therapist is there to provide professional guidance based on his or her knowledge base, experience, and philosophical perspectives on stuttering. Ultimately, it is the client's plan, and, as such, he or she must be in complete agreement with it (Manning, 1999).

As with any other general proposal, the treatment plan states what is *not* going to happen. It affords structure, a place to start, and a path to travel, but changes in direction and philosophy are inevitable. Some goals will not be necessary, others will be added, and still more will be altered. It is important, then, that plans be flexible. By way of example, prior to Behavior Modification therapy, Jaik was only interested in fluency. He gradually let go of that desire as he learned more and more about managing stuttering.

Although the actual goals vary from client to client, the primary objective of stuttering therapy should be effective communication. That is, regardless of the techniques learned, clients should be able to say what they want to, not what the stuttering allows (Conture & Guitar, 1993; Hood, 2003; Williams & Dugan, 2002). As the reader will see, there are different ways of addressing this goal.

When learning of the objectives of one treatment program, Jaik was told that the more regularly he attended, the more likely he would benefit from the treatment. This was the clinician's way of telling the clients to take some responsibility for therapy, an advantageous element to the initiation of treatment. If the plan is to become, as Jaik heard on another occasion, one's own therapist (a worthwhile goal), then the client has to be clear on the fact that therapy takes effort.

Of course, the need for effort is not ideally what a client wants to hear when starting therapy. It can feel as if one more weight is being added to the struggles, anxieties, failures, and embarrassments associated with stuttering, not to mention the tension that can be both physically and mentally exhausting.

On top of all of that add the length of therapy. Yes, it varies across clients, but, as Jaik came to realize, addressing the entirety of stuttering is not a quick endeavor.

A Running Speech Sample

Speaking of adult stuttering treatment...

A few years ago, I was jogging and felt a sharp pain in my knee. I assumed it was routine exercise soreness and attempted to run through it. My knee had other ideas. The pain not only continued throughout that day, but the next day as well.

Shortly thereafter, I asked the doctor. He felt around the knee joint a little, then suggested wearing a wrap (physician-speak for "I don't really know, but here's something"). I did so, but the pain continued. I tried making the wrap so tight it was practically a brace. Again, no relief.

My next step was to get off the roads and sidewalks and seek a softer track. I found a trail made of dirt and wood chips, but the new surface did not help.

It finally dawned on me that I had to change the way I was running. After all, other methods of ambulation were not difficult. I could walk without any pain. But there was something about the constant pounding involved with running that was hard on one knee.

So I tried relaxing my strides, first by making them shorter, then slower. I added more walking to each lap as well. And finally I was able to exercise without knee pain.

Then the problem became maintaining my gains. I became self-conscious about people seeing me run so slowly. Other times, my iPod would play fast songs and I would speed up. Then there were the occasions when I simply forgot and returned to my default position.

To remain pain-free, I had to run while thinking about the process of running. That is, I had to constantly coach myself to take short, slow strides. In time, this method allowed me to jog (with some walking) the same distances as before. That was six months after the day I first felt the knee pain. Habituating the new running style took several more months.

What does this story have to do with adult stuttering treatment? Well, keep a couple of things in mind:

1. Speaking is a far more complex task than running
2. All stuttering clients talk more than I run; thus, their speech motor patterns are much more ingrained than were my jogging movements

It took me ten months to find my new normal for a relatively simple and physiologically superficial activity. Given what SLPs are asking of stuttering clients—habituation of intricate, intrinsic movements—results are unlikely to happen quickly.

With that in mind, clients need to be realistic about the trials of both therapy and stuttering. Identifying stuttering's negative components can reduce anxiety in the short run (Cooper, 2003), and eventually lead to lasting change (Gregory, 2003; Guitar, 1998; Sheehan, 2003). This requires that the SLP and client discuss the disfluency, the concealed aspects that accompany it (Van Riper, 1973), and how ongoing treatment will address it all. Without identifying (and, eventually, addressing) the overt and covert behaviors of stuttering, the problem is unlikely to improve and may, in fact, degenerate. Ramig (2003) writes of a vicious cycle, whereby shame and guilt lead to avoidance, which, in turn, lead to more shame and guilt. And as was discussed in chapter 2, the increased avoidance can also result in added disfluency.

As the client's emotional baggage might be full of denial and shame, discussion about stuttering may not come easily. In these instances, clinicians can utilize activities designed to bring emotions to the surface. Writing letters to one's stuttering, for example, can be an effective discussion starter, as can reading essays that deal with pertinent issues (Williams, 2006). Clients are sometimes surprised at how identifying (or identifying with) the more covert aspects of stuttering releases emotions they did not even realize were there (Eldridge, 1997).

Counseling activities can help lessen the burden imposed by stuttering. The SLP's skills in this area can provide professional guidance to the clients toward resolving their personal issues related to communication. It is important for SLPs to remember that they are not there to explore all intimate issues, as those beyond communication are outside their scope of practice. But they can employ simple counseling techniques that will help to develop partnerships with their stuttering clients (American Speech-Language-Hearing Association, 2007).

Many of these techniques, in fact, are little more than active listening skills:

- *Attending Behaviors* - Communicating interest in what is being said, via eye contact, posture, verbal and non-verbal cues, and any other behaviors that indicate fine attention.

- *Empathetic Responses* – Responses that convey understanding on the part of the SLP and demonstrate to the client that he or she is truly being listened to.

- *Paraphrasing* - Repeating core aspects of the client's message in the SLP's own words in order to help the clients view his or her experiences from a different perspective.

Other basic counseling skills that can help clients address emotions and frustrations associated with stuttering are noted below.

- *Reframing* - Helping the client find opportunities he or she might not otherwise realize.

Client: A kid at school keeps asking me why I talk this way.

SLP: What a great opportunity to educate someone about stuttering.

- *Sharing self* - Revealing clinician experiences in order to empower the client and humanize the professional, e.g. the clinician says, "I'm not good at joining conversations. Do you have any ideas that might help me?"

- *Brainstorming* - Listing as many solutions as possible (no matter how crazy) to a problem, then reviewing the pros and cons of each.

In addition, limited research has identified Cognitive-Behavioral Therapy (CBT) procedures as promising toward reducing social anxiety in people who stutter (Fry, Botterill, & Pring, 2009; Menzies et al., 2008). Essentially, CBT involves identifying and modifying irrational thoughts and behaviors in gradual and systematic ways (Fry, 2009). For example, a client who avoids feared situations might be worried about listener reactions that are in actuality extremely unlikely. By exploring the client's thoughts and experimenting with new behaviors, the anxiety may decrease as more rational thoughts emerge.

Similarly, Acceptance and Commitment Therapy (ACT) is being applied to stuttering to reduce avoidance and improve self-acceptance (Cheasman & Everard, 2015). The philosophy behind ACT is that attempts to control a problem are often counterproductive whereas acceptance allows one to focus less on the minutiae of one issue and more on broader goals and dreams.

Of course, the activities listed in this chapter are by no means exhaustive. Interested readers can consult additional counseling-specific resources (e.g., Stuttering Foundation of America, 2006) for more complete information.

Whether accomplished via counseling or otherwise, improved identification of all aspects of stuttering is designed to expand the client's understanding of his or her speech-related attitudes (Sheehan, 2003), listener reactions (Cooper, 2003), and the actual disorder—what happens during disfluencies as well as how stuttering affects goals, ambitions, and quality of life (Cooper, 2003; Van

Riper, 1973). As a bonus, therapy is also likely to be better under-stood. In turn, the improved understanding helps to, as Jaik put it, "demystify" stuttering, that is, to change the common perception of it as unwieldy (see Corcoran & Stewart, 1998) to something that is manageable. As the disorder becomes less mysterious, the hope is that it loses its power. The client begins to figure it out. The value in that is significant. As Jaik noted:

> One benefit … was the knowledge that it if I got into a stammering situation, I could do something about it. This, as any stammerer will tell you, is more than half the battle.

Greater understanding of stuttering has additional advantages as well. The dangers of avoidance become clear. In addition, there may be an appreciation of the gradual nature of treatment and why it involves moving outside one's comfort zone.

Understanding one's own stuttering sets the stage for acceptance. Clients need to become comfortable enough with stuttering that change can occur. Fear of communicating must be diminished for any real improvement to take place. If problem words and situations can be approached without anxiety, attitudes toward speaking will improve and avoidance of speech (and life) will diminish. That over-all goal of *effective communication* becomes feasible.

People who stutter should become desensitized to feared words and situations (Williams, 2006) and the sound and feel of their own speech (Conture, 2001). This not only gets them talking, but also sets the stage for long term benefits. Treatment in any form in-volves changing one's usual speech pattern. However well learned the new pattern is, however, the client must still be willing to speak that way.

Should the speaker remain self-conscious about speech, such change will not come easily.

Some of the means of desensitizing clients include:

- *Open stuttering* – stuttering without accompanying secondary behaviors. That is, putting the disorder in the open, for all listeners to see and hear. In addition to being an effective desensitizer, this technique addresses secondary behaviors (by forcing the client to stop using them).

- *Voluntary stuttering* - stuttering purposely on a word that could have been said fluently. Again, the goal is to become accustomed to stuttering by, in this case, doing it more often. Although for some clients voluntary stuttering works well (e.g., Murphy, Yaruss, & Quesal, 2007), Logan (2014) advises against pushing this strategy with those who do not understand its purpose or do not feel comfortable attempting it.

- *Advertising* or self-disclosure – as discussed in chapter 2, this involves revealing one's stuttering. This revelation can be direct (saying "I stutter") or indirect, such as exhibiting stuttering-related buttons, cups, or posters (Hicks, 1997; Hood, 2003).

As a quick aside, notice that two of these techniques involve stuttering without secondary behaviors. Often, however, these behaviors require more focused treatment than merely open or voluntary stuttering, either because they have become habits or because the client feels such shame in stuttering that he or she continues to avoid it, even in therapy sessions. In such instances, the reinforcement being used for open stuttering can be coupled with mild punishers. For example, a game could be initiated in which the client earns a point for stuttering, but loses one for each instance of avoidance. The messages being sent to the client are 1) stuttering is not shameful and 2) secondary behaviors are unacceptable.

To be fair, sometimes avoidance really does seem necessary (not recommended or therapeutically beneficial, just momentarily helpful). Jaik related job interview experiences in which he was essentially told that fluency was a requirement for employment. Who would blame him for employing secondary behaviors in order to earn a living? There are other times that the costs of stuttering can seem too high as well: loss of opportunities, friends, or relationships, to name just a few examples. As noted in chapter 2, the problem is that if there are too many of these situations, avoidance increases and stuttering gets worse, leading to more avoidance.

Can such a vicious cycle ever be broken? Perhaps so, but doing so would be very difficult for a young man in London looking for a job.

Modifying Speech and/or Stuttering

As is the case for most clients, identification of and desensitization to stuttering elements would not have been sufficient therapy outcomes for Jaik. He also required goals that directly addressed speech production. At the age of eight, this was attempted via modifying the totality of his speech. Such approaches utilize physiological techniques to shape stuttered speech into a simpler and more fluent model. The preschool therapies reviewed in this chapter are based upon this perspective.

Speech modification therapy for older clients typically involves step-by-step instruction of fluency enhancing techniques, such as:

- Increased air flow at speech onset,

- Gentle initiations of voicing,

- Light contacts of the articulators during speech,

- Increased voicing, and

- Reductions in speaking rate.

The use of these and other techniques make speech easier (by increasing breath support, relaxing the musculature involved, and simplifying the speech physiology), allowing for greater fluency (Guitar, 2013). Justifications for such an approach include the beliefs that 1) what most clients want from therapy above all else is fluency (Schwartz, 1999; Shames & Florence, 1980; Shenker, Kully, & Meltzer, 1998) and thus therapy that teaches fluency-enhancing behaviors is motivating and 2) with sufficient practice, the learned behaviors of stuttering can be unlearned (Siegel & Gold, 1999) and replaced by those more conducive to fluency. Furthermore, studies of the effectiveness of such approaches (e.g., Andrews, Guitar, & Howie, 1980; Davidow, Crowe, & Bothe, 2004; Bothe et al., 2006) have been encouraging.

There are, however, concerns about focusing on speech behaviors to the exclusion of all other aspects of stuttering. Some (e.g., Ramig & Dodge, 2005) question whether the techniques will hold up in situations in which the client is apprehensive about speaking. Indeed, it appears that variables such as listeners' communicative behaviors and reactions to stuttering can make fluency more difficult for people who stutter (Bloodstein & Bernstein-Ratner, 2008). For example, many would find it hard to maintain a relaxed speaking model when joining a conversation in which all of the participants were speaking rapidly and interrupting one another. Such speakers might not display the requisite patience for comparatively slow or stuttered speech.

In addition to potential situational variations, many people who stutter report that fluency-enhancing speech is limiting (even "robotic") and/or requires too much concentration (Conture, 1996; Kalinowski et al., 1994; Manning, 2001; Starkweather & Givens-Ackerman, 1997). Despite the increased fluency, they eventually decide that they would rather stutter.

The majority of Jaik's adult therapy was grounded not in acquiring fluency skills, but rather in stuttering modification (which, he correctly noted, is based in large part on the writings of Charles Van Riper [e.g., Van Riper, 1973]). As Jaik described, stuttering modification approaches have traditionally been focused on managing (as opposed to eliminating) stuttering while directly addressing the secondary behaviors and negative emotions. Williams and Dugan (2002) phrased their modification goals as:

- "stuttering in a way you can manage,"

- "talking without tricks or avoidances,"

- "taking charge of the stuttering, rather than letting it continue to run your life," and

- "saying whatever you want to say, whenever you want to say it, even if you sometimes stutter" (which is basically another way of saying *effective communication*).

Or, as Jaik said it, he had to stop letting his stammer control him and instead begin "controlling it." These types of goals are not based on fluency, a drawback for some (Ryan, 2003; Shenker, Kully, & Meltzer, 1998). But stuttering modification advocates assert that, while stuttering is not curable (Conture, 2001), it can occur without shame, embarrassment, and avoidance. Moreover, clients can assume some control over *how* they stutter. Thus, Jaik learned to replace his tense disfluencies with those easier to produce.

During stuttering modification therapy, when Jaik was taught how to pause during speech, it was viewed as "vitally important" that the pause not be used as a secondary behavior. The reason for such a clarification is that a pause that allows the speaker to stutter his or her own way is a means of confronting the stuttering; pausing for avoidance, on the other hand, is retreating. How can a listener (or a therapist) tell the difference? Sometimes, it is impossible without asking the client. The key variable, after all, is what's going on inside the speaker's head. Is he or she challenging the stutter or running away from it? It is important to have open dialogue with clients about the affective and cognitive aspects of stuttering. After all, one cannot gain control of stuttering without corralling negative attitudes and emotions.

In *The King's Speech* , a movie Jaik mentions as an example of a positive stuttering portrayal, protagonist Prince Albert begins to make progress only after treatment moved beyond speech mechanics and included emotions and behaviors beneath the surface. Moreover, his definition of success turned out to be effectively communicating his message (in this case, a vitally important missive delivered under enormous stress).

At the end of this chapter in appendix B there is an outline of a stuttering modification program presented to the American Academy of Private Practice in Speech Pathology and Audiology (Sheehan, Williams, & Dugan, 2001). Those who review it will see that, although there are some differences between this program and the one described by Jaik, there are far more similarities. For example, both treatments include objectives to change "attitudes and feelings" via education about speech and stuttering, and a lot of work "on breaking habits and modifying…core stuttering." The actual modifications are the same as well, although the terminology is different (in-block modification is referred to as *pull-out* in the outline; pre-block correction as *preparatory set*).

The value of managing stuttering along with its associated affective and cognitive components is supported by data (McClure & Yaruss, 2003; Plexico, Manning, & DiLollo, 2005) that indicate client satisfaction with treatment objectives such as changing speech-associated attitudes and, to a lesser extent, modifying disfluencies. Furthermore, confronting stuttering may serve to decrease it, although the research finding are mixed on this point (Menzies et al., 2008; Murphy, Yaruss, & Quesal, 2007). The idea is that, as fewer words and situations become associated with speech failure, they no longer serve as stuttering triggers (Brutten & Shoemaker, 1967).

Although the bases for fluency and stuttering modifications are quite different, they are routinely combined within treatment plans (Dietrich, 2000; Gregory, 1991; Guitar, 1998; Latulas, Tetnowski, & Bathel, 2003; Ramig & Dodge, 2004). Fluency enhancing and stuttering modification speech targets are taught side by side with goals that address emotions and associated behaviors (Cooper, 1987; Dietrich, 2000; Donaher, 2003; Gregory, 1991; Guitar, 1998; Latulas, Tetnowski, & Bathel, 2003; Ramig & Dodge, 2004; Schwartz, 1999; Sheehan, Williams, & Dugan, 2001). So how do therapists decide what sorts of speech production goals to set? Some still advocate speech modification over stuttering modification or vice versa, but many more consider client factors before making their determination. For example, a client whose stuttering is mild and more of a nuisance than a disability may be unwilling to modify the entirety of his or her speech and instead wish to focus on the occasional disfluencies. On the other hand, someone willing and able to produce relaxed speech in all situations will likely spend more time addressing fluency modification goals.

As a final note on modifications, regardless of the speech techniques used, goals for self-monitoring should be incorporated into therapy. That is, the client should learn to accurately judge his own productions. The task itself is quite simple: The clinician periodically asks the client whether he or she used specific techniques correctly when producing a target utterance. The client's accuracy is the percent agreement with the clinician (who is, after all, the expert in the room). The desired eventual outcome of self-monitoring is self-correction, a crucial skill toward becoming one's own therapist. Taking this idea a step further, Harasym, Langevin, and Kully (2015) taught clients to video self-model—that is, to observe themselves performing targeted behaviors on video so that they could better imitate those behaviors—and found subsequent improvements in avoidance and stuttering expectancy.

Transfer and Generalization

Perhaps the most important, as well as most difficult, aspect of therapy is transferring skills to different environments (Conture, 2001; St. Louis & Westbrook, 1987). Clients can do magical things inside the treatment room but, too often, no place else. Real life, with all its reminders of past speech failure, is a tough place to implement new skills. As such, transfer is a part of therapy in which desensitization—to both the client's own reactions and those of listeners—is crucial. Of course, achieving such desensitization is easier said than done.

One reason that transferring skills is difficult is that clients often realize all of the ways that it can go wrong. Jaik could not bring himself to practice voluntary stuttering with strangers ("I was far too scared, self-conscious, and embarrassed") or to disclose his stutter to anyone, to name just two examples. So how can cautious clients be treated? On that topic, Williams (2008) offers some advice:

- *Define success.* It is not complete mastery on the first attempt. If the goal is worthwhile, success is a process that requires some failure along the way.

- *Set attainable goals.* Worries about failure can be diminished with objectives that are easily reached.

- *Model desired behaviors.* This allows the clinician to not only display the necessary skills, but also to show the client how to gracefully admit mistakes.

As part of therapy, Jaik was consistently given daily home assignments. This is a common and effective means of extending therapeutic goals to different settings. Home programs can take a variety of forms, from drill work to informal activities such as reading essays, watching videos, or searching for information on the Internet. Such assignments should begin early in the therapeutic process, to give clients practice between sessions and in novel settings.

Home practice of speech techniques, like the repetition of any motor act, is performed to develop the proper motor plans (Robb, 2012; Mass et al., 2008). Such practice requires more than repeated muscle actions, however. Fine attention skills are needed on the part of the client, as cognition plays a key role in the learning of novel motor skills (Starkes & Allard, 1993), particularly complex acts such as combining multiple speech targets.

Transfer of skills can also be aided by changing the session locale. If clients can employ speaking tasks in different places with a variety of listeners, they can learn to overcome communication barriers that exist outside the regular treatment room. In addition, various locations become associated with speech success.

There are also transfer activities that are possible inside the treatment room. Bringing in friends, parents, or spouses, for example, not only transforms the situation by changing the audience, it can help desensitize the client to the emotions involved in speaking to significant others.

The use of telephone calls is another way to add new listeners (Williams, 2011). SLPs usually set these up beforehand, so that the one who receives the call reacts appropriately. Sometimes calls are based on a hierarchy of difficulty. For example, the first call can be to a friend, then a friendly stranger, and so on, working up to calling a busy place of business. As with all transfer activities, calls work better when the SLP takes the first turn and models the desired speech for the client.

Role-play can also be effective with some clients (Susca, 1997). The therapist can take the part of the restaurant server, job interviewer, audience heckler, or whoever else is involved in difficult speaking situations for a particular client. This can help the individual to confront cues of past failure and develop strategies for addressing feared situations. Perhaps future role play will involve the utilization of virtual speaking environments to test therapeutic gains in approximated real world settings (Brundage & Hancock, 2015).

Another important component to skill transfer is development of a support system (Ramig, 2003; Trichon & Tetnowski, 2011). The SLP can encourage the formation of such systems by involving the client's family and friends in therapy (e.g., Boberg & Boberg, 1990). Caring listeners not only offer effective outlets for expressing the fears, emotions, and frustrations associated with stuttering (Hunt, 1987; Krauss-Lehrman & Reeves, 1989), they also provide an atmosphere of acceptance in which to practice speech techniques. Support groups (e.g. local chapters of the National Stuttering Association) can allow clients to witness the variety of people who stutter, and to learn about their strengths and successes. Perhaps because of these reasons, Boyle (2013) found stuttering support group experiences to be associated with lower internalized stigma (i.e., less acceptance of negative societal attitudes, such as stereotype agreement) and higher self-esteem, self-efficacy, and life satisfaction when compared to individuals with no such experience.

Completion of therapy

As noted, client goals can transform throughout the course of therapy. So too, then, can definitions of success. Jaik's journey went from a need for fluency to effective management of stuttering. In other words, his personal therapy goals changed over time. Such a transformation is not unusual (Plexico, Manning, & DiLollo, 2005; Pollard et al., 2009). In fact, stuttering clients can feel satisfied with their treatment even when formally stated goals have not been realized. For this reason, less formal indicators of therapeutic progress are also important to track. Jaik increased his confidence and identified barriers to recovery as a result of his therapy. It is likely that neither were treatment plan goals.

Once goals have been met or abandoned, it is best to taper therapy, as previously discussed in relation to preschoolers. If the client truly becomes his or her own therapist, there will be strategies available to help fend off relapse. For example, continued use of voluntary stuttering can help reduce secondary behaviors and sensitivity to listener reactions. Similarly, practice of therapy techniques can aid in their habituation. There are apps available to make such practice convenient. For example, the aforementioned *MyLynel* ® (e.g., Kale & Williams, 2014) offers lists, games, and activities that can be tailored to each client.

Despite attempts to maintain therapeutic gains however, clients may revert to old habits. For this reason, they should be encouraged to maintain contact with their SLP and schedule follow-up/ refresher visits as needed (Schwartz, 1999).

Group therapy

In most settings, therapy is individualized to allow focused teaching of new skills and discussion of personal information. However, group therapy can be advantageous as well. With children, there may be fewer stigmas associated with being in a group, as they discover that some of their peers also have communication problems. Members of therapy groups often experience a sense of belonging (Rollin, 1987), which aids in the implementation of many phases of treatment. For example, clients can practice therapy targets with more listeners (Ramig, 2003) and monitor each other's speech and secondary behaviors (Williams & Dugan, 2002). And once a client feels comfortable performing speaking tasks with a peer group, movement to other settings may be easier.

It should be noted that scheduling sometimes necessitates group therapy. For example, the caseloads of public school speech-language pathologists may require them to administer therapy in large groups.

Regardless of schedule or setting, therapy is more effective when a shaping group format (Leith, 1993) is followed. Under this format, participants are encouraged to offer feedback to one another and each client stays involved throughout the entire session. Because of the interactive nature of shaping groups, small ones generally work better than those larger.

Other types of management

In *The King's Speech*, early therapy attempts included putting marbles in the client's mouth or instructing him to roll around on the floor. Although these methods are, thankfully, no longer employed, there are some interesting means of treating stuttering aside from traditional therapy.

Portable Devices. In the discussion of fluency enhancing conditions (chapter 2), it was noted that interference with the auditory feedback system leads to greater fluency in some people who stutter. From those findings have emerged various portable electronic devices for stuttering. The basic idea with all of them is to change if and how speakers hear themselves. More specifically, by delivering the following types of feedback during speech, clients can speak under conditions known to enhance fluency:

- *Delayed auditory feedback*, or lengthening the time between the actual production of speech and when the speaker hears it (Goldiamond, 1965),

- *Masking noise*, which is essentially white noise that completely blocks out one's own voice (Block, Ingham, & Bench, 1996), and

- *Frequency altered feedback*, the electronic conversion of vocal frequencies to make one's own voice sound lower or higher in pitch (Howell et al., 1987).

Many electronic devices were designed to provide people who stutter with a solution that requires no training. In practice, however, they may work better in conjunction with traditional therapy ("Results of survey," 2004), a potential downside for clients who lack the time or means to attend regular sessions. The popularity of devices is further decreased by high cost, a lack of research demonstrating long-term and widespread effectiveness, and skepticism that they will work in the first place ("Results of survey," 2004).

Overall, success has been varied (Gallop & Runyan, 2012; Lincoln et al., 2010; Ramig, et al., 2010). In one survey, 38 percent of users indicated that their experience was not at all successful; 44 percent found theirs to be somewhat successful; and 18 percent reported their experience was very successful (Reeves, as cited in Kuster, 2004). This variance may be partly explained by severity; at least one study indicated that those whose stuttering was more severe experienced greater benefit from an altered feedback device (Foundas et al., 2013). Also, there are anecdotal reports suggesting that issues of background noise (Molt, 2002), waning effectiveness ("Devices are," 2004), and different levels of access to speech-language pathologists (to offer guidance) all play a role in effectiveness.

The bottom line, however, appears to be that electronic devices can offer hope to some people who stutter.

Pharmacological agents. For decades, people have been reporting on pharmacological agents and stuttering (Brady, 1991; Maguire, Yeh, & Ito, 2012; Meduna, 1948; Molt, 1998). These reports

have outlined the effects of such classes of agents as antipsy-
chotics, neuroleptics, and sedatives. While recent research shows
promise that some forms of stuttering may one day be treatable
with medication (e.g., Maguire, Franklin, & Kirsten, 2011), there are
several points to keep in mind:

- Much of the research involved small sample siz-
  es and soft science (Bothe et al., 2006; Boyd,
  Dworzynski, & Howell, 2011; Molt, 1998; Saxon &
  Ludlow, 2007), calling into question the quality of the
  evidence and the extent to which results can be generalized.

- Pharmacological agents can produce side effects
  (Maguire, Yeh, & Ito, 2012; Saxon & Ludlow, 2007),
  some more unpleasant than stuttering.

In a sense, the topic of pharmacological agents is similar to that of
electronic devices. No universal cure has been found, but it is nonetheless a potentially promising area of research.

Cultural Considerations

Many of the topics considered in this chapter (and indeed this book)
vary not just individual to individual, but culturally as well. For example, different cultures may demonstrate a wide range of beliefs regarding communication, therapy, use of medications, consideration
for listeners, how and with whom to make eye contact, parent-child
interactions, and presenting perceived weaknesses, to list but a few
examples of principles that could impact fluency and/or its therapy
(Battle, 2011; Cheng & Williams, 2011). Ideas about stuttering can
vary cross-culturally as well (Mayo et al., 2004; Nsabimana, 2011;

Ozdemir, St. Louis, & Topbas, 2011; Robinson & Crowe, 2002), including attitudes of the individuals who stutter (Daniels, Hagstrom, & Gabel, 2006). SLPs need to be mindful of cultural beliefs when evaluating and treating clients and counseling families.

Questions for Discussion

If you stuttered, would you rather no one knows, or be open about it? Why?

In order to diagnose stuttering, some or all of the following information must be obtained:

- Client history

- Sample of the client's speech

- Adaptation

- Negative speech-associated attitudes

- Effect of fluency-enhancing on speech

- Consistency

- Concomitant conditions

- Identification of communicative stressors

Place them in order of importance and explain your ranking.

Would adjustments such as relaxed speech and conversational turn-taking work in your household? If not, what sorts of adjustments would be needed to make them commonplace?

From an SLP's perspective, do you think you would prefer an in-direct or direct therapy model? Why? What about if you were a parent?

Why might a person deny the trials and tribulations associated with stuttering?

How do you define successful stuttering therapy?

In terms of their potential aid to people who stutter, what are the similarities and differences with respect to electronic devices and pharmacological agents?

As a client, would you prefer individualized therapy or group? What about as the SLP? Explain your answers.

Appendix A

Sample Assessment Protocols[4]

Sample Assessment Plan – Child

1. Parent(s) complete history form (see Williams, 2012 for example), along with attitude and secondary behavior tests, such as:

- *Communication Attitude Test (CAT)* (Brutten & Vanrycheghem, 2006) (speech-associated attitudes, trait) – for children aged 6 to 15 years.

- *kiddyCAT* (Vanrycheghem & Brutten, 2006) (speech-associated attitudes, trait) – for children under 6 years of age.

- *Speech Situation Checklist - for Children* (Vanrycheghem & Brutten, 2006) (speech-associated attitudes, state)

- *Behavior Checklist – for Children* (Brutten & Vanrycheghem, 2006) (secondary behaviors)

- *Overall Assessment of Speaker's Experience of Stuttering* (Yaruss & Quesal, 2010) (reactions to stuttering, impacts on daily communication and quality of life) – for children aged 7 years and older

2. History Interview with Parent(s)

---

4   These protocols are not complete or client specific. As such, they exclude tasks common to many SLP's usual speech-language evaluations, such as hearing screens and general motor testing. They are intended only as general guides.

- Can you describe your child's speech difficulty?

- When did the problem begin?

- Did it start gradually or suddenly?

- Has the problem changed since it was first noticed? How?

- How do people respond to his/her speech? How do you respond? Do you ever try to give helpful advice?

- Does the speech change in different situations? With different people? Are there easier and more difficult words for your child to say?

- Are there any other speech, language, or learning difficulties?

- Is there a family history of stuttering?

- Is he/she aware of the speech difference? Do you ever see signs of frustration?

- Are there any tricks your child uses in order not to stutter?

- Does he/she ever avoid speaking situations?

- Does the stuttering vary day-to-day? Week-to-week?

- Have he/she had therapy before? Can you tell me about it? Was it effective?

- Take me through a typical day in the life of your child, including who he/she spends time with.

- What does he/she like to talk about?

- What do you hope will result from this evaluation?

- Is there anything else I should know about your child?

3. Speech Samples

The child talks with the examiner and, separately, with parent or family. With children, different levels of language—e.g., single words, prepositional phrases, naming attributes, conversation, and story-telling (e.g., Stocker & Goldfarb, 1995)—may be assessed in order to determine the complexity at which breakdowns occur.

4. Fluency enhancing condition

Asking the child to sing or whisper is usually an easy way to obtain this.

5. Adaptation/Consistency

Depending on the age of the child, this can be a picture naming task, story retelling, reading single words, or reading paragraphs.

6. Assessment of Language and Articulation

Screening tools, such as the *Fluharty Speech and Language Screening Test* (Fluharty, 2000) offer quick testing (assuming the child passes the screen). Formal evaluation instruments, such as the *Preschool Language Scale-5* (Zimmerman, Steiner, & Pond, 2011) or *Test of Language Development-Primary* (Newcomer & Hammill, 2008) provide more detailed information.

7. Oral-peripheral and/or motor examinations

Often, these are informal structure and function tasks involving the articulators, although sometimes more complete assessments (e.g., Johnson-Root, 2015) are administered.

8. Recommendations

Sample Assessment Plan – Adult

1. History form (see Williams, 2012 for example), along with attitude and secondary behavior tests, such as:

- *Erickson Scale of Communication Attitudes* (or *S-24 Scale*) (Erickson, 1969) (speech-associated attitudes, trait)

- *Big Communication Attitude Test* (BigCAT) (Brutten & Van-ryckeghem, 2010) (speech-associated attitudes, trait)

- *Speech Situation Checklist - for Adults* (Vanryckeghem & Brutten, 2006) (speech-associated attitudes, state)

- *Behavior Checklist – for Adults* (Brutten & Vanryckeghem, 2003) (secondary behaviors)

- *Overall Assessment of Speaker's Experience of Stuttering* (Yaruss & Quesal, 2010) (reactions to stuttering, impacts on daily communication and quality of life)

2. History Interview

- Describe your concerns about your speech.

- When did the problem begin? Who first noticed it?

- Has the problem changed over time? How?

- Does it bother you? How?

- How do people respond to your speech?

- Does your speech change in different situations? With different people? Are there easier and more difficult words for you to say?

- Are there any tricks you use in order not to stutter?

- Do you ever avoid speaking situations?

- Are there any other speech, language, or learning difficulties?

- Is there a family history of stuttering?

- Does your stuttering vary day-to-day? Week-to-week?

- Have you had therapy before? What did you do? Was it effective?

- What do you hope will result from this evaluation?

- Is there anything else I should know at this time?

3. Speech Sample

4. Expectancy, silent reading

Client reads a passage to himself, marking words on which he believes he would have difficulty were he reading it aloud.

5. Adaptation/Consistency

3-5 readings of a passage

6. Fluency enhancing condition

Asking the client to read in unison with the tester works well with adults.

7. Expectancy, reading aloud

Client reads a clean copy of the passage he marked in step 4. This allows the clinician to see how well he could predict disfluent words and what types of words/sounds are feared.

8. Assessment of Concomitant Areas

Word-finding, receptive vocabulary, and/or expressive language may be assessed. Potential testing instruments include *Peabody Picture Vocabulary Test – 4* (Dunn & Dunn, 2007), *Receptive One-Word Picture Vocabulary Test-4* (Martin & Brownell, 2010), and *Expressive One-Word Picture Vocabulary Test-4* (Martin, 2010).

7. Oral-peripheral and/or motor examinations

These may be informal or formal (e.g., Johnson-Root, 2015) structure and function tasks involving the articulators.

8. Recommendations

Appendix B

Stuttering therapy: Treating the Whole Disorder (Sheehan, Williams, & Dugan, 2001)

Philosophy of treatment

I. What is stuttering?

Stuttering, as it is usually defined, consists of prolongations and repetitions. These speech breakdowns are what characterize the disorder. Without them, stuttering can not be diagnosed.

For school aged children and adults, however, stuttering is far more than disfluency. It is also anxiety, worry, guilt, shame, self-consciousness, and a lot of other baggage. It is energy spent trying to hide disfluencies, be it via bodily movements, the rephrasing of utterances, substituting words, or any number of other behaviors people who stutter have employed for this purpose. In other words, people who stutter deal with not only their speech, but also with secondary behaviors, emotions, attitudes, and fears about speaking.

II. Treating stuttering

A. Eliminating disfluencies

Unfortunately, the emotional and behavioral aspects of stuttering are often neglected in therapy. After all, if one defines stuttering as prolonged and repeated speech units, the job of the therapist treating this disorder would seem to be to reduce or, better yet, eliminate these disfluencies.

Predictably, techniques that focus on eliminating disfluencies have become popular. There are three likely reasons for this.

1. Logic

Stuttering is disfluency so treat the disfluency. This is not only log-ical, but also consistent with how speech-language pathologists operate. Problems are typically first defined, then solved. If the definition consists of overt

symptoms, the solution is to minimize these symptoms.

1. Efficiency

It is seen by many to be an efficient means of treatment in that the speech-language pathologist can focus on disfluencies only and still achieve satisfactory results.

1.Success

Some clinical reports are encouraging. With preschool children, for example, *fluency shaping*—techniques designed to eliminate stut-tering by teaching easier and more fluent speech—works so well that it has become the treatment of choice for most speech-lan-guage pathologists.

B. Treating the whole disorder

1. Stuttering as speech, emotions, and secondary behaviors

It should be noted that preschoolers do not typically present fears and negative attitudes about speech. This is a key point to under-standing the limitations of treating only speech breakdowns with other populations.

To elaborate this point, read these 2 descriptions and decide who has the bigger problem.

> *Client A presents one-second prolongations and/ or repetitions in 10% of speech when talking to his friends.*

Client B is afraid to make friends because of the shame he associates with speaking.

In other words, what is the real disorder? Is it disfluency or is it the anxiety, embarrassment, and other components that lead one to withdraw?

1. Education

It is important that the client understand his speaking behaviors—both the stuttering and the covert experiences that characterize it. This includes education about:

a) Fluent vs. disfluent speech

b) Types of disfluencies

c) Secondary behaviors

d) Any other stuttering-related behaviors specific to the particular client

1. Desensitization

Treating only the overt speech characteristics neglects important emotional and behavioral aspects of stuttering. Along with controlling the disfluencies, the well-documented fears and negative speech attitudes of stuttering clients need to be counter-conditioned in therapy. That is, the reactions that evoke anxiety should be replaced with those more neutral (or positive). If the client can approach problem words or situations without fear, his attitudes toward speaking will improve and avoidance of speech (and life) will diminish.

The client should also become desensitized to the actual stuttering. This is important because treatment in any form involves changing one's usual manner of speaking. However well the learned speech techniques are mastered, the client must still be willing to speak the new way. Should the speaker be at all self-conscious about speech, such acceptance will not come easily. Stated differently, if you take someone who is already anxious about the way he speaks and teach him techniques that seem unusual, don't be surprised if he is reluctant about employing those techniques outside the therapy room. Without desensitization to reactions (the client's and those of his listeners), there is little chance of long-term success.

The notion of stuttering as a cued behavior is also worth noting. Much research has supported the idea that, for a given individual who stutters, certain words and situations are more likely than others to trigger disfluency. There are clinical implications to this. For one thing, speech will be easy for a client in a clinic room that represents only encouragement, success, and a lack of communicative pressure. Second, once he exits this safe environment and faces the outside world (that has many times more cues of past failure), implementation of therapy skills will be far more difficult.

Facing cues of past failures armed with only speech techniques is a losing

battle. The client must be desensitized to these cues and willing to confront them.

2. Decrease associated behaviors

Associated behaviors are performed to avoid or escape stuttering. They include behaviors such as withdrawal from speech, peculiar phrasing, pitch changes, strange facial or bodily movements while talking, unusual speech patterns ("My name is um, um, um . . ."), and a long list of others. Unfortunately, the effectiveness of these behaviors is only temporary, but the behaviors are often maintained after their effectiveness has diminished. In the long run, then, avoidance and escape behaviors can become strange and seemingly purposeless maneuvers that serve to further complicate the stuttering problem.

Because their temporary effectiveness is seductive (social penalties associated with stuttering need not be paid when no one can detect it), associated behaviors are damaging in another way as well. Some individuals who stutter are quite proficient at using these behaviors to hide their stuttering. In doing so, they continually associate stuttering (and all the fears and emotions that accompany it) with new words and situations. For example, the client who uses the word "automobile" because it is easier to say than "car" will, in time, likely have difficulty with "automobile." If he continues to use word substitution as an associated behavior, he will eventually have a hard time with "vehicle," "ride," and every other synonym he chooses. Thus, he will go from one problem word to many.

3. Gaining control of speech

The preceding discussions of open stuttering should not be interpreted to mean that the client's speech behaviors are not changed. Nothing could actually be further from the truth. Speech is in fact the major focus of treatment. It is simply not the sole one.

As is typical of stuttering modification approaches, the speech goals are not based on achieving fluency but, rather, on learning to control disfluency. What we tell the clients is: *You take control of the stuttering, rather than letting the stuttering control you.*

This begs the question: Why controlled stuttering? Why not teach fluency-enhancing techniques with desensitization? Several points address this issue.

a) It's important that the client know that stuttering is not bad. As Joseph Sheehan said, "Your fluency doesn't do you any good. There's nothing to be ashamed of when you stutter and there's nothing to be proud of when you are fluent."

b) Many clients are uncomfortable with the controls that are necessary to speak fluently. These clients report that the resulting speech is limiting and requires too much concentration.

c) In order to decrease avoidance behaviors, the client must be open about what he is avoiding. One cannot confront what is hidden.

d) Fluency often improves as a result of stuttering openly. But it's a by-product of treatment, not a goal. The cruelest irony of stuttering is that it doesn't really start to decrease until the client stops caring whether it will.

e) Techniques designed to effect fluent speech need to be employed constantly. If the client uses them only when he is in trouble, they can easily become new avoidance behaviors (which make problem more severe).

f) Some clients will never achieve fluency, even temporarily. To suggest that all clients can is to tell these individuals that they are not working hard enough.

As a final note on speech targets, they should include goals based on client self-monitoring. That is, the client should learn to accurately judge his own productions. The desired outcome of self-monitoring is, of course, self-correction (i.e., the client corrects the errors without feedback from the speech-language pathologist).

1. Creating a support system

Living with a stutter is not easy. It can help a client immeasurably to know that he's not in it alone. Support groups also allow the client a place to discuss the fears and emotions associated with stuttering. Such groups also offer an ideal place to attempt therapy targets with new listeners.

2. Transfer

Given the fear associated with stuttering, along with the difficulty of employing therapy techniques outside the clinical setting, it makes sense that transfer of skills is difficult. Fortunately, all the aforementioned components of therapy can be incorporated into a program of transfer and generalization. Such a program should begin early in the therapeutic process. That is, the client should start right away attempting well-learned skills in different environments.

Treatment Methods

So what do we actually do inside the treatment room? The answers to this question, of course, depend on each particular client. Below are some general guidelines and ideas for each of the areas covered earlier. It is important to understand that this handout is not meant to be followed sequentially (i.e., education before desensitization; desensitization before associated behaviors, etc.). Rather, these are goals that are important throughout the therapeutic process.

I. Education

Hierarchies can help the client understand his speaking behaviors. Examples of lists that the speech-language pathologist can compose with the client include:

A. Situations where speech is easy and hard (this information can be taken from the Speech Situation Checklist if that was part of the evaluation protocol),

B. Words that are easy and difficult to say, and

C. Secondary behaviors that are effective and ineffective.

Then create hierarchies to use as a basis for discussion. Similarly, if you teach the client

A. Easy, normal, and stuttering disfluencies,

hierarchies can show you and the client:

1. Which disfluencies are easiest to control and

2. The disfluencies the client is most comfortable producing.

I. Desensitization

A. Open Stuttering

Early in therapy, open stuttering can be encouraged as a means of desensitizing a client. Stuttering without any attempt to hide it is reinforced. For some clients, the more severe the stuttering, the greater the reinforcement. The idea is to lift the shame normally associated with stuttering and replace it with a positive response. Also, this is step one toward giving the client the tool of voluntary stuttering, discussed in IV of this outline.

B. Making therapy fun

Similarly, the process of desensitization can be helped by making treatment a fun experience for the client. Don't be afraid to use humor in therapy. Depending upon the client's age, music, artwork, posters, literature, and other sources of entertainment can be incorporated into sessions. The idea, again, is to associate stuttering, temporarily at least, with positive experiences.

C. Demystifying stuttering

Learning about and becoming desensitized to stuttering make the disorder less mysterious and therefore less powerful. The therapist can design activities specific to the purpose of lessening the mystery of stuttering. For children, drawing pictures of stuttering is an effective means of opening discussion on topics such as fears and emotions. Letting the child tear up the picture can be a satisfying means of releasing frustration. For older clients, writing letters to their stuttering can have the same effects, as can simply talking about feared or embarrassing situations.

D. Transfer

The process of transfer also helps with desensitization. The more practice the client has using targets with different listeners, the more desensitized he becomes. Transfer techniques that allow the client to confront and address cues of past failure are discussed under VI of this outline.

I. Decrease associated behaviors

Generally speaking, associated behaviors are easier to treat than are disfluencies. This is because associated behaviors are voluntary and, as such, respond to reinforcement and punishment.

A. Open stuttering

Open stuttering (discussed under II. A.) is often the first step toward decreasing associated behaviors. The client is instructed to speak without using any "tricks" to not stutter. In this way, all the client's avoidance behaviors are treated at once. Education about associated behaviors and the problems they create is commonly included at this point.

B. Treating one at a time

Some associated behaviors are resistant to treatment. These may require focused treatment. For example, if a client typically uses the interjection "um" to launch a difficult word, the clinician can tell him to "speak without um's" and/or have the parents keep track of um's at home. Typically, when one behavior is focused upon, other associated behaviors are not addressed until later.

In our example, only speaking without "um" would be reinforced and the presence of other associated behaviors ignored until later.

C. Punishment

After the initial phase of therapy, when the client understands the danger of using associated behaviors, mild punishers can be introduced. A common game with adolescents involves assigning points for different therapeutic behaviors. Perhaps a point is awarded for a controlled stutter, no points for a hard stutter, and a point is taken away for each avoidance or escape. A more elaborate system is 3 points for a preparatory set, 2 for a pull-out, 1 for a cancellation (these targets are explained under IV of this outline), 0 for a hard stutter, and −1 for an associated behavior. Either way, the messages are clear.

1. Controlled stutters are best.

2. Hard stutters will not be punished (there is nothing to be ashamed of) **or rewarded** (they do not advance the client toward the goal of control).

3. Associated behaviors are unacceptable.

I. Gaining control of speech

A. Modifying the disfluency

Speech targets can be taught to help the client stutter more easily. Which targets to teach depends on the individual. For instance, if a client presents with unregulated speech breathing, he might need to be taught to speak after a full inhalation. Prolonging the first sound of continuant-initial words is a common first step toward learning easy prolongations (or "stretches"). Easy initiation of voicing helps the client start these prolongations with relaxed musculature. Light contacts of the articulators are necessary in order to learn the easy repetitions (or "bounces") necessary to easily stutter plosives.

Such targets generally have the effect of reducing the client's speaking rate. If not, the client may have to learn a slower rate that allows control. Along with practice speaking at the slower rate, the client will need to get used to hearing himself do so until it sounds normal.

Multiple targets are taught in cumulative fashion. Say, for example, the targets are prolonged initial sound, easy initiation, and light contacts. Prolonged sounds, as the first target, will be taught in isolation. Once mastered, easy initiation can be added. At that point, the client will be expected to produce prolonged sounds *and* easy initiations with each response. Similarly, when light contacts are added, the client will produce three targets at once.

B. Easy stuttering in everyday speech

Once the client can produce easy disfluencies—stretches and/or bounces—these need to be transferred to conversational speech. The conventional way to do this is to work through cancellations, pull-outs, and preparatory sets.

1. Cancellations

What are being cancelled with cancellations are the hard, tense stuttering behavior and the reward (relief, mostly) for blasting through the word. The technique of cancellation follows this sequence: hard stutter, pause, easy stutter. This is what is expected of the client. Therefore, if he stutters with tension and continues talking, the clinician must stop him and make him go back and say the word with a stretch or a bounce.

2. Pull-outs

The client next learns to pull out of the hard stutter before completing it. That is, he may begin the word with tension, but he changes to an easy stutter in order to finish the word in a controlled manner.

3. Preparatory sets

The ultimate goal for easy stuttering in conversation is to bypass the hard stutter altogether. Thus, the client must be aware of when he is going to stutter and do so easily. This involves preparing his articulators for the stretch or the bounce, and then producing it. In other words, with preparatory sets, the client does not even begin the hard stutter. All disfluencies are easy ones.

Why not just skip cancellations and pull-outs and teach preparatory sets? There are at least two reasons why this is not recommended.

a) Cancellation effectively counteracts the very human response of fighting through a problem. The client learns that struggle is not necessary and indeed can be counterproductive toward learning more controlled speech.

b) Pull-out, described above as a short-term goal leading to preparatory set, can also serve as a tool for the client to use as needed. Occasionally, he will forget or be unable to produce a preparatory set. In these instances, he should work to shape the hard stutter into an easy one.

1. Shaping everyday speech

Variations are possible and will necessarily be client-specific. For example, a client may be unable or unwilling to bounce. In this instance, stretches can be utilized in a slightly different way. The client may be able to stretch a phoneme previous to the feared sound, but, as long as he is willing to do so obviously (i.e., not use the stretch as an associated behavior), this is acceptable. Of course, such a speech pattern is not perfect: There will be those utterances that begin with a plosive, thus leaving the client without an effective strategy other than the bounce he dislikes.

1. Levels of communication

When teaching the client to use easy disfluencies in conversation, the clinician is advised not to start with long narratives. Rather, one can start with low levels of communication and work toward those more difficult. Examples of communication levels are:

a) One-word responses

The speech-language pathologist can ask questions requiring yes-no or other short answers (e.g., What color is this?). In this way it is the clinician, not the client, who has almost complete control of both the speech content and utterance length. Games such as memory or naming opposites can also be used to elicit single words.

b) Phrases and short sentences

A good way to elicit phrase-level spontaneous responses is to ask questions such as "Where were you?" and "When were you there?" Utterance length is, of course, longer than with one-word responses, but the clinician still maintains much control over length and content. Games such as go-fish also lend themselves nicely to this level of communication.

c) Listing

Asking the client to list attributes (of an object or friend or something else in which the client is interested) will result in longer speech strings than earlier levels, but not so long that the clinician cannot maintain some control over utterance length and content.

d) Structured conversation

With structured conversation (i.e., "Tell me 3 things about your teacher"), the client's responses are less limited than previous levels in terms of content, but the clinician still has some control over length of utterance.

e) Unstructured conversation

This is the highest level of conversational speech task, where the client is telling the clinician a complete story or conversing without restrictions on length or content. Unstructured conversation is elicited with statements

such as "Tell me about school."

1. Self-monitoring

As they progress through the hierarchies of easy stuttering and conversation, the clinician should periodically ask the client whether he used the targets correctly on the last attempt. The client's accuracy is the percent agreement with the clinician.

2. Voluntary stuttering

Deliberate use of the easy stutters (i.e. stuttering purposely on a word that could have been said fluently) helps some clients maintain their therapeutic gains. That is, should hard stutters or, worse, associated behaviors, become more prevalent, voluntary stuttering can return the client to the therapy mindset. As such, it can be viewed as another tool for the client to take from therapy.

3. Modeling appropriate speech

The clinician's speech can have a major impact on therapeutic gains. Early in therapy, it is recommended that speech be relaxed:

slow rate (not unusually slow, but on the lower end of the normal range) with a lot of pausing. The clinician should be willing to listen without interrupting or hurrying the client in any way. The message this sends is that the speaker has as much time as he needs to say what he needs to say. Targets are easier to learn and practice in this type of communicative environment. Only when the targets are mastered should the clinician add disrupters (increase speech rate, interrupt, etc.).

I. Creating a support system

There are a variety of options available for support.

A. Group therapy

Even on an inconsistent basis, group therapy can show a client that he is not alone in what he faces. Therapy groups offer good opportunities for activities such as letter writing or discussion of fears (discussed in II. C.). Clients are often more willing to discuss the emotional aspects of stuttering in the presence of others who face the same obstacles.

B. Support Groups

In most geographic areas, support groups exist. The National Stuttering Association is a good place to start looking for one.

1. NSA phone: 1-800-364-1677

2. NSA web site: http://www.nsastutter.org/

A. Internet

Also, there are a variety of internet sources available for support. The following resources can be used to find them.

1. Stuttering Home Page: http://www.mnsu.edu/comdis/kuster

2. National Stuttering Association: http://www.nsastutter.org/

I. Transfer

There are many transfer activities that are consistent with the treatment plan being offered.

A. Home Programs

Home programs should begin as early in the therapeutic process as possible. There are 2 reasons for this:

1. The client can start practicing therapeutic tasks at home and

2. The client and significant others become accustomed to the idea of outside work as a part of therapy.

Homework tasks are typically one level behind tasks done in therapy. This is to assure that the correct targets are being reinforced. That is, if the client is practicing what he has mastered for the therapist, chances are good that he is not performing incorrect behaviors. In fact, it is a good idea to have the client or significant other keep track of performance and, if it is not at or near 100%, make adjustments in the home assignment.

Keeping the homework one level behind the current tasks begs the question of what to assign before the client has met any goals. Some ideas include sending home the Speech Situation Checklist or other attitude scale (assuming it was not used in the evaluation), asking the client to construct hierarchies (see I of this outline), and having the client locate information on the recommended internet sources.

As with any home program, the speech-language pathologist must instruct the client and/or significant others how to differentiate and response record correct vs. incorrect answers. Reinforcement must also be taught.

B. Role play

1. Confronting cues of past failure

One reason transfer is so difficult with fluency clients is that cues of past failures are hard to overcome. The client must be made aware of these cues and confront them. Role play is one effective means of doing so. The therapist can take the role of the teacher, interviewer, boss, parent, or whoever else is involved in difficult speaking situations for a particular client.

2. Pragmatics

A related reason for engaging in role play is to teach the client about language pragmatics. For example, if the client has difficulty entering conversations because he cannot match the rate of speech already set by the participants, he can learn new means of getting the listeners' attention (e.g., gestures, verbalizations, expressions).

A. Altering the communicative environment

Throughout therapy, and within the home plan, it is possible to alter the listeners and the setting in which communication takes place.

1. Within the treatment setting

a) In some therapy settings, it is possible to hold sessions in different rooms, which can help with the problem of one and only one location becoming associated with success.

b) It is also possible for the clinician to move the client through hierarchies of increasingly difficult listener situations. For example, a family member can be brought in to witness a client's use of easy stutters in conversation, then a second clinician or someone from the office staff, then a stranger, etc.

c) In or out of the treatment room, it is important for the speech-language pathologist to be the leader in all transfer activities. That is, the clinician should model easy stutters first when new listeners are involved. This shows the student that the teacher believes in what he or she is teaching and that there is nothing shameful about stuttering.

2. At home

a) Once it is established that home assignments are being carried out, the clinician can instruct the client and/or client's family to practice in different parts of house (or elsewhere). This avoids the potential problem of having a single setting that the client associates with fluency.

b) Home assignments can specify that targets be practiced with different family members, or with friends, or (later) with strangers.

B. Taking chances

As the client begins to habituate the therapy targets, he should be made aware that mistakes will be tolerated. The client will make far more progress if he is willing to take chances than if he always plays it safe. The clinician should talk to the client about how the fear of making mistakes holds back improvement. If the client can embrace difficult situations, if he can view them as challenges, he can progress beyond them. Conversely, it is impossible to improve without trying new skills.

C. Completion of therapy

Because relapse is high with stuttering, it is not recommended that the client be dismissed from treatment as soon as preparatory sets are mastered. A better course of action is to reduce the frequency of therapy and monitor conversational goals in order to assure that performance can be maintained without regular therapy. Thus, a twice-a-week client might be asked to start attending therapy once a week. Then, frequency can be reduced to once every 2 weeks, then once a month. Should gains be maintained and the client discharged, it should be with the understanding that the therapist be contacted in the event of any relapse (e.g., more avoidance, inability to stutter easily). Follow-up telephone calls are recommended as well, to help monitor the client's skills

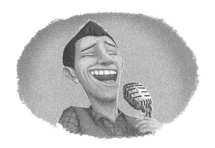

Chapter 7: Why I Became a Comedian

I don't think humans are born happy. Most of us, in fact, enter the world crying. From that fateful beginning, a supportive, kind, and loving environment gradually teaches us happiness. As far as I can see, my 5-month-old daughter Emma is happy, especially when I smile at her. The audience is indeed a mirror.

But what about people whose surroundings are better described as adverse, punishing, and distant? Well, some of them become comedians.

To be clear, discontent wasn't the sole reason I went into comedy. It's more complicated than that. But I don't think it was something I was naturally born to do. According to my mother, I was a fairly shy child, too scared to go into nursery at the age of 3. Still, a streak of gregariousness has always been present. Perhaps being a middle child deprived me of the attention I later sought.

Early Influences

The comedy seed was planted early. Due to having busy, self-employed parents, I probably watched too much TV growing up. My parents were fairly relaxed about me going to bed at a set time, and around age seven, I was regularly allowed to stay up and watch a popular and very funny adult BBC2 TV comedy program called *Not the Nine O'clock News*. I remember wondering how these people could be in a comedy show and avoid doing a normal job. It just looked totally glamorous and fun. A few years later, when I was entering my teens, I read about Rowan Atkinson, one of the stars of the show (later famous for his Mr. Bean character). Rowan had a stutter, which I found quite inspirational.

My brother Guy was four years older than I and into music, sports, TV, and films. Thanks in part to him, I remember watching many American movies starring actor/comedians such as Robin Williams, Steve Martin, Dan Aykroyd, and Chevy Chase, all of whom started out on the US stand-up circuit. For Guy and me, comedy films were an escape into a fantasy world of laughter and self-assuredness. They still are today. I would also see stand-up comedians performing on TV and was probably overly-influenced by the praise and respect they received from the media and the general public. It seemed like an interesting and exciting way to make a living. The ability to stand up in front of an audience and take control appeared to be an almost magical skill. I wanted to learn how to do it. I guess I thought it would be a perfect way to show the world that I wasn't just some average chap with a stutter.

Although I was never the class clown or even particularly adept at making people laugh at school, I believed that comedy was my destiny from the age of eight.

However, I'm certain if I had watched less television, my young brain wouldn't have become quite so obsessed by the need to make it into the worlds of comedy and TV.

It could be argued that my fascination with comedy also stemmed from feelings of inadequacy and insecurity, plus a need to prove myself to a generally disapproving and overly critical father. In other words, the seeds all consisted of negative feelings. If so, I was hardly alone. Many comedians I have met over the years displayed some degree of negativity in their personalities.

Criticism

One way to cultivate pessimism is to come of age under constant criticism. I realized at a young age that whatever I did was never going to be enough in my father's eyes. But it was not just paternal disparagement that helped my inner seeds of negativity grow. Looking back, many of my memories involve disapproval, searching for attention, or both. Maybe everyone eventually views life negatively, I don't know. In any case, the ability to flip that and count my blessings has always been difficult for me, despite being lucky enough to live in a highly developed Western society.

As noted in chapter 3, my home life and schooling both had their negative moments. My lack of confidence with girls was also frustrating, and despite having 2 or 3 very short-term girlfriends as a teenager, my self-consciousness definitely hindered the development of these relationships. My first girlfriend stayed with me about three weeks, then never spoke to me again. The negative effect of being ignored lasted an unrealistically long time. (Interestingly, I met her 19 years later and she said that she regretted the way she had acted, blaming it on being "precocious and flighty at 13, a different manifestation of self-consciousness").

Unfortunately, our time together was pretty representative of all of my adolescent romances.

Bristol University

By the time I entered Bristol University at the age of 18, my search for fulfillment became, if not mature, at least more adult-like. Bowing to peer pressure, I reluctantly played rugby and discovered some extra motivation from being watched by girls on the side of the pitch. And although my dating luck remained the same as before, I was able to obtain the odd drunken kiss here and there. In fact, I won a prize at the end of the first year for being the "biggest shark" in my hall of residence, an award that probably lowered my chances of actually having a girlfriend. After all, who wants to go out with the guy who chats everyone up? It was a victory attributable to college drinking, which made me flirtatious, attention-seeking, and more confident with the opposite sex.

Overall, the college lifestyle had a negative impact on my speech. The lack of sleep, poor diet, sparse exercise, high workloads, and stress of trying to talk as fast as everyone else all combined to destroy my speech fluency. My stutter often made me feel like the odd one out among my housemates. Because of this, I enrolled in group therapy. Due to embarrassment, I stupidly didn't tell my housemates why I disappeared every Saturday. I would make up a story, such as I had spent the day writing an essay, which likely did not fool anyone.

Toward the end of year 2, there came a time, sudden and largely unannounced, when my housemates explained that they'd be going to different houses in year 3. When only two of us remained, we had to quickly scramble to find a new place to live.

Due to the time constraints we were under, we took a convenient 2-bedroom flat without considering what it would be like to live together.

There were problems from the start. Firstly, we were very different people. He was focused on his accountancy studies and rugby, whereas I was into geography, music, and writing. On the plus side, the flat was close to campus, which meant I could remain there for a few weeks over the summer holidays to finish my year 2 dissertation and stay out of my father's way in Suffolk. Also a quieter flat meant that I could focus on my studies a bit better, with fewer distractions. I also had my first proper girlfriend that year. The times spent with her were the happiest in that place.

Her stays were short-lived, however, and I spent far more time dealing with roommate differences and the large amount of work needed to graduate. I was also losing touch with many of the friends I had lived with during my second year. These factors all combined to bring me down a little.

My 21st birthday party

One of my university friends was a very outgoing and funny chap who everyone seemed to adore. Most of the time I envied him, but his confidence seemed to rub off on me when we were together. I remember he gave a witty and confident speech at my 21st birthday party which (of course) made everybody laugh. After he was finished, it was my turn to speak. It was a tough act to follow, but I did OK. It was probably the first time that I was able to make a small audience laugh, which was an uplifting experience. It was also the highlight of an otherwise disastrous event.

The party took place at my parents' restaurant in Suffolk. It was an occasion I never really desired in the first place, but felt pressured by the importance my parents placed on the event. Life would have been much easier if I had simply been assertive and said no.

My birthday is 31st December, which meant that New Year's Eve business was sacrificed for me, an expensive decision. On top of that were the costs of the live band, marquee, food, free drinks, and invitations. Between 60 and 80 people attended, including many of my parents' friends. It had the potential to be a good night, except that my father could not relax. The fact that the restaurant wasn't big enough to hold so many people seemed to be a primary source of his agitation. So too were my friends' excessive New Year's Eve drinking and rowdiness (the latter keeping my father from being the center of attention). At one point, a university friend broke his ankle when he was pushed off the roof of car. Unfortunately, this mishap was not the worst moment of the night.

My father was wearing a kilt, about which some of my friends commented. Many didn't even realise he was my father, as he was so busily picking up wine and beer glasses that he appeared to be part of the waiting staff. His actual intent was to limit any damage and, when a friend accidently broke a glass in front of him, he went over the edge. Pinning the friend to a wall, my father then pulled a *skiendoo* knife[1] from his sock. Fortunately, all he did from there was to throw my friend outside, an act for which my father received a punch in the face.

As bad as all of that was, the incident was still not over. A few days later he made an impromptu visit to the father of the person who hit him, calling his son "arrogant and uncontrollable." As the father

---

1   A *skiendoo* knife is traditionally worn with a kilt, tucked into the right sock.

happened to be the vicar at my old school, it was all very embarrassing.

The repercussions from that evening were lasting. For one, I haven't spoken to the friend since. It also isolated me from some of our mutual friends. It was 17 years before I bumped into the vicar and his wife, at which time I apologised for my father's actions of that evening. Both remembered it all as though it were yesterday.

Graduation Day

What kept me going during the final year at university was a desire to graduate with honours. This was so much of a goal in fact that I even ended things with my girlfriend. I told her that I "needed some space" to focus on my exams, which was true, but still hurtful to her and regrettable for me.

My focus paid off, as I received a 2.1 (honours) at Bristol. I invited my parents to attend graduation, a milestone event that quickly turned distressing. It began with a 4-hour drive from Suffolk to Bristol with my father talking non-stop the entire way. After the ceremony, we ran into a friend who mentioned that he was going on to do a Master of Science (MSc). My father then announced that we must all get back to Suffolk that evening so that I too could apply for an MSc. Despite my wishes to stay in Bristol for a couple of days and attend a few graduation parties, we drove home that afternoon. I told my father about an MSc course in which I was vaguely interested, so the next day he directed me to apply for a self-funded MSc by Research at Edinburgh University, to start in October of that year. It was rushed, but not all bad; I no longer had a girlfriend in Suffolk and the course was a way to move out and do something positive with my time. There was still an opening, but I felt that with more time and research, I could have applied for a course with funding attached to it (not to mention one I actually wanted to take). Receiving money from my parents for another year was painful, given my desire for independence.

That summer was a disaster. I lived for a few weeks at my parents' house and then moved in with my brother, three miles away. If I went out at night to a pub, I would sometimes run into the ex-girlfriend and her new boyfriend, always a less than comfortable situation. By the time I drove up to Edinburgh at the end of September, I was happy to get away from Suffolk. The MSc was serious work, but I could handle it and found renewed confidence on both personal and academic levels, despite at times still totally regretting the course I had chosen.

Edinburgh University

Edinburgh was at times a dream-like experience. It was not only exactly what I needed at that stage of my life, but turned out to be an important stepping stone into becoming the person that I wanted to be.

When I first arrived, I lived in a large shared flat with 11 other guys, nearly all of whom were starting MSc courses or PhD's. It was an enjoyable and stimulating time meeting so many intelligent people of different nationalities. I was also a tutor to two groups of 18 year-old first-year geography students, which with my stutter presented quite a challenge, but an experience that I nevertheless found rewarding. I had to prepare an hour's class to two groups each week, which tested me more than anything I had done before in my life. I also had postgraduate presentations to do and course work for the five geographic information system (GIS)/Geography "training courses" I was doing for the MSc.

I found the keys to the presentations were preparation and having the confidence in knowing what I was talking about.

An old Bristol University friend lived in Edinburgh. Because he also had a stutter, I found being with him to be quite comforting, as it made me remember that I wasn't the only person in the world to have this impediment. Together, we occasionally made use of the fine Edinburgh pubs to have some laughs. I remember once an American man asked if he could have whatever drugs we were on, not realising that we both stuttered.

I watched my first live stand-up show at the Edinburgh Fringe in August 1996. I remember walking out of that show having not laughed very much and telling my friends that I've got to do stand-up one-day. That show reignited my interest in performing comedy. (I didn't know it at the time, but I was still four years away from actually getting on stage.)

By the end of the MSc, I had run out of money. My last week was spent sleeping in the geography department or on friends' floors.

It was time to look for a job.

Job interviews

I quickly secured various interviews. Unfortunately, they normally ended with the words, "We'd like to give you the job, but the stutter is too much of a problem." I still remember one CEO asking me if I was "going to jump off a bridge" due to what she had just told me.

"No, don't worry," I replied. "I'd probably jump off a bridge if I worked here."

I returned back to Suffolk to write job applications. Oddly enough, given that I was out of work, out of money, and back with my parents, I met someone. It didn't end well—unbeknownst to me, she eventually started dating someone else—but at the time her positive influence on me was a godsend. My confidence and self-esteem shot up, especially when I was with her.

Despite feeling better about myself, however, the job interviews were not improving. In fact, they normally ended like the first one had (variations of the directive "Come back when you've lost your stutter"). I joined a small temping agency and eventually got a job doing data input for an engineering firm. I immediately hated it and soon moved on to a 6-month GIS digitising contract, which wasn't much better, plus it involved moving. I found a small uncomfortable flat in Aberdeen, one best described as depressing. The way in which the relationship with my girlfriend ended further accentuated my feelings of dejection, destroyed my confidence with women, but, oddly, made me think more about being a comedian.

My solace at the time was that life's negativity had to taper off, if for no other reason than the law of averages. Then, however, came London to prove me wrong.

London

I could tell from the start that London was a competitive environment (just *how* competitive I would learn later, when I performed on the city's comedy circuit). Surviving any entry-level job there required hard work and an acceptance of the mundane. One also needed a quality self-assessment of his or her own strengths and limitations. Any company in London expected high productivity levels in exchange for paying a decent monthly salary.

But I was never very good at filling roles void of creativity and, as a result, found most office environments fairly restrictive.

My first proper job in London was at Brent Council, which is a local government organisation managing the Borough of Brent, in North-West London. My job was crime mapping officer, which involved mapping and analysing high volume crime data for the Police and the Council. I was using a GIS to identify crime hot spots, along with other trends and patterns. This helped the police and council evaluate projects and allocate resources, such as CCTV camera locations and street lighting, more effectively. I actually quite enjoyed this job but found the office far too noisy to concentrate properly. Moreover, I wasn't disciplined enough on the weekends, due to excessive alcohol and late nights, and so my stress levels and stutter were not kept in check. One night in Brixton I was mugged at knifepoint, which didn't exactly help my positivity. When the mugger asked if I had any money on me, I blocked. Then I silently gave him a £20 note and he ran off. I used to joke in my comedy routine that after seeing me stutter, he ended up giving me £20.

Even without the distractions, the crime-mapping job had been a little out of my depth, as I had naughtily embellished my information technology skills during the interview. It ended after 18 months due to what can only be described as "management wanting to get rid of me." I ended up in a rehab centre in Wembley with two speech therapists, practicing how to say my name. It was probably not how the average person ends a contract.

Although I had talked about being a comedian before, it wasn't until I left the crime mapping position that the idea really started to take hold. During the speech therapy sessions I attended and within the books on stuttering that I was reading, public speaking was viewed as a good idea. So I thought that going on the comedy circuit could help improve both my self-confidence and speech. I felt that I needed to teach myself how to speak without fear. Therefore, while I job hunted, I also looked at ways of getting into comedy. The first jokes I wrote were related to confidence issues.

> *As a teenager my biggest fear was a lack of confidence. But then I grew up and I realised it was actually the French.*

and

> *I went to my speech therapist. I said "How do you get more confident?"*
>
> *She said, "Act like Arnold Schwarzenegger. Speak to people in authority."*
>
> *So I walked up to a Police Officer. I said, "I want your clothes, I want your boots, I want your motorcycle." Totally fluent. I was arrested. I couldn't even say "I'll be b- b- b-back."*

OK, they needed work. In my defense, however, I was hindered by never getting a good night's sleep, as the man next door would always blast his TV late at night (despite my banging on the wall between us). Fortunately, I was able to move out when a friend of my brother said that there was a spare room in his flat.

I stayed with my new roommate for most of the following year. Once, over a drink, he asked me what I really wanted to do with my life and I remember saying "I'd like to be a comedian."

His reply was "Well just do it then!"

Up until then no one had ever asked me that particular question. It was a memorable moment in an otherwise dismal situation. The rent was expensive, the flat had basically no furniture, and my roommate smoked constantly. He was going through a rough time himself, having lost a job and a girlfriend, and stayed up late at night playing music and watching TV. Going to comedy shows in the evenings was basically a way to get out of that flat.

I needed one more catalyst to enroll in a comedy course. This happened on my 26th birthday when I ran into an ex-girlfriend on New Year's Eve 1999. She ignored me in favour of another ex of hers, which bothered me enough to get very drunk. This solution eventually led to me falling over and hitting my nose on the dance floor, causing blood to flow everywhere. Determining that I had just hit the lowest point of my life, I decided it was time for a change.

I considered simply moving out of London and going travelling, or becoming a tour rep in the Mediterranean, or even returning to Suffolk. But I felt I wasn't finished with London yet. It's funny how the more one is driven to despair, the harder one rebounds to attempt to find justice. If life is over-privileged and comfortable, what stimulus is there to bounce back from it or create anything?

My strategy for beating London was to throw myself into comedy. Watching, performing, and writing became my means of dealing with the daily annoyances of home. The more flatmate issues that arose, the more I immersed myself in comedy and, as a result, I gradually became better at it.

London relationships

I can't blame my inability to attract a girlfriend on becoming a comedian. My vain attempts at meeting the women of London normally involved drinking and smoking too much, followed by horrendous hangovers. Even when I was able to secure a woman's phone number, calling her back was a disaster because of my stutter. The sad thing is that if one of the girls I met had requested a long term relationship, I can almost guarantee that I would not have gone on the stand-up comedy circuit. My reason for frequenting dodgy and noisy nightclubs was to find my soulmate. The problem, I'm sure, was that my real soulmate was sitting at home, quietly reading a book.

Once I chose comedy as my maverick career path, I instantly reduced my chances of finding a typical girlfriend. Who wants to go out with a poor, mildly alcoholic, semi-egotistical wannabe comic? I had no career or proper job that I liked doing, but with respect to comedy, I was very ambitious. I liked the idea of being in a relationship but also liked my own company. At that time of my life, I wasn't ready to settle down and any sort of deep bond would have been distracting. Besides, finding true love takes time. My attempts can be summed up in two clichés: the grass is greener on the other side and you don't know what you've got until it's gone.

The succession of failed relationships forced me into self-examination. I thought that I lacked decisiveness, assertiveness, and confidence, but now I could add patience to the list.

Achieving anything worthwhile requires a great deal of time and focus, but I wanted each new connection to be "the one" instead of just letting things develop.

Because of the way I threw myself into relationships, I subsequently had difficulty letting go, no matter how broken they became. Then I would feel like a lesser man than the bloke who followed me.

My frustrating love life did motivate me to practice communicating with people, especially women. So too, did my day jobs, which consisted in large part of sitting in a room and staring at a screen. Going home to watch a different screen was largely unappealing and so a comedy course where I could practice speaking became a far more attractive way to spend my evenings.

Breaking up is also hard to do, especially, I think, for males. Women get their hearts broken, phone all their friends, and then seem to move on reasonably quickly. Men can take years to get over it; sometimes they never do, especially those with deep insecurities. Men go on dates with other people and just see the ex-girlfriend sitting there. We hear our date's voice, but hear only the ex talking. We can't eat, sleep, or even listen to music the same way for years. The dating game would have been much simpler for me if character traits such as desperation, anxiety, and lack of self-discipline were seen as attractive.

Fame

Stand-up comedy put me amongst other comedians who were as insecure and self-doubting as myself. We weren't all there making people laugh to become rich and famous, but like many media-obsessed, TV-watching would-be entertainers, I'd be lying if I said the concept of fame—how it occurred and what it would be like—didn't interest me.

I remember in 2000, writing a list of all the pros and cons of being famous and I decided that at the time, being famous had more pros. These included:

- Exciting lifestyle,

- Improved self-confidence,

- Being interviewed for radio/TV, which would be exhilarating,

- The knowledge that I've done something noticeable and memorable with my life,

- Being recognised on the street would be an ego boost,

- Going to cool parties and meeting famous people, and

- I would show my school and my parents that I wasn't lazy, or a failure.

The possible negatives to fame I listed were:

- Stress,

- Having to be funny every time you get on stage or are interviewed,

- Lack of privacy,

- Being recognised could be quite annoying and make it difficult to relax anywhere in public (this obviously depends on your level of fame),

- The competitive and tough nature of the comedy business,

- Extra pressure on my relationships with family and friends, and

- Wondering if people liked me for who I am and not what I had become.

I had heard about the trappings of fame and my response was, "What about the trappings of everyday life?" People fall in love, get married, get tied down to jobs they secretly hate, and spend their lives with partners they tolerate, potentially navigating life through someone else's constraints, constantly compromising and trying to avoid arguments. Fame and success to me were like going on holiday by yourself—that is, doing exactly what you like, when you like, where you like—compared to travelling with someone else who has different interests and priorities, and having to make sure that person is happy.

There can also, of course, be financial benefits to fame. Comedy in the UK is big business these days, especially on the live circuit, with big-name tours and comedy clubs large and small spread across the country. A top circuit act can make over £80,000 a year from playing gigs seven nights a week and making TV appearances, while the crème de la crème of the comedy world can rake in a cool quarter of a million pounds from tours, corporate appearances, TV, radio, and endorsements.

Overall, I think I wanted to be famous because I watched too much television growing up, which instilled in me an admiration and awe for TV celebrities and personalities. I also heard that having a narcissistic father leads to obsessions with abstract escapes, such as movies and comedy, as well as a need for more material objects.

My brother's high profile position—reporter for BBC local radio—also played a part.

I often heard my father regretting that he had not been a famous actor or singer, and this definitely had an effect on me. It made me grow up thinking that fame was important. If someone he knew had a small part in a TV show, it was talked about for weeks. If a friend or work acquaintance of my father's was in the paper, it was a major issue for him.

Living in a British/western society also gives more credence to becoming a famous actor and comedian, rather than becoming a doctor or lawyer, for example. But this is purely a relative concept. To farmers living in the countryside without access to television, radio, or newspapers, fame no longer exists. To them it means nothing. When the world ends in 5 billion years' time (or no doubt much sooner due to dwindling world resources, water shortages, climate change, nuclear war, or asteroid hits), all of man's inventions, creative work, and lists of famous people will be gone.

To me, however, fame seemed like the answer to many of my problems, especially my relationships with women and my father. Being famous seemed like the cure for my stutter and insecurities too, and thus the key to a better and happier world. I have since changed my views on this, realizing that 1) our society is too obsessed with fame and 2) I was too obsessed with fame.

Just think of the thousands of people around the world who perform selfless and important deeds every day to help others. Nobody has even heard of them, yet their lives are worthy of recognition.

I believe that a small desire for fame exists in all of us; it's just some people want it more than others. It seems that those who achieve it often experienced negative events during childhood, such as the loss of a parent or rejection from a key figure in their lives. They were told directly or indirectly that they would not achieve anything. They set out to prove their doubters wrong and have the last laugh.

Conclusions

I acquired much comedy material during my years of young adult struggle. I met some interesting people and had the opportunity to live in different places. Yet when I think of those times, my mind goes to the hassles of London, relationships ending badly, jobs that seemed hopeless, an interfering father, and, of course, my stutter. From these depressing points emerged comedy, as a means of both developing confidence and following a dream.

Overall, comedy was an enlightening experience. Moreover, making people laugh and helping myself at the same time has been quite satisfying.

Most men wake up each morning with decisiveness and confidence. They decide what they want and then confidently set out to achieve that goal. They are in control of their lives. By this standard, it is embarrassing to lose a job or to end up in a rehab clinic unable to handle the emotional stress associated with stuttering. Even now, despite years of work on my speech, there are fears that go through my head, such as whether I will ever:

- Stand in a church and declare "I do" with control, and conviction;

- Say my name without hesitation in a crowded room or on the phone;

- Use plosive sounds without speech breakdowns; or

- Meet my partner's significant others and not feel like a stuttering moron or an outsider.

Yes, my stutter still gets me down.

As noted, I am glad that I got into stand-up comedy. It is, however, a very difficult and competitive business. Moreover, it's a role that can take one outside of basic humanity and reality. The average person sees tragedy on the news and thinks, "How awful. That's just terrible." A comedian thinks, "How awful. Now where's the joke in that?"

A comedian always tries to finish his routine with his funniest gag in order to end on the loudest laugh possible. Similarly, people want life to end in a crescendo. But we can't always expect the show to get better (especially with my comedy routine). When the jokes are there, laugh. When the opportunity arises, seize it. Life is short. Sorry—another cliché.

As you've just witnessed, there weren't many things in life that made me particularly happy. And I still believe that, ultimately, happiness is the key to life. Our short time on this planet shouldn't be spent going around looking miserable all the time.

For me, happiness hasn't been easy to find. I will admit that there were times that simply ending the story seemed like an easier option. But then, as Al Pacino is told in the film *Scarface*, "Everyday above ground is a good day!"

Questions for Discussion

Rank order Jaik's early comedy influences—television, movies, his brother Guy, insecurities, criticism, and feelings of inadequacy— from most to least influential. Explain your rankings.

What was Jaik's biggest social barrier at Bristol—stuttering, shyness, or low confidence? Explain your answer.

Does it surprise you that a shy, stuttering child who was good in school and looking for stability ended up in stand-up comedy? Why or why not?

What are your feelings about an interviewer overtly rejecting a prospective employee because of stuttering?

Jaik's first jokes were about confidence issues. Is there any significance to that?

Jaik writes that "(b)eing famous seemed like the cure for my stutter." How would fame cure (or even help) stuttering?

On the topic of fame, Jaik stated, "I often heard my father regretting that he had not been a famous actor or singer, and this definitely had an effect on me. It made me grow up thinking that fame was important." His father's regrets could have been utilized another way too. Gaining more fame than his father had may well have struck a hurtful blow against the man who had tormented him. Could this also have been a motivator for Jaik to seek fame?

He also wrote that,"Most men wake up each morning with decisiveness and confidence." Do you believe that statement to be true? Is
it less true for those who stutter? What is the relationship among
the three variables of stuttering, confidence, and decisiveness?

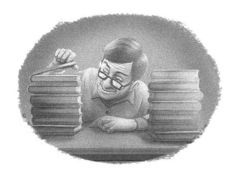

Chapter 8: Attitudes, Risk, and Relationships

When I read Jaik's belief that a "desire for fame exists in all of us; it's just some people want it more than others," I remembered a show I once saw about celebrity. It was supposedly an impartial look at the topic, hosted, of course, by a celebrity. Some of the probing and "objective" questions asked were, "What sets celebrities apart?" and "Who are the people who attain fame?" The premise was clear: We should all strive for celebrity and celebrate the special people who achieve it.

I didn't take the show very seriously. By that point in my life, I already knew plenty of people for whom fame would have been their worst nightmare, most of whom were far better at what they did than celebrities are at their chosen vocations. Nevertheless, it was a clear illustration of Jaik's point that society's celebration of fame is quite real and even influential.

Attitudes of People Who Stutter

For his part, Jaik viewed celebrity as a remedy for the *negativity* that is a constant theme throughout chapter 7. As noted earlier, the association of stuttering and negativity has primarily been investigated via studies of speech-related attitudes. Such is not always the case, however. General attitudes of adults who stutter have been investigated for decades (e.g., Blumgart, Tran, & Craig, 2010; Griener et al., 1985). Some investigators have utilized attitude scales to assess traits such as general anxiety, social isolation, and, one that is particularly pertinent to Jaik's story, confidence (among others). Those who stutter were typically found to be on the negative end of such scales (that is, more anxious and isolated, less confident) in comparison to non-stutterers. However, the relationship of such broad differences to communication is ambiguous. Separating generalized and speech-related attitudes is very difficult with people who stutter. For example, asking subjects to rate how often they "experience humiliation" (Wolpe, 1982) may, on the surface, appear to address general socialization skills (i.e., those unrelated to speech). For the young adult who stutters, however, humiliating experiences may very well be interrelated with communication. Thus, that subject's rating may not reflect the general attitudes sought by researchers.

The data on speech-associated attitudes are clearer. Group differences emerge in preschool years (Clark et al., 2012; Vanryckeghem, Brutten & Hernandez, 2005), based on speech difficulty. That is, children beginning to stutter sense that speech is harder for them than it is for their peers, but this realization does not necessarily change their speaking behaviors.

Speech attitude differences have been found with school-aged children (Bernardini et al., 2009), adolescents (Beilby, Byrnes, &

Yaruss, 2012), and adults (Andrews & Cutler, 1974; Erickson, 1969) as well. As Jaik's experiences suggest, these differences are likely based on affective and cognitive stuttering factors. After all, Jaik's emotions, fears, worries about listener reactions, and attempts to hide stuttering were as big a part of his story as his speech break-downs.

The results of at least one study (Manning, Dailey, & Wallace, 1984) indicate that older adults who stutter (defined as ages 52 to 82) self-report greater acceptance of stuttering in comparison to their younger adult years. To the extent that this is true (one always wonders with self-reporting), it is difficult to say why. Do they stutter less? Do they care less? Are they less often in the types of anxiety-producing situations (e.g., job interview, first date) common to younger adults? Unfortunately, there is not enough research to adequately answer these questions.

All in all, then, it appears that negative attitudes about speech emerge early with stuttering children, continue (and perhaps even worsen) throughout adolescence and early adulthood, but eventually become more positive. From the research done to this point in time, it also seems that it is an overgeneralization to assume that the negativity goes beyond speech.

Regarding confidence, it is difficult to determine whether Jaik's perceived deficiency is only related to speaking. He states that most men wake up each morning with confidence, decisiveness, and control, a questionable assertion but one that likely reflects his frustration in the area of self-reliance. After all, it can seem that everyone else is confident in situations where we feel the opposite.

Expanding the Comfort Zone

With clients school-aged and older, negativity toward speech (with or without a corresponding lack of confidence) usually needs to be addressed in therapy. As noted in chapter 6, even the best learned speech techniques are useless for clients who are unwilling or unable to employ them when they are actually speaking. Simply stated, to move beyond situations in which the use of such techniques is easy (e.g., the treatment room), clients must expand their zones of comfort. They have to shape uncomfortable situations into comfortable ones via direct experience, a struggle that understandably feels risky.

In one sense, Jaik seems well-suited for risk-taking. He came from family of entrepreneurs and entered stand-up comedy, a precarious endeavor by any standard. On the other hand, he generally seemed to want to play it safe with relationships, hoping his "soulmate" was right around the corner and displaying a propensity to hold on to memories of happiness well past the time had come to let go. More to the point, there were some definite fears about divulging his stutter, which is exactly the sort of risk that helps expand the comfort zone.

Moving beyond one's comfort zone is challenging because clients feel as if they are facing the unknown. For Jaik, there are speech situations—for example, interviewing for a job or simply joining a conversation—fraught with potential perils. The problems with taking risks in such feared circumstances are 1) by definition, they sometimes go wrong, leaving the risk-taker with a sense of loss, and 2) individuals tend to overestimate the probability of failed risks (Kahneman, 2011). Perhaps because of these reasons, people are generally risk averse (Worrell et al., 2013). Exceptions to this aversion seem to occur in instances in which we have given ourselves permission to fail. Jaik tells a risky joke and there are two possible outcomes—outright success or failure balanced by the poise of an experienced comic. It's easy to take risks when the cost of failure is nothing more than a moment of awkwardness one can easily move past. However, such is not the case when, say, a speaker has no idea how new listeners are going to respond when surprised by a speech difference. In that scenario, the fear of failure is pronounced and taking risks can seem exceedingly difficult. After all, speech is an activity that should be routine. Performing it poorly can be embarrassing. It follows, then, that granting oneself permission to stutter in all situations—job interviews, dates, telling jokes to an audience—is a great challenge. Hopefully, examination of therapeutic risk-taking can help speech-language pathologists address this challenge with their stuttering clients.

What risk-taking is and is not

In the interest of operationally defining terms, let us first discuss what risk-taking is not, as well as what it is.

For purposes of this chapter, risk taking has nothing to do with race cars, mountain climbing, or parachuting. The purpose goes well beyond an adrenalin rush or change of pace to make life more interesting. The idea that when confronted with two choices, one should always take the riskier one is not advocated here.

Rather, this is about the kind of risks that people such as Jaik take every day, for example:

- Advertising their stutters without knowing how people will respond.

- Voluntarily stuttering with strangers in order to desensitize themselves to listener reactions.

- Stuttering openly during job interviews rather than resort to harmful secondary behaviors.

In other words, this is about taking risks that help with the attainment of personal goals. For clients, these goals can be desensitization to stuttering, making speech easier, or others, such as implementation of speaking techniques, granting oneself permission to stutter, or learning to communicate jokes to an audience.

Why do stuttering clients need to get outside their comfort zones?

As alluded to in chapter 6 (and elsewhere), for a given individual who stutters, certain situations and words are more likely than others to trigger disfluency. Once that person can enter these situations or say these words without anxiety, their power diminishes. That is a foundation of desensitization. And if the fear of these words and/or situations can be removed by confronting them, they can, in a sense, become disassociated with stuttering. Ideally then, they would no longer serve as triggers.

Speech is easy in a clinic room in which there is no history of speech failure. However, once the client exits this safe environment and faces real life, with all its reminders of past setbacks, implementation of therapy skills is far more difficult. Viewed from another perspective, if the speech-language pathologist teaches only novel speaking patterns to someone who is anxious about the way he or she speaks, the SLP should not be surprised when the individual is reluctant about employing those patterns in other environments.

Jaik's development as a stand-up comic can serve as a parallel to the idea of communicative risks. He could not learn to get up in front of people and tell jokes without actually getting up in front of people and telling jokes. In other words, he had to place himself in that uncomfortable situation in order to learn how to handle it. Similarly, the stuttering individual who wishes to face down an unpleasant aspect of communication must at some point place him- or herself in circumstances that are personally risky.

Is getting outside the comfort zone, in and of itself, enough?

Let's take Jaik's story about job hunting. He was told that he couldn't have the job because of his stuttering (i.e., a reason out of his control), an obviously hurtful comment that even the interviewer herself realized was insensitive.

Jaik was feeling rejected (mainly because he *was* rejected) after putting himself in an uncomfortable interview situation that did not go well because of stuttering. At that point, how would he have responded to advice that taking risks—for example, stuttering openly in new situations—is a key to success? At the very least, it would be difficult for him to buy into the idea.

The question for the SLP is how to keep the rejected client from retreating back to the safety of avoidance, old speech patterns, or other ineffectual behaviors. Post-interview Jaik could be told that taking risks leads to long term success, but such a declaration would likely sound trite. Besides, he needed a job right then, not at some undefined point in the future.

A more practical solution might be to start expanding his comfort zone a little at a time. He could, for example, practice answering interview questions in therapy, then try mock interviews with strangers, and so on until he was confident meeting an actual employer. For Jaik, jumping into a stressful interview at that stage of his life was akin to putting someone who just told his first joke into the *Stand-Up Britain* final. As you read in the opening chapter, that final was even difficult for a comedian as seasoned as Jaik. Reductions in comfort are rarely easy.

Unfortunately, there are no shortcuts to improving desired skills, be they speech, comedy, or otherwise. Risks are necessary, and so is failure. I am certain that all of the greatest comedians in history have felt the humiliation of a joke unexpectedly falling flat or being bested by a heckler. Not only that, all accomplished businessmen, musicians, educators, athletes, speech-language pathologists, and anyone else can tell you about their failures as well. Many reached their present statuses by continuing in uncomfortable situations until those situations became part of their comfort zones. In other words, they learned and moved on, trading short-term setbacks for long-term success.

Weighing the risks

As noted, no one always takes the riskier option when confronted with choices. To do so would be foolish. But what about situations in which risk is called for, but the protagonist simply loses his or her nerve?

The quick answer is that clients need not beat themselves up for playing it safe now and then. I remember watching a hockey game in which the winning team's goalie was the star. As he was skating off the ice at the conclusion of the game, he was stopped by an interviewer and cameraman. A crowd gathered to watch him speak. He could not have been any more center of the spotlight. He was entering a doorway into the fame that Jaik claimed everyone desires.

Like Jaik, he was a person who stuttered. The difference was that the goalie wanted no part of this type of attention. Almost from the start, one could see him lapse into avoidance behaviors. He gave only short answers, substituted words, rephrased his utterances, changed his pitch, and basically anything else he could do in order not to stutter. And I did not really blame him.

I like to think that I would not have handled the situation better, but I don't really know. What I do know is that there are consequences to playing it safe. Perhaps the goalie knew it too, but determined that in this instance the costs of avoiding were outweighed by the immediate benefits.

There is another aspect to this question of too much risk taking: the client for whom failure affects his or her very livelihood. Over the years, I have heard a half dozen versions of the following story:

> *I have a job where if no one wants to partner with me, I'll be out of work. So I can't let potential partners see any weakness. If they see me stutter, they'll want to partner with someone else. Word will get around.*

First of all, it is important to realize that there are some people who are in positions in which stuttering truly does limit their aspirations. However, it is also true that clients often constrain themselves. They play it safe, making assumptions about policies and attitudes that do not exist. Indeed, a study by Bricker-Katz, Lincoln, and Cumming (2013) suggests that the workplace self-stigma of people who stutter originates from past negative experiences more so than from any actual events that occurred on the job. As self-stigma can lead to reductions in self-esteem (Boyle, 2013) and empowerment (Boyle, 2015) which, in turn, can negatively impact goal achievement, it appears that such fears are potentially very limiting to the stuttering employee.

All of this is not to say that discrimination against stuttering is non-existent. Hurst and Cooper (1983a) found that more than half of employers surveyed would choose a non-stuttering candidate over an equally qualified stuttering one. Still, I am confident stating that most people who stutter are not in positions where their speech affects their ability to make a living. Like Jaik, they can do their jobs and stutter.

Ideas to help clients expand their comfort zones

If we truly believe that the primary goal of stuttering treatment is effective communication in all situations, taking risks will be of utmost importance toward recovery. Again, clients need to shape feared situations into ones that are more comfortable. But how? The types of transfer activities discussed in chapter 6 (home programs, talking to new listeners, etc.) are effective ways to begin widening the zone of comfort. Exactly what is being transferred, however, depends on the client's personal objectives. His or her goals might be to diminish the power stuttering has over everyday life, to stop avoiding, to speak up more in class or at work, to make more friends, to communicate effectively during a job interview, to impress comedy club audiences, or others unique to a given client.

Once a set of goals is in place, the person who stutters needs to determine what risks make sense for him or her. That is, goals can be matched to actions such as:

- contributing more to conversations,

- ordering the difficult-to-say menu item,

- introducing him- or herself to a stranger, or

- offering a comment in a group setting.

Of course, because the goals are individualized, so are the activities. Thus, the list above is only a small sample of potential risks. It is also worth noting that the immediate goals might not be the final goals. Perhaps—taking the last activity as an example—a client could first make a comment to two listeners, then three, and so on, gradually working his or her way to the desired group setting (similar to the job interview preparedness sequence noted earlier).

Again, during the process, clients must understand that mistakes are inevitable and necessary toward achieving meaningful goals. Thus, setbacks should not be discouraging, but instead viewed as part of the process. The key is to learn from temporary failure and then move on to the goal that needs to be accomplished. Just because someone cannot handle an interview for an entry-level position today doesn't mean he won't be making large television audiences laugh tomorrow.

Relationships

With the help of alcohol, Jaik took risks in the pursuit of women. However, risk-taking was less evident once relationships were established. As a young adult, he seemed so intent on finding his one true love that he had difficulty accepting any other result. Even the one time that he broke off the relationship, his regret was almost immediate. Did stuttering play a part in his tendency to cling? Was there, perhaps, a fear that girlfriends would not come along that often and thus he had better latch on to those who did? Given the likelihood that the relationships were more complicated than that (relationships generally are), it could well be an overreach to say so. Still, the realm of interpersonal relationships is one in which stuttering can create barriers. Someone interesting happens along and the stuttering is or is not noticeable. In the latter cases, the individuals who stutter might continue to use avoidance behaviors in order not to drive away a potential partner. There are several possible reasons for this:

- The shame involved with an inability to perform an everyday function such as speaking fluently,

- The person who stutters views his or her stuttering as unattractive[1], or

- Convenience (that is, the stuttering individual simply wants to talk without interruption).

Once a relationship has been established, the significant other presumably has seen and accepted the stuttering. It may even be viewed positively, as a sign of vulnerability or a challenge to overcome. Nevertheless, it can still be a source of conflict. If, for example, the onus of communication falls on the non-stuttering partner and he or she must make all of the telephone calls and handle most public communication, such unbalanced responsibility can lead to resentment (Kendall, 2000), particularly given that partners of those who stutter tend to underestimate the adverse impacts of the dis-

---

1   There is some evidence suggesting that stuttering could detract from perceived attractiveness, at least in the eyes of adolescents (Van Borsel, Brepoels, & De Coene, 2011).

order (Wilder, 2013). That is, they may view stuttering as an inadequate reason for speaking fears.

Resentment can stem from other sources as well. If the stuttering becomes a bigger issue between two people, either because of a change in severity or in the partner's attitude, the partner may resent the imperfect life he or she now has to lead. Kendall (2000) noted that spouses of disabled individuals may actually experience a period of grieving over the loss of their dream lives. And, as with all grieving processes, it might not be pretty. Although uncommon, anger may arise when spouses feel cheated. Depression can also result.

While grieving is a normal process that, hopefully, leads to acceptance (Crowe, 1997), it still needs to be monitored. It is a good idea for partners to be a part of the recovery process (Boberg, 1997). This involves everything from learning about stuttering to helping the client generalize speech modifications, with home programs, support, and numerous other therapeutic aspects in between.

Jaik made no mention of stuttering discussions with girlfriends, so it is difficult to say how accepting they were. Then again, Jaik's overriding negativity at that stage of his life may have served as a barrier to their involvement. Fortunately, he seemed to realize the importance of confronting this lack of self-approval, however difficult that process can be.

Questions for Discussion

How do you differentiate generalized vs. speech-associated attitude differences?

Why do you think older adults report improved speech-associated attitudes in comparison to their young adult years?

Think of an endeavour in which you had to take risks to improve. How easy/difficult was it to do so? Describe the process.

If you were treating an adult client who had just been told that he was not hireable because of his stutter, how would you convince him to take some risks?

Think of a risk you took that backfired. Are you glad you took it anyway? What would you change is you could do it over again?

Can you think of a circumstance in which a speaker really cannot afford to stutter? Explain.

Explain how you as an SLP would guide a client through the process of risk-taking for each of these stuttering issues:

- Excessive avoidance behaviors

- Difficulty meeting people

- Desire to use learned speech techniques in all situations

If you met the love of your life, how anxious would you be to divulge something like stuttering? If that person stuttered, would you want to know about it right away?

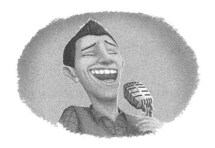

Chapter 9: How I Became a Comedian

As I noted in chapter 7, my negativity in London served as a catalyst to search for local comedy clubs. After watching a show one night, I asked one of the performers, "How does someone become a comedian?"

He answered, "There's a comedy course here starting soon. Call this number."

So I telephoned and, despite my obvious stutter, a man named Michael Knighton pleaded with me to join his class and even made me promise to turn up for the first session. I didn't know it at the time, but joining this course would help me to improve my speech and my life.

Michael Knighton's Course

A month after the phone call, I attended my first comedy class along with five other men and two women, all roughly the same age and level of education. It is said that one gets out of comedy courses what he or she puts into them (apart from the cash, which is non-refundable) and I found Michael's to be exciting and a useful introduction to comedy. I looked forward to it every week.

From the start, however, the stutter was a definite problem.

The first time I went on Michael's stage to tell a joke, I was looking at my feet, noticeably self-conscious as I struggled to get out a single word. Overcoming my fears and insecurities was going to be difficult. Worse yet, I hadn't been in control of my speech since the age of about six. Fortunately, the instructor was up to the challenge.

Michael Knighton had studied acting before performing several hundred stand-up gigs on the London comedy circuit. He therefore approached comedy with an acting bias. Because he was honest, direct, informative, and inspiring, he motivated and brought out people's comedy personas in a positive, calm, and supportive way. It was a fun night out each week, despite knowing that the course would culminate in a "showcase" performance before a proper audience.

Many of the techniques we learnt were based on developing confidence, that same old issue in my life. For a 5, 10, or 20-minute spot, the comedian has to convince the audience that he is funny, even if he is really shy, reserved, and lacking self-esteem (which a surprising number of comedians are). I gradually learnt how to do this, aided by many hours of stage time and, regrettably, by alcohol.

On stage, we were taught to react to anything that happened, such as a glass breaking or someone coughing or sneezing loudly. If an audience member left his or her seat or if a mobile phone rang, we were to make a joke out of it. If someone heckled, we dealt with it. We were also told to mention anything that the audience couldn't miss. For example, if there was a piano on stage, the comedian could walk on and say "Hello, we've got Elton John coming on next!" That isn't a particularly funny line, but it establishes control of the room. The comedian has to be in command.

Therefore, I had to avoid displaying any insecurity in myself or in my material, which was a challenge, considering at the time I could hardly say my own name or write a funny, original joke.

Stand-up comedy was therapeutic in a number of ways. It forced me to cut out the "ums" and "errs", something my speech therapist had also told me to do. I also learnt that using hand gestures and physically expressing myself whilst talking not only helped me to get the words out, but also held people's attention. Finally, pushing my communicative comfort zones, along with the decreased self-consciousness and improved self-control, helped me reduce my stutter. I used to start my act by telling the audience that I had a stutter, an action that relaxed both them and me. Telling my secret to so many strangers also made me less sensitive about having a stutter, which gradually led to improved speech.

Persona

Comics are not born funny. There's a long course to getting there, and it wasn't the one I expected. As Michael told us, "Comedy is 90% persona, 5% material and 5% the (courage) to get on stage and do it." This was bad news to me— *bad*, because I was relatively shy and normally exhibited a narrow and reserved emotional range, and *news*, because I always thought the words were the jokes, and thus I concentrated solely on writing.

Being a comedian obviously requires jokes, but it's more about how they are told. We were taught to deliver the punch lines with confidence (there's that word again) and believe in what we were saying 100%. Otherwise, the audience would lose faith in us and our material. What mattered was not necessarily the substance, but the style. For example, Steve Martin's famous *A Wild and Crazy Guy* tour in 1978 wasn't actually full of the most brilliant or memorable jokes, but he was having such a great time on stage and looked so confident and funny that it didn't really matter. The tour was still a great success.

Top comedians can tell almost any joke and get a laugh. They have a big advantage over unknown comics, in that the audience already knows their reputation and humour, and therefore are primed to laugh. Unfamiliar acts, on the other hand, have to start from scratch every time they step on stage, subtly persuading the audiences to believe in their acts through performance skill, charisma, charm, and quality of material. If a comic shuffles nervously on stage, fiddles with the microphone, and then speaks in a quivering voice, the chances are good that the audience will produce nothing but embarrassing silence. But the comedian who swaggers onto the stage, grabs the microphone as if it is his or her own private property, and tells the same joke in the most confident tone possible will probably get a healthy laugh.

Stand-up comedy, and perhaps even dealing with everyday life, is therefore a bit of a confidence trick. In reality, I am no funnier than the average person; I just learnt how to make the audience believe in me. It was, however, not a skill that came easily. By trial and error, for example, I realized it was not a good idea to apologise if a joke flopped, as this made the audience uneasy and started to destroy whatever faith they had in me as a comedian. I also learnt I could rescue a joke which had flopped with a bit of cheeky self-deprecation, but this only worked if the audience was already with me.

The importance of appearing mentally relaxed and remaining alert were additional lessons learnt, as was showing my personality and vulnerability on stage. If the comedian is tense or uptight, the audience will be too. I also needed to speak more precisely, as the audience had to fully understand the joke in order to laugh. Stuttering on punch lines could ruin everything.

At the time, I was reading Paul McKenna's (2006) book *Instant Confidence* and I realised I needed a more commanding voice. I tried to imagine how my voice would sound if I were totally self-assured. I visualized passionate people I had seen in the media and attempted to match my voice to whatever confident example occupied my mental image. For example, the imagined voice might say, "This is how I sound when I am confident," and I would try to repeat the same phrase out loud many times until I started to feel comfortable using this more confident tone of voice.

On stage, I tried to perform with no expectations about the material, and thought of the audience as old friends (until I got heckled). Another trick was to remember a time when I was talking with good friends, feeling relaxed and at ease, and then transferring that feeling to the stage. But this association did not extend to practicing my material with friends or family. The environment was never the same as a comedy club and they normally didn't laugh, causing me to wonder whether the joke would work in front of an audience.

The relaxed persona could take me only so far, however. I had to learn to balance it with sufficient passion. I found that if I were enthusiastic about what I was saying, the audience responded to it. For example, the following joke did not look like much on paper, but it normally raised a laugh because I delivered it with abundant emotion.

I went speed dating, which was a disaster.

You only have three minutes with each person.

It turned into lots of mini hostage situations!

Everything was linked to keeping the audience's attention because without that, the routine was doomed. If I felt I was losing their interest, I would step forward and accentuate my conversational style with gestures and make sweeping eye contact with everyone in the room. I might also change my vocal pitch or speed of delivery. When I had their attention, I could step back and relax a little.

Another important persona tip was to look at the crowd, and not my feet. The audience needed to be respected and acknowledged, while still being controlled. However, eye contact was something I had generally avoided since the age of six, and so I found this instruction very difficult. And frankly, remembering my next line was easier when looking at my feet. I clearly had to know my script better.

Michael taught us that when the laughter went from 100% to 95%, it was time to start the next joke. This kept the laughs flowing and avoided pauses between the jokes. We were also taught to act larger than life without being arrogant, which was a difficult balance to achieve.

Writing

The setup of a joke, we learned, must be edited to be as concise as possible. It was then important to emphasise the punch line, so that the audience would know when to laugh. Jokes also needed to be rewritten and edited until they were as funny as possible.

The key was to not stop editing when people were simply laughing, as the final tweaks were the ones that turned a great joke into a fantastic one. Often one word, facial expression, or gesture made all the difference. Any "chuckles" in a routine needed to graduate into "laughs" and "laughs" advanced to "big laughs". Material that was confusing to the comic or the audience, or that had become tiresome to say, had to be cut. The key was to keep it simple, and as funny as possible.

In order to write comedy that actually makes people laugh, one must be in touch with his or her own comedy instincts. Therefore, I tried to write material that I found funny. I figured that if I laughed reading it, the audience should too. I also tried to maintain my comic authenticity and originality by not watching too much TV and absorbing any subconscious inspiration it might offer. Keeping my mind different and developing my own unique comic vision was imperative. I only deviated from that philosophy to watch stand-up, as often as I could. This helped me to see the type of material audiences liked and improved my chances of producing usable jokes. It was also good to see how professional comedians worked the room and delivered their material. Once I had analysed why material worked, I tried to come up with jokes using the same mechanics, and then tested them out during open mic nights.

Alcohol

One of Michael's key points was to enjoy being on stage (or at least pretend to).

"The audience is a mirror," he said. "If the comics enjoy themselves, the audience will too; if you smile sincerely, they will smile back."

Michael told us to give the performance a great deal of energy, and to use our own unique styles. I tried to greet the audience positively at the start, such as saying, "How are you all? Are you well?" and then reply, "Jolly Good."

After the greeting, however, I found high energy difficult to muster. Unfortunately, I turned to alcohol for help.

I think the reason anyone drinks is to liven up life. Suddenly everything becomes a mini-adventure and all things seem possible. Horizons are instantly broadened. On stage, alcohol increased my enjoyment. I wasn't perhaps quite as alert, but I still viewed it as a helper. Popular UK comedian, Bob Monkhouse once said, "I never go on alone," and for hundreds of gigs I too brought along my aide. My natural persona was, and still is, fairly sullen, shy, and quiet. A pint of lager improved my mood, made me temporally forget my worries, lowered my anxiety levels, reduced my self-consciousness, and helped my speech. It brought out the extrovert in me, a trait normally in hiding.

I realised that to be good at stand-up comedy, I had to turn my monitor down to zero whilst still being in control. That is, whatever filter prevented me from acting clownish had to be removed. For me, this often required one to two pints of strong lager. No more than that because pre-show was a time to rehearse, rewrite, and exhaustively prepare the material. Besides, I needed to be in command of myself during the routine and not slurring words or forgetting lines (and, of course, I wanted to avoid any of the long-term damage—e.g., liver disease and cancer—associated with drinking).

The need for alcohol beforehand became a big concern for me and even led me to perform less often. As bad as that was, however, the period after the shows may have been even worse. If I had a great gig, sometimes the promoter or audience member bought me a drink to celebrate. If I had a bad gig, I drank to get over it. I got a lot of laughs, but some of the hangovers were horrific.

I tried to do gigs without alcohol, but my own perception was that I wasn't as funny. My naturally self-conscious, shy, and nervous persona came out on stage, which in comedy terms was disastrous. What concerned me most was ruining paying gigs. When comedians do that, promoters won't ask them back as paid acts. Considering how many years it takes to get those shows in the first place, going back to solely unpaid gigs would essentially amount to starting over.

Eventually, the drinking moved beyond performance nights. I didn't go out drinking (much) when I was not doing a show, but amidst the hustle and bustle of London, finding work, women not returning any calls, and all the other life stressors, I began to view alcohol as my true, and sometimes only, friend, one I turned to whenever I needed a boost.

There is a stereotype of the "depressed alcoholic comedian" and I guess I fitted that profile. Whenever I had a drink, it felt like a sort of chemical equation inside my head was completed. The real me functioned more happily with alcohol, but without it I was a depressed, sad, old soul. In fact, one date I went on ended with the woman saying, "I think you are the most miserable man I have ever met."

Cigarettes were another friend I made to help deal with the stress and anxiety. By the time I started smoking, I felt I was unduly relying on vices to please audiences. After a while, I used up so much positive energy trying to make people laugh that the only way to recuperate was a quiet week or two on a beach in the Canary Islands.

243

Nerve Control

There are many variables with stand-up. It's a high-octane experience and a medium so volatile that it is impossible to walk off stage
not having learnt something. But the stresses involved are constant
and unhealthy, as it takes a long time to get noticed and even longer
to make any money. If I didn't have a stutter, I don't think I would
have bothered with it.

However one reduces stress, it is important not to go too far. A bit
of nerves is good. It produces the adrenaline that drives the routine.
The problem is when nerves cross over to fear. Fear and comedy
don't mix and audiences can smell fear a mile away. They will not
believe that a frightened comic has the power to make them laugh.

I found that practice was the key to controlling my nerves. The more
I practised, the less nervous I was the next time I performed that
material. I learnt and practised my set as much as I could, often
whilst out walking or jogging. Ideally, I got to know my material so
well that I was sick of saying it. Or, as Jerry Seinfeld put it, I would
have been able to say it if I parachuted from a plane. I would aim
to practice it five times a day, then 3 to 4 times quickly on the day
just before the performance, and relax as much as possible on the
day of the gig. If I had any free time, I was normally practicing the
set. There was a potential problem with this schedule, namely the
potential to over-practise the lines (rather than writing better, newer
quality material), but I did know my routines well.

Once I knew I had a good set, the nerves diminished. The practice
also helped to improve my speech. Having a script meant that I
didn't need to think about what I was going to say, so I stuttered
less.

Keeping still on stage, speaking slowly, breathing deeply, expressing myself when I was talking and being "in the situation" helped me both on and off stage.

I tried to arrive and check into gigs on time and practice walking on stage and taking the microphone out of the stand, to be certain I did so correctly at the start of the routine. I didn't want to be fumbling about with the mic, looking lost and out of control. I also tried to chat with the promoter and the other acts, which normally calmed me down a bit.

Unless the comedian throws up on stage, most people can't spot how nervous he or she is. Part of my daily schedule was finding ways of alleviating my anxiety, such as jogging or seeing friends or eating healthily. Slowing down my delivery and speaking carefully helped me to disguise my nerves and be understood. The use of pauses also gave the audience time to laugh. I also used a vibrating watch, which told me exactly when to get off stage, as it was not a good idea to overrun. Effective time management also helped reduce the stress.

Pressure

Comedy is a pressure game and even for the most stage-loving individual, a degree of stress is part of the job and hard to avoid completely. With each rung up the comedy ladder, the pressure increases. I experienced stress from a young age (see chapter 3) and that perhaps worked to my advantage, as I don't remember feeling all that nervous, even in front of large audiences. I'm sure that if I had not had the father I did, stand-up comedy would have been too much for me. Maybe his upbringing was designed to teach me how to deal with pressure. If that was the rationale, it eventually backfired. In any case, for me, talking to a room of 100 people was less pressurised and stressful than a one-on-one chat with my father. Perhaps real pressure is sitting in a noisy office, trying to concentrate and having to do complicated data analysis to a set deadline.

Being able to control the audience reduces the pressure in a comedy club. If a young comic asked me for advice on how to accomplish that, I would say, "It starts from the moment you walk on stage: Acknowledge everyone as you walk on and look people in the eye. Know which parts of the audience are not responding too well, and try to get laughs from them too. You must also believe that you can cope with the gig every time you walk on stage, and that hecklers will be no problem. If you think you can't do the gig, you will probably have a bad performance. If you walk off to cheers every time, then the promoter will have you back again, but accepting that one gig a month will be bad is also part of reducing the overall pressure. Professional comics can never be flawlessly funny time after time, but they do their best, which is normally good enough."

Stuttering on Stage

It should be evident by now that, even without a stutter, comedy is a nerve-wracking process. But the angst increases exponentially when there is uncertainty about talking.

It's interesting: Part of stuttering is the constant dread of becoming stuck on a word and essentially exposed as being different. Up until that point in my life, I had tried to hide my stutter, as I was so embarrassed by it. It's not like being in a wheelchair or holding a white stick, where something is obviously atypical. Stuttering is a hidden impediment until it's time to speak. As such, it takes audiences by surprise. On nights I thought I was going to be word perfect (not often), I didn't reference my stutter. To do so confused the audience and a confused audience is a resentful one. I used to make a joke about doing a comedy routine at the British Stammering Association conference and speaking too fluently, which was a mistake as everybody thought I was mocking them with my stuttering jokes.

But when I did stutter, I had to mention it and laugh at myself. Doing so relaxed the audience, and also helped me become more desensitized to my speech. Of course, addressing it necessitated having stuttering comedy material. In that regard, I had to be careful. Since about 2007, I felt that audiences have become more "politically correct" and so have laughed less at disability-related jokes. In fact, some comedy promoters warned me that doing a whole routine about stuttering wouldn't work, and I agree with that. I had to move away from just doing stuttering material. The highly respected UK comedian Daniel Kitson, for example, did quite a bit of material about his stutter when he first started, and then moved on to more diverse subjects. In the end, audiences appreciated him for his versatility of material.

The comedian Jerry Sadowitz once said to me "The more you can cheat the stuttering, the better. But you must keep control of it." Useful advice perhaps, but I didn't want to be known as a comedian who puts on a stutter to get laughs, an impression already held by some audiences. Alternatively, there were times I spoke too fluently, which also made people wonder why I was making jokes about stuttering at all. On those occasions, I tried to make sure I worked in some voluntary stuttering. Sometimes, however, the more I tried to stutter, the less it actually occurred!

Michael hypothesized that the day I didn't have to wonder whether I was going to stutter was the day when it would disappear. He also said, "Talk about the stutter until it goes away." Unfortunately, stuttering isn't quite as simple as that and besides, there were benefits. Although I didn't want to become known as "that comic with a stutter" (my aim, after all, was to reduce my stuttering), there is no denying that it was a unique selling point, something that made me stand out from the crowd. It certainly made some of my initial performances distinctive, and audiences' attitudes to it were normally very accepting, tolerant, and respectful. Moreover, I was turning a life-long negative into a positive.

When I first tried to write some stuttering material, I found the process difficult and frustrating, mainly because I couldn't construct a funny and original joke. I tried to follow my instincts about what I thought was funny, to wit:

> *I made a mockery of my school's tough anti-drug policy called "Just Say No". I was told to "just say something."*

> *I tried to get married last year, but by the time I said "I d-d-d-do", my wife was already filing for divorce.*

From there I moved to short stories, which gained more laughs. They sounded original and real, although I normally exaggerated the experiences for funnier punch lines.

> *I was stopped by the police last week. He said, "You've got the right to remain silent."*

> *I said, (pause) "That sh-shouldn't be a problem."*

> *No seriously, he asked me what my name was, what my address was, and where I was going.*

> *F-F- Fifteen minutes later, he charged me with wast-*
> *ing police time.*

I tried to avoid telling the same type of stuttering joke (for exam-ple, following this line with another joke about taking a long time to speak). I didn't want the audience to find me repetitive, even if my speech was.

Of course, there is a fine line between making a joke about stutter-ing and simply mocking a speech impediment. As someone who stutters, I could be light-hearted about it, but I didn't want to confuse the audience. I needed to convey my material without stuttering too much or too little, a task that required me to be totally alert and well-practised.

Mental Imagery

Michael advised us to regularly picture the best, most enjoyable routine of our lives taking place in the very club in which we would perform (particularly for the big gigs). Even seeing the venue be-fore the gig was advised in order to calm the nerves and aid "pre-gig confidence." The idea was that thinking of the ideal performance— complete with the desired experiences of confidence, laughter, and enjoyment—would help turn the hypothetical into reality. Apparently when David Beckham (or any other top striker) attempts to score a goal, he is focused only on the ball going into the back of that net. As comedians, we were to picture our routines going very well without worrying about cameras, the audience, other comics, or the promoter standing at the back.

Onstage, we were taught to enjoy each gig more than any other we had ever done. Michael felt that the best performers are often the ones who enjoy themselves the most. At the same time, however, it was important to keep to the prepared set. The moment I started to improvise, I usually lost confidence on stage, and the audience noticed this. My experience is typical. Even UK acts such as Eddie Izzard or Ross Noble, who seem to be improvising constantly, are in reality doing highly scripted and learnt material.

Michael also taught us not to change too much of our material in the last two weeks before a big gig or a competition, as we wouldn't be 100% confident with it. We could make one or two new tweaks, but the aim was to look self-assured and comfortable on stage. The comedian has less than a minute to make the audience laugh (ideally, this is done within 15 seconds), so at the start it is very important to use a lot of quick, easily comprehendible, funny gags. Mentally, one must be 100% settled in before going on stage. Life's anxieties have to wait. "Sorry, I'm not feeling very well," even if true, will not be appreciated by the audience. Better they later think, "Wow, he was good and he had a sore throat".

Social Control

I believe that many people are trapped inside comfort zones and social controls, which can govern our lives and influence how we speak. At work we think, "I'd better not say that in front of my manager" or at home it's, "I'd better act like that in front of my father-in-law" and it sets up potential pressure and stress, which in my case increases the likelihood of stuttering. To stay with my latter example, the first time I met my potential father-in-law I was a stuttering wreck!

Humans are generally more comfortable blending in than they are suffering the consequences of being different. The part of me that is always trying to be polite and say the right thing is the easiest persona to be, but also the least funny and most unsure. As a student, I had been fairly introverted, for fear of being kicked off my course or my friends thinking I was too over-the-top. Entering the work force was another emotionally controlled experience for me, trying to get on with new people and to fit in the room by being appropriately reserved, rather than risk losing my job or obtaining a poor reference.

When I first told jokes on stage, I was restricted and inhibited, employing the same social behaviours as everywhere else. Comedy club audiences, however, needed to see the part of me that took risks, moved emotions, and said unspoken or socially awkward thoughts. I had to learn to play the fool, to be flippant and inappropriate. I had to reconsider my take on various subjects and move to a new, more maverick level in order to get laughs. In a way, letting go of my social controls helped me let go of my stutter a little, in that I became less concerned with pleasing people and always trying to fit in. On the comedy stage, one can be celebrated for not fitting in, as longas the audience is laughing. It was a refreshing change.

As the months on stage rolled by, fuelled by alcohol and my competitive desire to get more laughs, I realised that I could have a bolder persona than I previously thought possible. I began to exaggerate my responses because doing so got bigger laughs. For example, I found that playing with extreme actions and attitudes, such as shouting at hecklers, making silly facial expressions, and generally acting in an unrestrained manner was not only funnier, but also very liberating. Some of my best gigs were when I had been in a confined office all day, and then let loose in front of an audience where, for 10 or 20 minutes, I became a free speaking and uninhibited being. The moment I learnt to do this, I was on the way to better stand-up. But I was on another path as well: one toward desensitisation and better communication.

Being reserved and shy were no longer positive traits. By exaggerating my emotions and showing my personality, I was releasing all those feelings kept hidden by my stutter. I was communicating effectively whether I was fluent or not. For the first time in my life, I was thinking, "Maybe I'm not such a quiet, unconfident, and reserved person after all." The anger and frustration that my stutter had created became a driving force for my comedy and an engine for my creativity. Had I simply stayed confined to my controlled office environment, leaving only to watch spirit-crushing TV shows in the evenings or to hang out with friends who quite rightly had their own ambitions and agendas, my stutter may never have improved.

Loosening the social controls also helped me to think faster and discover more entertaining ways of talking about a variety of subjects. For example, my original material about relationships was quite reserved. But then I decided to approach relationships using a more self-deprecating angle, but making sure it wasn't too negative. My tragedy became comedy, so I learnt not to be shy about how I was feeling inside and try to speak from the heart, for example:

> My last girlfriend said that because of my stutter I embarrassed her at parties.
>
> "P-P-People just laughed at us."
>
> I said "Yes, b-b-but you are seventy three."

I felt that I also became more engaging off stage. Replacing my self-consciousness with smiles and an easy-going manner relaxed listeners. Conversations became more comfortable. For the first time in my life, I believed in myself and began to understand who I was. Additionally, I stuttered less.

Robbie Pointer Advice

In 2001, club promoter Robbie Pointer told me that I performed a relaxed and well played routine, one on par with the closing act. He had positive things to say about my material and asserted that I made "good use" of my stutter. He then offered me some useful feedback and advice as to how to improve my act, which I also noted down and kept. Some of his suggestions were:

- Earn every single laugh.

- Be wary of tough gigs.

- Quicker material will get more laughs.

- Mention the stutter early to relax the audience.

- Take your time.

- Maintain a good persona.

- Make the opening words fit how you come on stage (i.e. be nice to yourself and to the audience).

- Do less self-deprecating material. The audience doesn't want to feel sorry for you.

- Every word needs to be chilled.

- What you say has to make sense to the audience.

- They need the joke immediately. Do not waffle.

- Get to the point as soon as possible. Be very concise.

- Personality is very important. Stand-up is less about material, more about personality.

- Learn to deal with the drunk 1 a.m. crowd.

- Mention the stutter as soon as you stutter.

- Show people that you are having a good time.

- Do not laugh too much at your own jokes, especially if the crowd isn't laughing with you.

- Don't lose your power on stage.

Amused Moose Course – 2002

After Michael's course, I joined an advanced comedy course in London. This class was run by the "Amused Moose" and met for weekly 3-plus hour sessions for three months. It was mainly taught by Logan Murray, who had been a comedian for two decades, having performed in many venues and written for both TV and radio. He had also appeared in variety shows, sit-coms, documentaries, panel programs, and game shows. His courses are still highly regarded in the UK, where he is acknowledged as one of the best comedy tutors. Martin Beaumont, another fine comedian, helped Logan out during the course.

On a basic level, many of the points covered in this course matched what I had learnt from Michael. In some areas, however, it went deeper. For example, Martin explained that comedy is a "can do" business. That is, you must believe that you *can do* the gig; otherwise it will not go well. When an Olympic sprinter kneels down on the starting blocks, he intends to win. If he instead fears failure, he will have no chance. Similarly, I had to get rid of any negativity by reminding myself every time I walked on that stage that I *could do* this. Failure was not an option.

Logan told me that one of the main advantages of performing with a stutter was that it made the audience warm to and like me, as well as probably remember me. He felt that comics needed to be charismatic, have pathos, and sound honest, and having a stutter made these traits easier to access.

My persona in 2002 was a stuttering, shy, endearing, and slightly confused character, who talked about having a stutter and life's other complexities. My mind, like my speech, sometimes seemed to work in starts and stops, so this persona worked well for me. It provided me with a funny delivery that kept the audience engaged. As such, it was the most positive and upbeat part of my personality. Most comedians have a comic flaw which they can tap into, and mine was not being able to speak very well. The trouble was that I had to present this flaw positively, which was not easy, given how complicated it made my life.

A persona also needs dedication. A comedian is selling an idea to an audience and needs to be totally committed to that idea for it to work. I was taught to celebrate each joke as though it was the best one ever told. I also had to make thoughts sound playful, not laboured and tired. The problem with the filter of critical thinking I had learnt from university was that there were times I would read my material and think, "That is terrible," leading to a fall in the commitment level. If this fall was reflected in how I said the joke on stage, the audience would not laugh.

Most people, if pushed, can probably walk on a stage and tell a joke. But having fun up there is far more difficult. I had to access the part of myself that enjoyed playing around and being a fool, because that generated laughs and made the audience feel relaxed.

It had to start from the moment I walked on stage. Achieving this level of enjoyment was based largely on preparation, focusing on my own persona, and being able to read the audience. Once I had my own style, it was just a matter of communication. I would shake the hand of the compere as I walked on stage and ask the audience to give him or her a round of applause, as this made me look warm and generous and got the crowd clapping (the hope being they were more likely to do so during my act). I also tried to be open and spontaneous with the audience, and not simply recite my material and walk off. The act had to be more than jokes to look professional.

There's no feeling as good as a gig going well, but conversely, there's no feeling as bad as one bombing. Failing on stage is not fun, and something I tried to avoid at all costs. It may be as close to going down with all guns blazing as most of us ever get.

Writing

We also covered new (to me) writing techniques. One of these consisted of writing down something we wanted, something we'd settle for, and something we get. For example:

> *"I want to speak perfectly, I'd settle for speaking with a slight stutter, I get to have to ask my friend to order me a curry on a Friday night."*

Or

"I want to film five action movies with Universal Studios. I'd settle for being a presenter on a shopping channel. I get to tell a room of five people in pub about being hopeless with women."

A list of all the statements I never want to hear could also lead to some funny ideas.

- *"Sorry, Sir, you're in the wrong queue. The rear of the queue you want is back there."*

- *"You know how you said to me that you never wanted children…?"*

In time, I learned that an audience normally laughed at a joke if they could easily relate to the situation, but are then taken someplace bizarre.

"Absurd logic" was therefore the basis of some of the material I wrote. For example, one joke I used was:

I was at the airport and I had packed a bomber jacket.

The security guard said, "What's in the bag?"

I got stuck. I said: "It's a bomb, it's a bomb, it's a b-b-bomb, it's a bomber jacket."

I continued to avoid improvisation, but reached a point where I could get memorable reactions on those rare occasions I went off script. For example, I had a joke about checking into the airport and stuttering.

I delivered the set up line as, "I was asked at the check-in desk, 'Have you p-p-packed your bags yourself?'" Rather than allowing the disfluency to ruin the joke, I ad-libbed, "Sorry, she didn't have a stutter" and got a big laugh.

We were told that ninety percent of general comedy writing will not be useable, but is necessary to do in order to dig out the 10% that's gold. I found that the routine's first five minutes were reasonably easy to write, the second five minutes more difficult, the third five minutes very difficult, and the final five minutes impossible! We were told to be truthful with our writing and stage persona. Amidst the wash of media and political information people are fed every day, they like to hear the truth with comedy.

One problem I found is that life just isn't that funny. Most of us wake up, go to work, tolerate our day, come back home to our friends, families, or loved ones, try not to upset anyone, have a meal, and go to bed. Humorous material is not that prevalent. So I tried to look within myself and my previous life experiences and write from the heart. But if I channelled my emotional problems into a piece of highly personal material and it died on stage, it felt as if no one cared about my innermost thoughts.

On the other hand, if the same material got a great response, I then felt the need to keep dredging up those emotions at every gig, which can be quite painful!

Another issue was my insecurity, as I had a bad habit of distancing myself from self-deprecating gags, keen to let the audience know that the story never really happened, for fear they might think less of me. Unfortunately, doing this demolished any sort of flow or rapport that would convince the audience of my abilities as a comedian. For example, I used to make jokes about being hopeless with women, and then say, "Ladies, of course that's not true," which defeats the object of saying the joke in the first place.

Overall, comedy became the outlet for anything that was wrong or annoying in my life, such as failed relationships or my stutter. It was like a composter, breaking down emotional waste and turning it into something useful. If I started to notice that comedy itself was dragging me down, then I tried to step back and change my perspective (i.e. learn to enjoy it more).

Stuttering on TV

As with Michael Knighton's training, the Amused Moose course also ended in a showcase evening. This one was seen by a producer interested in creating a TV idea based on my act and persona. I was somewhat surprised by this, as I didn't think producers were on the lookout for stutterers. I assumed they needed people who can speak fairly precisely, due to the short attention span of viewers and the need to avoid any "dead air" that causes people to switch channels. After all, there are currently few TV celebrities who stutter.

Like many stand-up comedians, I was interested in performing on television. Finding something that a producer liked, however, required more than interest. I spent many, many hours brainstorming ideas.

One concept we discussed was to use me as a kind of stuttering reporter role, as an insert into an existing comedy programme. A bit like the "Stuttering John" personality on the Howard Stern show, who asked celebrities rude, impertinent questions. The ideas considered (but unfortunately never accepted) included the following:

- I could interview a famous celebrity or politician and ask some borderline offensive questions. The person would have to keep a straight face whilst I stuttered. If I were culturally or socially clueless but overtly disabled, the interview subject would have to be kinder to me than he or she is to the typical interviewer.

- Alternatively, this persona could participate in a crowded press conference. I could use a loud, ranting voice (much like my father, in fact).

- Along the same lines, I could interview a blind politician, with my deaf comedian friend (Steve Day). Steve would ask the question, but couldn't hear the reply. I could hear the reply, but couldn't tell Steve what it was. The blind politician couldn't see what was going on as I looked at Steve in bewilderment. If done correctly, this skit could show all three disabilities in a positive light.

- Strange nervous mannerisms could develop during interviews. For example, when talking to a politician, I'd suddenly say, "Shhhhh." The politician would likely respond with something like, "I'm sorry, do you want me to be quiet?" I would answer, "No, sorry, it's just a nervous mannerism. Please continue. Shhhhh."

- Serious interviews with famous people who stutter (e.g., Rowan Atkinson, Nicholas Parsons) could help demonstrate how stuttering can be a spur to success.

- Outdoor reporting in cold, wintry locations would increase the tremors in my speech to comic effect. (I was getting a bit desperate with this one!).

We also moved beyond the reporter characters and considered additional ideas:

- I could be filmed with a hidden camera testing people's patience with my stutter while buying train tickets, asking directions, and speaking to policemen, among other situations.

- Hidden cameras could be used to film reactions as I answered want ads for an auctioneer, bingo caller, or race track commentator.

- A regular "topical stutter rant section" could outline heretofore unknown predicaments associated with stuttering, such as:

Having a stutter makes you very critical of yourself, as well as making you critical of everyone around you. For example, I organise old school reunions and then don't show up. If everyone from back then is in one place, I know I won't bump into any of them when I'm out!

My main priority was to make sure that stuttering was put in a positive light, so as not to offend other stutterers who may be watching and to avoid letters of complaint from the general public. The main aims of the sketches/interviews were therefore to:

1) Lighten the negativity associated with stuttering in today's society.
2) Educate more people/increase public understanding about stuttering by showing what it means to have a stutter.
3) Provide hope to other people who stutter who may be watching.
4) Show that people with stutters must be respected in today's society.

Condensed into one thought, what I'd like to be saying is that a stutter shouldn't stop anyone from doing what he or she wants to do (even becoming a comedian), which surely is an encouraging message. Part of the reason these ideas didn't get used was because it was difficult to hold stuttering in a positive light. I didn't want people simply to tune in and laugh at someone with a speech impediment, and neither did the producers.

Other Parts of the Business

Booking gigs

To obtain a spot at an "open mike" comedy club, a would-be comic has to find a club's number from the Internet or in the *TimeOut* magazine comedy listings, and then confidently ring up, selling himself as a reasonably experienced comic looking for an unpaid 5 to 10-minute open spot. I invariably stuttered doing this, but I think this probably helped me to get spots, as the promoters were likely taken by surprise that someone with a stutter would want to be a comedian. They were probably interested to see what would happen if they put me on stage.

In terms of finding an agent, a Catch-22 applies: You can't become a star without an agent and you can't get an agent unless you're a star. As a new comedian, then, I had to book my own gigs. I therefore quickly had to resolve my fear of the phone if I ever wanted to develop my act in front of live audiences. Unfortunately, speaking to promoters on the phone or leaving voicemails on their mobiles was often a total disaster, sometimes hearing the end beep before I had finished saying my name. On the plus side, a stuttering voicemail message was probably more memorable than the standard "Hello, can I have a gig message" that promoters must receive several times a day. One promoter used to joke that he would phone me up to book a gig and pray it would go onto my voicemail because it was too expensive for him to speak to me.

Overall though, I realised that I had to sound confident when phoning up promoters, especially to obtain paid work. Once again, being shy, reclusive, and stuttering was of no advantage, so I had to force myself to improve my telephone manner.

Dealing with hecklers

At open mic nights, there was normally very little heckling. If people tried, the MC usually told them not to butt in or simply asked them to leave. At bigger gigs, however, hecklers were more part of the show and therefore nerve wracking. I soon realised that they could collapse an entire routine if not dealt with correctly, swiftly, and confidently. Michael Knighton said that dealing with a heckler was a matter of not showing fear and remaining in control of the situation. Of course, a stutter doesn't exactly help with that.

To make the heckler feel uncomfortable, I was taught to put all of my focus on them, and say something such as, "Where are you, you coy heckler, you!" Or "Right, I see you. In that slightly offensive coloured shirt." Any unacceptable comment had to be dealt with. Even if someone quietly muttered "This is terrible" I would pick up on the comment and deal with it. Ignored, it could unbalance the rest of the performance, as the audience could lose faith in my ability to control the room. Therefore, I practiced and learnt put down lines until I could say them with as much confidence as possible. Most of these lines are not appropriate for a textbook, but some of the cleaner examples included:

- "Can you say that in English? I'm sorry I don't speak drunk. Actually I just d-d-don't speak."

- "I'm sorry?" (The heckler repeats his line.) "I heard what you said, I'm just sorry."

- "Look, I get paid to look an idiot. You're doing it for free!"

- "Look the purpose of a heckler is to make m-m-me look like an idiot, so well done, you've completely succeeded."

Comedians have to be careful not to be excessively rude to hecklers and accidently turn the whole audience against themselves. They cannot overact to provocation or become angry. It's all about maintaining control of the room. Another key is to maintain more power than the heckler. For this reason, I was taught to never, ever give the heckler the microphone, as to do so would take away my power. It helps to be speaking louder than the heckler!

Having a tight material-based routine was almost a necessity for me, as I didn't want to allow hecklers in. Because of my stutter, I worried that I couldn't deal with them confidently. Hence, I concentrated on the material and did not encourage hecklers, unlike some of the comedians who seemed to enjoy them.

Compering

I never did much compering (i.e. hosting), but it's a good way to try out new material, as it doesn't really matter if it bombs. After all, the compere is not specifically there to make the audience laugh, but, rather, to hold the night together and bring on the acts. But it's not an easy job. The journey from a cold and quiet room to a warm, laughter-filled one can be long, and the compere leads the way.

The responsibility to control the proceedings may involve telling the audience to keep quiet or to turn off their mobile phones. The host must also address comedians overrunning their time on stage. One has to communicate effectively, something it never hurts to practice.

Conclusion

In this chapter, I have tried to show how difficult it is to become a comedian, let alone make any money out of it. It's not a typical 9-5 job. Rewards are potentially few, and complications many. It impacts not only relationships with people, but quite likely also general health, social life, and mental well-being. Sometimes if there is payment involved, promoters can wait weeks or even months before getting around to sending the check (if they remember at all). There are many, many comedians and not that many paid gigs. It was probably easier in the 1980's/90's as there were fewer people wanting to be comedians and more opportunities, as TV channels were on the lookout for new talent.

Today, 5 to 10 years is seen as the average time it can take to start getting regular paid work. Frank Skinner, a successful UK comedian, once said that it takes "ten years to be any good" which seems about right. The comedy circuit can be a cruel and unrewarding place. Progression up the career ladder is more difficult now than it ever was. The bigger clubs don't really need more comics as they can repeatedly book the established acts. The smaller clubs can pay what they like, as there's potentially another performer who will gladly do the spot for free (and is probably no less funny). In addition, fewer people are venturing out to comedy clubs due to the downturn in the economy, an increase in home entertainment systems, and the ease with which entertainment can be downloaded off the Internet. All of this prevents newcomers from easily being noticed. It is important to stay focused on being funny, writing quality material, getting gigs, and networking. Comedy in the UK always needs fresh material. What it's not crying out for, unfortunately, is someone with a pronounced speech impediment.

Questions for Discussion

Jaik writes of a "confidence trick" in which poise and self-assurance keep listeners from focusing on the speaker's miscalculations. Is there an application of this "trick" to stuttering therapy?

Do you believe mental imagery could work to transfer stuttering treatment skills? Why or why not?

Were you surprised when Jaik stated that if he didn't stutter, he would not have pursued comedy? What do you think he meant by that?

When practicing his comedy routines, Jaik found that he stuttered less when he "didn't need to think about" what he was going to say. Would you expect the same phenomenon to occur with the use of therapeutic techniques? Explain your answer.

Jaik experiences more pressure talking to his father or trying to work in a noisy office than he does telling jokes to large crowds. What does this say about the individualism of stuttering?

How would you explain the statement, "the more I tried to stutter, the less it actually occurred"?

Why was it important that Jaik's audiences know that he stutters when he's telling stuttering-related jokes?

Jaik writes that "letting go of my social controls helped me let go of my stutter." Is there a clinical application to this? How about when he later wrote that changing his routine led to improved speech? Explain your answers.

Do you believe Jaik's love of performing to captive audiences is related to growing up with a stutter? Why or why not?

Do you believe Jaik's more confident persona helped his communication? If so, how?

A producer told Jaik that he made "good use" of stuttering. What do you think that means?

In comedy, failure has a high cost, but the potential rewards are so great that the risk of failure is taken. Do you believe a lifetime of stuttering helped or hurt Jaik in his pursuit of comedy rewards? Explain your answer.

When discussing television show ideas with a producer, Jaik's "main priority was to make sure that stuttering was put in a positive light." Which of the listed ideas accomplish that?

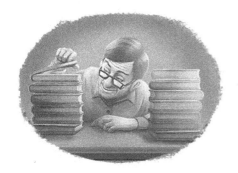

Chapter 10: Listeners, Humor, Jobs, and Advantages of Stuttering

Jaik chose to seek his fortune via stand-up comedy. I ask the reader to think about the courage needed to attend a comedy course—performing original and novice material for judgmental listeners, all the while knowing that a real audience is in the very near future. Now to that mental image add a stutter. When one considers how stuttering can lead to avoidance of speech and, not incidentally, of life, Jaik's story is quite remarkable. In telling it, several themes emerged which require further examination. One of these is listener reactions.

Listeners

Jaik writes of a "confidence trick," in explaining how audience reactions differ based on the attitude of the comedian. That is, the nervous and unsure comic gets heckles while the one who "swaggers onto the stage" and practically dares his or her listeners not to laugh gets the desired reactions. This contrast may have an application to stuttering therapy. Although there is little research literature on confidence and stuttering, clinical reports and support group discussions have provided me with a recurring theme related to this so-called trick. Many clients report a decrease in teasing post-therapy, regardless of whether fluency improves. It seems possible that when clients become desensitized to listener reactions, they present themselves differently, perhaps reflecting less vulnerability and greater speech confidence. As a result, listener reactions change for the better. In a sense, they are swaggering onto a metaphorical stage to the desired effect.

(It is also worth noting that the biggest change might actually be in the *perception* of basic listener reactions [Kuster, J. personal correspondence]. For example, whereas in the past blank stares might have been interpreted by the stuttering speaker as, "Oh no! I just made a horrible impression!" now they are viewed as, "She's thinking carefully about what I just said.")

Although confidence is important to comedians, it has limits. Jaik writes, "We were also taught to act larger than life without being arrogant, which was a difficult balance to achieve." That may be true of comedy, but I believe avoiding arrogance is less important for stuttering individuals dealing with listeners. While common courtesy should not be relinquished, the truly desensitized client places relatively more value on what he or she has to say and less on what listeners might think. Doing so not only improves speech-associated attitudes, but can also make stuttering easier to manage (Plexico, Manning & DiLollo, 2005). In this sense, a certain amount of arrogance can be beneficial.

One of the listener reactions that concerned Jaik was the thought that he was feigning a stutter for laughs. Strangely, this is a perception reported commonly by comedians who stutter (Williams, G, & Campbell, 2015). I use the word *strangely* because of an experience that seemed to indicate to me that listeners can tell the difference between disordered speech and mocking. I routinely direct graduate students to pseudo-stutter with strangers. Some worry that they will end up talking to listeners who stutter. In such an unlikely event, they believe, the listener will think that he or she is being ridiculed. When I brought this concern to a support group meeting, however, there was universal agreement that derision is pretty easy to identify (and thus the students could rest easy). Perhaps the contrast is easier to spot for those who stutter than it is within general audiences.

In addition to instilling some overt confidence, comedy also gave Jaik a lesson in language pragmatics. To regain the attention of the audience, he would "step forward and accentuate (his) conversational style with gestures" or change his "vocal pitch or speed of delivery." In other words, the ways in which language was used—not just the words themselves—impacted the effectiveness of communication.

Pragmatics came into play off stage as well. Interpersonal dynamics became less stressful via the use of smiles, gestures, and "physically expressing" himself. Not only did Jaik report greater self-assurance and increased control over communication situations, but also more fluency (see chapter 6 for a more detailed description of how changes in language pragmatics can impact the speech of people who stutter).

Another listener issue mentioned in the story is relatively minor, but nevertheless worthy of comment: the obvious difficulty with stuttering on punch lines. On an occasion when I had the good fortune to speak to Dr. Frederick Murray, one of the forefathers in the study of fluency disorders, I wondered aloud how realistic it is to expect clients to stop using secondary behaviors altogether. After all, I haven't stopped completely myself. Dr. Murray admitted that he has not either (which made me feel better about my own slips). Some of the difficult situations we discussed included occasions when words needed to be uttered rapidly, talking to people who are quick to interrupt, and, yes, ruining the punch line of a joke. Silly reasons for avoidance perhaps, but reasons nonetheless. Sometimes the monster is tamed but not broken. As noted in chapter 6, clients are taught that they eventually have to pay for the secondary behaviors they use. Nevertheless, we sometimes choose that option.

Treatment Applications

In keeping with the subject of stuttering clients, there were numerous other treatment-related experiences in Jaik's tale. For example, teaching himself to speak in a passionate and self-assured voice required much desensitization. Once he had the desired model in his head, he practiced until he became comfortable with it. It is much the same with clients learning fluency or speech modification techniques. Knowing the methods is not the same as habituation. One has to move past the idea that the new speech is foreign and uncomfortable.

In discussing this generalization process, Jaik noted that "practice was the key...The more I practised, the less nervous I was the next time I performed that material." Similarly, with stuttering clients, we ask them to complete home practice not only to habituate therapeutic skills, but to transfer them to real world situations.

One item that helped Jaik to communicate with audiences—eye contact—requires some explanation. Some people—SLPs and stuttering clients included—confuse everyday eye contact with staring. Normal conversational eye contact is occasional, enough to regard, to let the speaker know that he or she is being acknowledged

(Cummins, 2012; Miller & Sammons, 1999). Unwavering stares are less engaging than they are creepy.

Two treatment-related items discussed in previous chapters were experienced during Jaik's climb up the comedy ladder. On stage, he found advertising his stutter to be both liberating and empowering. Similarly, he discovered that "the more I tried to stutter, the less it actually occurred," another way of saying that once he gave himself permission to stutter, the less power it had over him.

He also stated, "...I didn't need to think about what I was going to say, so I stuttered less." This thought is consistent with some therapy experiences in which people focus less on controlling speech than on communicating naturally (e.g., Dahm, 2015). That is, clients are freed from their tendencies to exert more control over all elements of speech whenever it breaks down, and instead practice behaviors that allow speech to flow more naturally.

Finally, there was one strategy mentioned that might appear to be applicable to therapy, but probably is not. On stage, Jaik was successfully able to recreate feelings of relaxation and ease by thinking about conversations with good friends. In my experience, this type of transference is difficult for stuttering clients to accomplish. The reason for this difficulty might lie in the neurological mechanisms of speech. Within the human brain lie literally hundreds of neural sites and generators involved in language production. Which ones are involved in a given speech sample depends on the circumstances surrounding it—the phrasing, emotions, body activity, and numerous others (Webster, 1999). In other words, speech may be neurologically different enough from one setting to another that recreating the same motor patterns across situations is challenging. It is akin to the difference between making a free throw when playing around with friends in an empty gym vs. doing so during a game with an arena full of people watching. Perhaps conveyance of moods works better with comedy because it is scripted. Or perhaps Jaik was merely recreating a very general feeling of repose.

Stuttering Humor

Perhaps even more so than listeners and therapy, the topic of stuttering-related humor was heavily woven through Chapter 9. The difficulty of making a disability funny is age old, yet people continue attempts at this balance (some with more success than others).

My local support group once met with an acting troupe to discuss ideas for a stuttering video. Some of the suggestions were quite similar to those Jaik kicked around with the television producer. I remember at one point during the meeting proposing a firing squad scene in which the victim would be given a blindfold and cigarette, then placed against a wall. The squad captain would bark, "Ready! Set! F-f-f-f-f-f…" The cigarette would burn low as the accused fearfully awaited his fate. The camera would switch back and forth between the doomed and perspiring criminal and the struggling captain trying to release the key word. The soldiers would glance about in confusion as the scene faded to black. I probably remember the discussion mainly because all of the people who stutter laughed at the idea but none of the non-stutterers did.

Perhaps the line between funny and offensive has much to do with who is telling the joke. Had a non-stutterer voiced the same idea, would the support group members have laughed? Did the non-stutterers stay quiet because they found the skit offensive? Or were they uncertain whether it was appropriate for them to laugh along?

In addition to who's telling the joke, of course, offensiveness also depends upon the joke itself. *A Fish Called Wanda* was a comedic movie in which a stuttering character was routinely demeaned and this drew many protests from the stuttering community (Feinberg, 1990; McLellan, 1989). When the controversy reached Saturday Night Live's *Weekend Update*, Dennis Miller's joke was the following.

> *The National Stuttering Project, protesting the portrayal of stuttering in the film* A Fish Called Wanda, *has received a contribution of $2,500 from MGM/UA. The payment was made in small amounts at irregular intervals* (Takahama, 1991).

Instead of protests, the National Stuttering Project (now the National Stuttering Association) applauded the joke. Why, I'm not certain. Perhaps they just appreciated any stuttering humor that rose above playground level. Historically, stuttering humor in movies and TV has been of the slapstick variety. It was comedy rooted in the speaker's struggle. Stuttering also offered an easy target in that those suffering from the disorder grew up ashamed of it and thus were unlikely to protest. Then in the 1980s, something amazing occurred. People who stutter began to speak out. The NSP and other groups launched media advocacy efforts to combat negative media portrayals on the bases that they were inaccurate and seemed to legitimize making fun of stuttering.

Predictably, there was backlash to these efforts. Advocates' complaints were dismissed as "hypersensitive" (or that other favored copout phrase—"politically correct"). Essentially, critics were offering a 4-pronged argument (Williams, 2006):

1. I am sensitive.

2. Therefore, anything that does not offend me is not insensitive.

3. By definition, then, anyone who is offended is hyper-sensitive.

4. And, finally, if they can't take a joke, they are certain-ly not worthy of sympathy, but are instead deserving of ridicule.

For the purposes of this chapter, let's ignore the illogic and even the arrogance of this argument and focus instead on its superficiality, the willingness to dismiss the issue before delving deeper. Rather than arguing about who's right and who's wrong, maybe we should be looking at *why* some individuals are so sensitive to stuttering media portrayals. If we consider their experiences and the impact of stuttering on their lives, we might find a perfectly logical basis for their sensitivity.

Insensitivity of a different sort emerged from a study of stuttering comedians (Williams, G, & Campbell, 2015). All of the comics sur-veyed stated that, like Jaik, they addressed stuttering in their acts, but many changed the focus of their humor from themselves (i.e., making fun of the stuttering itself) to mocking the ignorance of their listeners.

With all of this in mind, Jaik's ideas can be viewed as landing throughout the entire span of the funny-to-insensitive continuum. As this is largely a matter of perspective, I will offer my own views on how well he accomplished his goals of lightening the negativity of stuttering, educating the public, providing hope to people who stutter, and cultivating respect for these individuals.

To my mind, three of the ideas offered in chapter 9 achieve these objectives quite successfully:

- Serious interviews examining how stuttering can be a spur to success,

- Interviewing a politician who would have to be careful not to react and appear insensitive, and

- Organizing reunions for the sole purpose of avoiding people from the past.

Many of the other ideas risk protestations. This is not to say that they shouldn't be tried, just that, based on the brief descriptions offered, they are unlikely to find universal appeal. Examples of such ideas include the following.

- Joint interview of a blind politician by Jaik and a deaf co-median, i.e., one asks the question, but cannot hear the reply; another can hear, but not communicate the message. Meanwhile, the interview subject cannot see what is happening.

- Outdoor reporting in cold locations to increase the vocal tremors.

- Hidden camera situations in which listeners' patience is tried or a stuttering individual seeks speaking-centric jobs.

- Stuttering at an airport desk in a way that results in arrest.

Jobs Incompatible with Stuttering

The humor inherent in ideas such as the stuttering auctioneer or interviewer stemmed from individuals performing tasks for which they were ill-suited. This raises the question of whether there are jobs that people who stutter simply cannot do. After all, there are limitations with other disabilities. Someone who is blind cannot drive a taxi. Cognitive impairments can keep people out of professional programs. Sometimes accommodations are simply not feasible.

What are the limitations of having a stutter? Can someone disfluent be a disc jockey? An air traffic controller? Can he or she be on TV and risk, as Jaik stated, the dead air that causes people to change channels?

Although it is likely that every job noted in the previous paragraphs—from auctioneer to television personality—is right now being performed by people who stutter, sometimes the stuttering is severe enough that opportunities will be limited. This is not to say that people who stutter cannot have lofty aspirations or follow their dreams. It is just that, like most of us, their roads to success will include some detours. It is not that unusual for people to end up in jobs other than the ones they sought when they were younger. Different people are suited for different tasks. Some traits may be outside an individual's control, but they are still factors in determining such suitability.

Advantages of Stuttering

As Jaik noted, stuttering can make one memorable, which in a competitive business like comedy can lead to more opportunities. This is an idea that has been expressed by other disfluent comedians as well (Williams, G, & Campbell, 2015).

But are there real benefits to stuttering for those who aren't on stage?

When that question is put to people who stutter, the responses generally center on the good people they met within the stuttering communities and the sensitivity they developed toward others with overt differences. But there are other potential advantages as well, some of which stem from stuttering *dis*advantages. For example, some have said it improved their determination because there was always an extra barrier to overcome.

Additional benefits I have heard people list (some more serious than others) include:

- It keeps me humble.

- No one asks me to say grace at Thanksgiving dinner.

- It serves as an extra filter before stupid things come out of my mouth.

- As a salesperson, customers gravitate toward me, assuming I won't give them a hard sell.

- A woman I wanted to meet took me on as a project even though she was out of my league.

Perhaps the best answer came from a school-aged child who stutters. He said, "When the rest of the class has to prepare a 6-minute speech, I only have to prepare a 3-minute speech."

And by the way, is that funny or insensitive?

Questions for Discussion

How do you feel about the concept of increasing clients' arrogance? Should a different word than *arrogance* be used when discussing this with clients?

You have been told to spend a day talking differently (e.g., with more confidence, more disfluency—any way you want to imagine). What are your thoughts? What might be difficult about this assignment?

Where do you draw the line between funny and offensive?

Jaik's television ideas were classified into those potentially positive, educational, hopeful, and respectful vs. those less likely to be viewed as such. Do you agree with how they were divided? Why or why not.

Aside from those noted in this chapter, can you think of any other potential advantages of stuttering?

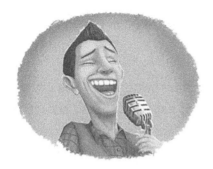

Chapter 11: The London Comedy Circuit

Hubert Gregg wrote *Maybe it's Because I'm a Londoner* in 1941, apparently after seeing German doodlebugs over the city. The song is about how much he loved London, and I can see how people born and bred there would feel very proud of their city.

These days, I find London to be a very diverse and cosmopolitan place. It has a thriving multi-cultural society which, unfortunately, brings with it a share of religious, cultural, and racial prejudices. For the most part, however, London moves along without too much friction or discomfort, although there are exceptions (notably, the 2011 riots).

In addition to cultural separations, I believe that London presents a distinct class system, characterized by old boy and old school networks, with everyone assessing one another on fairly superficial levels. People are far more likely to be judged by what they wear or which cars they drive than by any important measure.

Those who can endure the city's noise, stress, crowds, public trans-portation, density of closed circuit security cameras, and sheer expense will find London tolerable. Those raised in the countryside (say, in Darsham), however, might view such hassles to be never-ending nightmares. In fact, my brother lived in London for eight months and couldn't wait to leave.

This is not to say there aren't rewards for living there. The city possesses some interesting architecture, excellent tourist attractions, and world renowned museums. There are numerous opportunities to make money and a thriving night life. There is also a comedy circuit like none other. In fact, becoming a comedian in the UK necessitates making it in London.

And so I went.

Working life in London

Of course, no one moves to London and immediately pays the rent through comedy. Thus, the first order of business was to find real work.

When I interviewed for jobs, often everything was fine until my speech broke down. At that point, stuttering prejudices cropped up and I was treated as if I lacked either intelligence or whatever other attribute was needed to do the job. In a capitalist mecca such as London, openings available to newcomers typically involved serving customers in some capacity. Anything that might prevent sales is a deal breaker. I once rang up to apply for a telesales job, and the manager who picked up the phone genuinely thought that I was joking. He said on no account could he possibly employ me. Then he told me to get lost.

Despite such difficulties, I did find a variety of employment in London. Due to my stutter, I favoured jobs that didn't involve speaking too much, such as information technology positions or movie extra (called "background artist") work. In general, I found my colleagues to be enthusiastic and hard-working, despite paranoia about their job security, safety, and personal property.

Hearing "Please take all your personal belongings with you" on a continual loop when traveling around London probably didn't help, nor did the media's constant need to highlight potential terrorist threats to the transport network.

Many people I met dreamt of working "in the media," but that industry was competitive and difficult to break into. Entry level positions were usually not very well paid, given how replaceable they were. "Don't give up your day job" is a heckle many comedians learn to deflect, but in London it's sound advice. It's a high-cost environment, and it sometimes seemed people's precious lives were slowly ticking away amidst all the noise, expense, and stress.

While I did not relinquish any wage-paying employment, I did find London to be a big enough place to take some risks. After all, if they fail, how does it matter? If I go up to a woman in a bar and try and speak to her and she walks away, who cares? No one will ever know anything about it and I will never see her again. On the other hand, if she is willing to chat, as many were, interesting things can happen. Even employment rejections didn't faze me after a while. I just applied for the next opening.

My first stand-up gig

My first performance was at a comedy club in Woking, England in April 2000. I travelled there on the train with Mark Dolan, a friend from a comedy course who later went on to star in various television shows, most notably *Balls of Steel*.

The promoter had also attended the same comedy course and asked if we were interested in performing at his club. I remember being quite nervous before the gig but it was a relaxed audience and it went quite well.

While travelling back with Mark, I remember thinking that stand-up comedy was quite fun. Little did I know what I was getting into.

My first review

About nine months later, I received my first published review (Bennett, 2001). It wasn't so bad—certainly kinder than some that followed (more on that later). Anyway, here is what the reviewer had to say:

> *A bizarre act, this, and one that works better when he isn't delivering jokes. Campbell's stuttering, nervous character is enough to generate laughs from an audience unsure if it's an act or if it's natural. The first two minutes as he nervously struggles to get going is hilarious. If he were able to create a routine based on his own shortcomings, it would be a sure hit. Let's see...*

The circuit

The London Comedy circuit is essentially a collection of back room shows in drinking venues. In keeping with the predatory nature of the city, the shows are run by promoters who make a large portion of their money from free labour.

The average employer can't legally do this, due to the 1998 UK National Minimum Wage Act. Unfortunately, comedy clubs are exempt.

Some comedians run their own clubs in the back rooms of pubs. Although that should be an improvement, it is more often the case of the exploited becoming the exploiters. In their defence, however, those running their own shows have to make sure comics turn up, attract a suitable (and hopefully paying) audience, and serve as hosts. Even seemingly simple tasks—mailing out show information, posting flyers in the streets nearby, asking friends to attend—all have their own stresses and costs.

These numerous smaller gigs are often started by acts fresh off a comedy course who want to compere and obtain stage time. In theory, this should be great because they and other young comics have the chance to perform. In practice, however, it results in a string of badly run gigs where the promoter takes all the money and the audience members are confused as to why they paid £5 to see new acts trying out untested material about relationships or why they hate the world.

The main circuit is better organized and more stable, a system effectively designed to sell drinks. Comedy is just the means to herd the buyers to the alcohol. If they are having a good time, the club makes money. On the other hand, if the paying audience doesn't laugh enough, they won't return or recommend the place to their friends. The lone problem with that, from the club owner's point of view, is that fewer drinks are then sold from the bar.

London has more comedy clubs, comedians, and promoters than any other city on the planet (Hay, 2007), and probably contains more comic talent per square metre than anywhere else on Earth. As a result, it also features experienced, critical, and demanding audiences expecting to hear astute performers from all over the English-speaking world. Given the competition and performance level needed, success on the London circuit is not easy. I estimate that only about 10-15% of performers get paid work. I was lucky enough to be in that group, but felt trapped by my success. Once I was in the comedy loop, with some prominence and gigs booked in advance, I was afraid to leave that status behind.

I always had a love and hate relationship with London. Some days I enjoyed it immensely, other days I loathed the dog-eat-dog mentality. Without the comedy circuit, I would have probably left earlier and gone travelling. That may well have been a more constructive use of time than drinking too much and writing silly, self-deprecating jokes.

Comedy promoters

To get paid work, comedians have to satisfy the promoters. Without them, it is impossible to get the all-important "stage time" needed for career advancement. As noted, comedy promoters are looking for acts that sell drinks. For them, a perfect comic is original enough to be distinctive, but won't stray beyond the "mainstream."

Most up-and-coming comics working the circuit perform in small venues night after night, often for no fee, just to get noticed by a promoter or agent. Many of today's top names started out this way. The easiest point of entry into the world of comedy is the "open mike" spot. Many pubs and clubs run such comedy evenings, where hopefuls turn up, take to the stage, and try to make people laugh. If a promoter likes an act, the comedian might get booked. Once that happens, by the way, the comedian better show up for the gig, regardless of where and when it is. If the comic cancels for any reason, chances are good that the promoter will not call back again.

Few promoters want to pay a comedian who performed for free somewhere else the previous week. Fee-paying gigs are few. Given how necessary stage time is, unknown comics often end up doing one unpaid performance after another, a cycle that is difficult to break.

In my experience, comedy promoters are a mixture of enablers and exploiters, disguised as friends. They can be harsh critics as well, but I suppose they have to be. After all, they've chosen a fairly precarious way to make a living. I tried to remain on good terms with promoters, but it was not always easy. Disputes with comedians are common, usually for reasons of payment or billing. If promoters perceive a gig as substandard, they can remove the comic from their paid spots.

One would think that such individuals would have little patience for a stutter, but most promoters found it beneficial because it was different from the other acts. It also allowed them to make jokes, such as: "Next up is Jaik Campbell. Please don't worry if the microphone starts cutting in and out. It's just Jaik – he's got a stutter."

The stuttering outsider

A stutter can be a problem when trying to fit in. Too much prejudice against it (or any difference) can turn someone into a recluse. In London, I always felt like a bit of an outsider until I joined the comedy circuit. There, being an outsider was applauded. In fact, it was almost a necessity. Comedy turned my stutter from a negative into a positive.

Before starting stand-up, I'd be out with friends but lacking the confidence to join in properly with the conversation. People we met up with must have assumed that I preferred not to take part, was too arrogant to speak, or even that I was a bit stupid. None of that was true, of course. I just communicated differently.

There is perhaps a growing need to develop a more humanitarian approach to the world's diversity, and understand the benefits of being open about it. We are all the same human race living on a planet travelling round the sun at 75,000 mph, in a universe so big that our brains can't comprehend the size of it. The fact that we are here at all, in a stable orbit (thanks moon) within the habitable zone round the sun, with the right percentage of oxygen in the air, is an absolute miracle. It's enough to make even me both religious and health-conscious, as life seems too precious, and certainly too short. We're surely just all lucky passengers on spaceship earth and hence should be part of the same team. Where and what we are, even what football team we support, is pure chance. We have no choice in the matter; maybe we don't need to take it so seriously.

The other acts

In general, there was an enjoyable level of camaraderie between the comedians, and I met some interesting and colourful characters. Some were extroverts and others were introverts, but most had a fairly high amount of self-confidence and self-belief. A successful act needs a particular set of character combinations. They generally disclose a great deal about themselves and it takes commitment to do so. Everyone thinks comedians are insecure but actually they're no more insecure than the average person. In fact, we normally hide our real insecurities.

Comedians actively show their vulnerabilities on stage in order to charm the audience. Some are brilliant gag writers and deliver the material very well, but never made it big because they did not have any warmth about them.

Even comics who perform dark material have to have that twinkle in the eye to get the audience on board.

I made and lost more friends as a comedian in London than during the rest of my life combined. But the comraderie was nearly always positive. There was a general feeling that we were all on this long journey together. We all knew the challenges related to making the audience laugh, as well as getting paid for it. When I did receive advice or correction from another act, it was normally constructive and helpful, and I tried to act on it. It was far easier to accept than criticism from reviewers.

In general, most of the comedians on the circuit were good fun to be around, especially after the gig, when everyone could relax. It was interesting to meet so many talented and funny people from different nationalities and backgrounds. There were Indian, Iranian, Dutch, Swedish, American, Canadian, Australian, New Zealand, Scottish, Irish, Welsh and of course English comics working along together with normally good comradeship and support.

We all shared a common destination and the road there was so rocky and twisted that we all developed a similar mentality and out-look. It was an intriguing and inspiring experience.

I found the female comedians particularly interesting, as they usu-ally had very insightful and stimulating material about relationships. Their jokes actually helped me to better understand women. I guess I learnt not to be as scared or intimidated of them as I was prior to doing stand-up.

Show nights were exciting because we never knew what was going to happen. Who would get laughs and who wouldn't? What unex-pected events would occur? There was normally someone in the venue who drank too much, either a performer, an audience mem-ber, or the compere (and no, it wasn't always me). The larger the audience, the higher the level of enthusiasm. Not only was it always interesting, it offered a chance to learn from the other acts. I spoke to many of my comedy heroes, and sometimes was even on the same running order as them.

A bit like at work, sometimes a comedian friend would be "promoted" to doing longer sets. There were normally good feelings about this. It showed that there was a ladder in the comedy world that could be climbed with enough talent and hard work. Sometimes it was obvious that a certain act had star quality, like the first time I saw Alan Carr in a small club. He is now a UK household name, no surprise to anyone who saw him that night.

The audience

Varied is probably a good word to describe my audiences. Sometimes I performed to three people above a pub in Soho and other times found myself in front of a hundred students at a London university. Some nights I could make people laugh uncontrollably, and then there were the shows where people nearly walked out in disgust. The crowd could consist of sixth formers (high school students), university students, young professionals, families, couples, stag parties, and/or tourists who didn't speak English. I once even did a gig in front of a group of catholic bishops.

My material had to be as diverse as my listeners. I tried to find humour in anything, with topics that included relationships, love, friends, stuttering, university life, politics, philosophy, and even my cat.

The late nights

Two conditions that stress me out and exacerbate my stuttering are lack of sleep and hangovers. Unfortunately, both had become part of the routine. Given my speech and overall lack of attention, holding down full time jobs was difficult. My professional career, not to mention my bank balance, would have definitely been more stable had I not gone down the stand-up comedy path!

When I first started, I would typically do two or three gigs a week. As I was also working a full time day job, I would then have to get up the next morning. That part was fine, but the late nights would often catch up with me during the work day. Sometimes I'd be so tired that I wouldn't be able to keep my eyes open and would have to fall asleep in the men's toilet for half an hour or so. Admittedly, that wasn't very responsible, but it seemed like the best option at the time.

I used to share an office with a chap who often worked at home. Then my boss was fired and there was literally no one overseeing (or, for that matter, even paying attention to) my work on a day-to-day basis. I was able to spend large amounts of time editing comedy scripts and using the telephone to obtain gigs. Again, naughty but fortuitous. There came a time, however, when the management finally realised what was happening and I was asked to leave. No hard feelings. I even gave a short stand-up comedy routine on my way out, which in hindsight was probably a mistake. My reference probably read something like "Jaik gradually slacked off during this year in his quest to be comedian, but gave a solid, funny stand-up performance on his last day. What an asset to my company. Good riddance to him!"

The following year was a frustrating one, not only in terms of my speech, but also socially, artistically, and vocationally. I was lonely, my performances were inconsistent, and the daytime work was boring. Management knew my crazy schedule and moved me onto less complicated (and more tedious) tasks. Stand-up comedy was now seriously affecting my career path. I was clearly suffering for my art.

The travelling

I didn't have a car in London for seven years, so getting to gigs always involved tubes and trains. Most of the time I enjoyed this, as I could read and practise my lines. And if I had a drink (or two) during the show, I would not have to worry about being over the limit when driving back home. However, there was often a mad dash to try to catch the last tube home. I and everyone else wanted to avoid having to take the perilous night bus through the streets of London, which took forever and made getting up in the morning a night-mare. In addition to being slow, it involved riding with many drunken people leaving the pubs and clubs. At times, it was quite stressful to avoid potential trouble, pick pockets, or even fights. I remem-ber once having my tape recorder pinched from my jacket pocket. When I noticed it was missing, I accused the people around me of stealing it (and of course no one owned up). In my confident and highly annoyed, alcohol-filled state, I even started frisking random strangers to see if it was in their pockets. (I didn't find it.)

Emerging stress

Stuttering was not a major stressor until I landed bigger gigs. I over-practiced those to compensate for my speech and to be cer-tain I remember the script. But there were other pressures early on.

Although the first few gigs went well, it was a case of style over substance. It took me a long time to develop a script of sufficiently high quality material, as one early review noted:

"Jaik Campbell's biggest handicap as a comic is not his stutter, which is actually hardly noticeable, but his complete lack of funny material, stage presence, audience control, self-awareness, discipline or delivery" (Berkowitz, 2005).

Obviously, that was not the best review I could have received. I should have responded by doing fewer gigs and more writing, but that meant less of that all-important time on stage.

The stress of inducing laughter in a group of strangers night after night was high. Unlike most jobs, comedy successes and failures are very much in public view. It's like being a politician but is even more of a publically accountable experience, with laughter levels, rather than polling numbers, being the measure of achievement. Going home at night to a cold and empty bed after being rejected by an audience is a soul destroying experience, and one I tried to avoid.

Another problem was getting the words sorted out and clear in my head before going on stage. Often I had to do this while standing outside (sometimes in the pouring rain) and shouting the words out. Because this possibly looked a bit odd to any passers-by, I learnt to hold my mobile up to my mouth as though I was making some very irate phone call to someone.

Other strains included weight gain—due to the lack of exercise and too much fast food, alcohol, and late nights—and just getting home safely. Sometimes the tension on stage was matched by that from worrying about being mugged or pickpocketed getting back to my apartment.

I don't quite know the exact reason, but the stresses of performing, learning lines, living in London, and stuttering on stage eventually resulted in obsessive compulsive disorder (OCD) tendencies. I spent too much time checking that I hadn't left the stove on or the door unlocked. So, of course, I joked about it on stage:

> There are certain jobs that aren't very suitable if you have OCD.

> Like being a burglar.

> Because you'd burgle a house, and then have to go back a week later to check that the oven was off.

I also read up on OCD, which helped somewhat. Basically my brain was overestimating fears. It was like a more generalized version of stuttering—getting stuck and searching for perfection. The key was not to worry too much, advice easier to read than follow.

Finding a toilet

I almost forgot to mention the worst part of the London circuit. It wasn't the heckling, the constant late nights, or the tiresome female groupies (I wish!). No, rather, it was the pub toilets.

I normally tried to use the toilet before going on stage. However, many comedy nights were in small pubs, where the toilet was basically a confined hell hole. Now it would seem that getting a bathroom right is fairly simple: install a toilet and stall (preferably with a seat and a door), put on a lock, and add some toilet paper. But most London pubs couldn't seem to get this combination right. Permutations included a toilet with toilet paper, but no lock; a lock on the door but no toilet paper; or, on really unlucky nights, a toilet with no seat or door. Hovering over a toilet like a ninja, with one hand on the door, praying that no one pushes it open, is no way to begin a work night. Some places didn't even have a toilet, forcing me to make a mad dash to the nearest fast food place, hoping to get there and back before being introduced by the compere.

Payment for stand-up gigs

Even for professional comedians, earning a living from stand-up is difficult. As noted, I had to supplement my income with IT jobs and film extra work for five years.

Payment for gigs depended on status of the act (headliner vs. other), how big the club was, audience size, and length of the performance slot. Comedians are only as good as their last gig and a terrible one could result in an unpaid spot. Most new acts don't get paid. Payment for an average 20 minute stand-up gig was quite low, ranging from about £10 to £80. Established London venues could pay between £80 and £160, but getting these required a very strong routine. And even then, an individual comedian would only be given a spot once every 6 months or so.

Out of London gigs could average about £120, with headlining at about £150 and opening at about £100 or so. These were also competitive and did not pay the comic's travel costs.

High end sums were £200 per night plus hotel for a club and £500 or more for corporate work. Christmas shows usually paid double for the night. As a guest comic on a cruise ship, the figures were about £800 - £1500 for one 40 minute set and a free cruise for the comic and partner.

Generally speaking, established comedians commanded between £50 and £75 a night. To put these figures in perspective, in London at that time a fast food meal and a pint of lager would cost around £7, a restaurant dinner at least four times that. The national UK mean wage today is about £26K gross (i.e. before tax is taken off). So a comedian earning £72 a night would have to work 365 nights a year to hit the UK average. And that's without any agent fees.

Variability of income is also an issue. For example, a stable salary is necessary to convince a mortgage company to provide a loan, and, understandably, stand-up comedy isn't viewed as such. Most comics therefore have a day job for security. Interestingly, the acts that were successful were often the ones who quit their day jobs and focused solely on comedy. That, however, is a risk most cannot take.

So yes, it is possible to make a living out of comedy. But it's less a career choice than a life choice. It requires a love of performing, not for wealth but for comedy's sake. Riches and fame can be by-products of success, but that success requires dedication to the craft.

Comedy gets *really* competitive

In June of 2001, I performed in a heat for *So You Think You're Funny* at the Amused Moose Soho. Luckily, I managed to be selected for the semi-final to be held at the 2001 Edinburgh Fringe. That was quite a confidence boost, particularly when I was asked to record a 15-minute interview about "stuttering and comedy" for Sky TV. It was my first TV interview and was quite exciting. It also justified my decision to work part-time and slowly develop a niche in the comedy world.

A month later, I attended a morning audition for an ITV (Independent Television network) comedy programme called *Take the Mike*.

I had to compete against four other comics. Feeling not funny at all at 9 am, I decided to drink a pre-show can of lager whilst sitting next to a vagrant on a city bench. It worked, but at a cost.

The show involved an established comedian, Junior Simpson, coaching five new comedians, who then took his advice and performed 7-minute spots in front of a live audience that same evening. Fortunately for me, the workshop-style format was something with which I had previous experience, thanks to Michael Knighton's course.

I remember at the start of the filming, Junior came in and shook everyone's hand and asked us our names. When it was my turn, I blocked and nothing came out of my mouth. The director told me to silently repeat my name over and over so that when Junior came up to me on camera, I would be able to say it. So while the other four people were smiling and looking relaxed, I was full of tension and silently mouthing, "Jaik, Jaik, Jaik, Jaik, Jaik, Jaik, Jaik," which must have looked a bit odd to anyone tuning in. Even following this strategy, the introductions required four takes. When I finally did say my name, it popped out of my mouth inappropriately loud. My introduction was never seen on air.

From there, fortunately, things got better and I gave a confident and funny morning performance. I tried another lager before the evening act, but the morning alcohol kept this one from having the desired effect. Combined with a lack of funny material, the end gig wasn't that strong.

Shortly thereafter, I entered the *Hackney Empire All-Star Talent Quest* at the Bullion Room Theatre, and made it into the final. This was somewhat surprising in that the large and culturally diverse audience didn't seem to fully appreciate my stuttering act. Again, the later stand-up session was less effective, although parts of it were televised on a Saturday morning TV programme called *The Best of the London Comedy Festival*. Interestingly, that night's winner, Shazia Mirza, went on to big things in the fields of journalism and television.

The following night I won the *Amused and Abused Talent Stand-Up Contest*. Overall, I was pleased with my performances that summer. My plan seemed solid and I was focused on me. However, one never knows what life will bring.

September 11th 2001

As was the case with many, many people, the tragic events of September 11th 2001 had quite a big effect on me. Of course, life changed for many that day, even those not directly affected by the tragedy. The world seemed less controlled, and this undoubtedly troubled many people. I remember reading that one woman in England hung herself a few days later because of the anxiety and depression caused by the terrorist attack. It was a reaction that seemed extreme, but on another level understandable.

Part of my introspection was the realization that life is short and fragile. In October 2001, I quit my job to focus on being a comedian. On my last day there, my boss suggested that becoming self-employed was an idea that I should consider.

I said, "Yes, I agree. I'm becoming a self-employed comedian."

King Gong

The rest of 2001 was spent doing various unpaid open spots, attending speech therapy classes, and practising and writing lines.

In October, I did a 5-minute heat for the *Daily Telegraphy Open Mic Award* at Brunel University, which went badly and made me again realise that I needed sharper and funnier material. So I began making daily trips to the British Library to do stuttering-related research and writing. This was partly for material, but I was also hoping to find information to help my stutter. I remember it being a very happy time in my life, as I was doing something interesting and worthwhile, with few interruptions and distractions. In December I did a gig for the Soho Laughter Lounge to a packed audience and the promoter told me that I must continue with comedy as I was on par with the headliner. My comedy was back on track.

The new year started with the usual speech therapy courses and comedy gigs, but also a week in Gran Canaria, a very relaxing vacation (particularly for someone who grew up with chaotic ones). I returned for scheduled ten minute spots in new clubs such as Up the Creek, the Chuckle Club, Comedian's Graveyard and the Comedy Pit. In addition, I entered numerous "new act" competitions, making the finals of the *Laughing Horse* and the aforementioned *Stand-Up Britain*.

My dream, like most London comedians, was to perform at the London Comedy Store, a venue of 360 seats and an electric atmosphere. The audience anticipation for each act is palpable. It is accepted (and expected) that all of the performers there are top notch and will, one by one, keep the crowd laughing heartily. I felt I was up to the task, so I regularly rang up to book a slot at the club's infamous *King Gong* show on the last Monday of each month. This show involved performing until three people in the audience held up red cards. Three red cards and the compere bangs a gong, signifying the end of the routine. Those who last five minutes put themselves in the running for a coveted Comedy Store gig.

Over time, I learnt that by stuttering and doing some stuttering related material during the first minute, I could grab the attention of the
audience. My route to this realization, however, was rather slow:

1) April 29th 2002 – I lasted 21 seconds.

2) May 27th 2002 – I lasted 2.5 minutes.

3) June 24th 2002 – I lasted 21 seconds.

4) July 29th 2002 - I lasted 2.5 minutes.

5) September 30th 2002 - I lasted 50 seconds.

6) January 27th 2003 - I lasted 40 seconds.

7) February 24th 2003 - I lasted 1.5 minutes.

8) May 26th 2003 – I finally lasted the full five minutes!

My reward for not being gonged was to stand on stage with the other comedians who had also managed five minutes. The audience
then cheered for their favourite act of the night. I was thrilled when
the loudest cheer was for me!

It was a rocky road to the Gong Show win. Yes, it took me over a
year to compose the right material and to learn how to successfully
play that venue, but I truly believe that having a stutter also helped.
In addition to helping me stand out from the other comics, it made
me likeable enough for at least some audience members to root for
my success.

Continuing my hot streak, my first 5-minute spot at the Comedy
Store went very well. To stand in front of over 300 people and, de-

spite a stutter, make them laugh for the full length of the spot (which, after all, is what's expected there) is a scary prospect. It also was a real confidence test for me. I convinced myself that I had a right to be on that stage, that I could hide my considerable fear and successfully play a top venue.

Comedy is, however, a series of ups and downs. My fortunes stayed up long enough to reach the London regional final of the *BBC New Comedy Awards*. However, by (bad) luck of the draw, I had to go first on, which was always my least favourite spot, mainly because I wasn't relaxed enough and the pre-show alcohol hadn't taken much effect. For those reasons or others, the routine didn't work very well. I was in a very depressed state for a few days after that, wondering if I couldn't perform without drinking.

The reviews I received reflected my struggles. It takes a stout heart and a balanced mind to be able to cope with negative criticism, especially if it's published in a newspaper or on the internet for everyone to read. With comedians, these attributes are in short supply. Still, the negativity can serve as a wakeup call, a reminder that no string of success is permanent.

Lessons learned

Hopefully, this chapter demonstrates that persistence and hard work can make an impact on the London comedy circuit. Maybe the impact will be small, but it is there.

I don't know what my influence was on the London comedy scene, but I can speak to its effect on my speech. As a result of performing so much stand-up comedy before large audiences, I experienced a gradual desensitisation to my own stutter. I felt I controlled it, as opposed to the other way around. In my early twenties, I tried to cover it up and avoid talking about my stutter, strategies that only made it worse. When I started being open about it every day, I pushed my comfort zones to the extreme (it helped that it was a subject that audiences found funny and interesting). Comedy is an industry that consciously encourages experimentation with new identities and boundaries. Before, openness about stuttering was beyond my limits. When my boundaries expanded to include it, my speech became better.

The highly tensed and adrenaline-filled seconds before I first stepped out on stage in front of 360 people at the London Comedy Store was genuinely a feeling I will never forget and was probably the most desensitizing moment I have ever had. I faced my stuttering demons totally head on and did so with a smile.

In front of a packed house, I was saying, "Look, I have a stutter, but it's fine. I can still do stand-up and get laughs. I can still get on with my life. And no, I'm not a rap artist."

I not only routinely disclosed my stuttering, I also used various points in my routine to voluntarily stutter. This purposeful stuttering was mostly done to reinforce the joke or accentuate the punch line. But the desensitization

benefit was a major bonus. The following joke serves as a good example:

> Someone with a stutter came up to me once after a show
>
> He said, "You're a shhhh, you're a shhhh. You're a shhhh, you're a shining example. Well done!"

I told him to f-f-f, I told him to f-f-f, I told him to f-f-fol-low the advice of his speech therapist.

The voluntary breakdown got bigger laughs than a straightforward punch line. It also put me in control of the stuttering.

As touched upon in chapter 9, a potential result of stuttering humour is crossing the line into mockery. Bill Hicks famously said, "It's always funny until someone gets hurt. Then it's just hilarious" (Hicks, 2005). While I'm not sure I totally agree with this analysis, I have laughed at potentially hurtful punch lines. For me, a joke is acceptable as long as the boundaries of maliciousness are not pushed too far. For example, I sometimes used the following joke in my routine:

I have a stutter. I don't know if anyone else here has a stutter? It does sometimes happen.

(Pause.)

They don't normally call out.

It is certainly not a kind joke, but because a stuttering comedian was the one saying it and it did not come across as nasty, I think it was suitable. It normally received a healthy laugh. At the end of the day, jokes are simply jokes and not heartfelt opinions. There aren't many subjects at which comedians don't poke fun these days. The important element is where the jokes are coming from – a good thought or a dark place; a creative, original, and questioning mind, or a childish, lazy, and simple one.

My only regret with respect to stuttering-related humour was being too self-deprecating. For one thing, I worried about how audience members would treat people who stutter after I had portrayed myself as the fool. I found it difficult to tell a joke that made the stuttering speaker look like the winner.

> *Asking out girls at school was tricky. Lots of heavy breathing involved.*

> *The girl just thought I was some kind of sad pervert.*

> *And that's before I had even phoned them.*

> *Singing actually helped my stutter.*

> *So I sung everywhere, and my friends heard me singing.*

> *And they said* 'Jaik, go back to the stuttering. (Pause.) We'll wait.'

I would have preferred to use cleverer jokes that could make the audience laugh *and think* at the same time, as well as put stuttering in a more positive light. Maybe I should have tried to persuade an audience to look at their own prejudices through my own, unflinching, critical deconstruction of society's view of people who stutter. That, however, would have been extremely difficult in a comedy club environment.

All told, it's hard to add up the number of hours I spent on the London comedy circuit writing, practicing and performing material about my life and my stutter, but it must have run into the hundreds. The buzz of making people laugh, of having a sort of control over them for 10 or 20 minutes, became an addiction for me. The more I spoke about my stutter, the more accepting I became of it. I realized that it wasn't a shameful disorder, but, rather, a character trait that could be celebrated and applauded.

Rather than trying to fool listeners into thinking it didn't exist, my stutter became an overt and important part of me. It's interesting: By confronting the problem, it improved. Ignoring it only made it worse. No wonder the speech therapist had advised me to tell as many people as I could about my stuttering. I bet she had no idea I would do so to large audiences all over London. But I did and lost a great deal of the shame, secrecy, and seclusion in the process. Interestingly, I also increased my fluency.

Another desensitisation activity, one I simply stumbled upon, was recording my gigs. I did so to tweak my comic delivery and to see which jokes worked (and which didn't), but repeatedly hearing my stuttering made it seem routine, less powerful. I learned how noticeable my stutter was and the key words I had the most trouble producing. I later videoed some of my gigs to observe the types of facial expressions I made, which desensitised me even further.

Comedy is like stuttering in the sense that one has to get out there and say what he or she has to say. Of course, the audience is important too. Listening and reacting to their needs is as much as part of the communication as my delivery. Yes, I talk the way I want to, even pausing for long periods of time to improve my timing. But I still have to consider my listeners and make sure that my message is received. On stage, I am never just reciting jokes. I am telling people my thoughts, and checking in with them now and then to see if they are still with me. The best comedians have a relationship with the audience and are very attentive to them. A speech flaw just means finding other ways to project my point of view.

Questions for Discussion

Do you believe that a large city is either a better or worse place for a stuttering adult to live? Explain your answer.

How do you think working with promoters, finding agents, and the other behind-the-scenes tasks needed to become a comedian can be impacted by stuttering?

As a "stuttering outsider," Jaik describes life as "too precious" to waste, then concludes that people need not "take (life) so seriously." How do you make sense of these seemingly contradictory ideas?

Why do you think comedy audiences are interested in stuttering?

Jaik stated that his stuttering improved as a result of confronting it. Explain why that could have occurred.

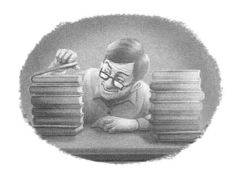

Chapter 12: Finding and Maintaining Employment

Jaik hit London and had to find work and, just like when he grad-uated from college (see chapter 7), it was a task made more un-pleasant by his stutter. Although cold calls and job interviews are stressful for anyone, most do not have to additionally experience mockery about their speech. Could Jaik have handled the process better? I do not believe so, at least not in any meaningful way, given that he persevered and found work. But his story does touch on an interesting topic: that of stuttering and job hunting.

A central question with prospective employers parallels one that Jaik addressed when discussing his comedy—when to let the lis-teners know about stuttering. That is, should the disfluent applicant self-disclose right away or wait until the disorder is obvious?

My clients have handled this issue in a variety of ways. Although none have acknowledged their stuttering on the resume, some have referred to it indirectly (for example, *Member, Boca Raton Stuttering Support Group*). One could argue that such a reference lessens the surprise for the interviewer.

The majority of stuttering clients, however, did not divulge stuttering during the application phase at all, agreeing with Jaik that such a disclosure would limit their opportunities. There is certainly sound-ness to this approach. Given that prospective employers actually interview only about 2% of candidates from the stack of resumes they receive (Harris, 2014), one could argue that it is ill-advised to list traits that are potential deal breakers. Not only does stuttering make some people uncomfortable, but as Jaik noted, the stereo-type associated with it does not necessarily match that of an ideal employee (see chapter 2). That is, many employers are searching for people who are energetic and effective communicators (Arthur, 2012; Robles, 2012); thus, applicants deemed as timid and poor speakers are at a disadvantage.

In the US, the 1990 Americans with Disabilities Act makes it is ille-gal to deny a position because of a disability, assuming reasonable accommodations can be made. In federal courts, the question of whether stuttering constitutes a disability under the ADA has been ruled on a case-by-case basis, with severity being a key determi-nant (Parry, 2009). Even if one's stuttering is severe enough to be considered disabling, however, such a law will not necessarily help an applicant if those interviewing are uncomfortable with his or her speech. They can always find another reason to hire the competi-tion. But the point is that they have to deny the disfluent candidate on another basis. They cannot overtly state that stuttering is the reason, as prospective employers did to Jaik.

I asked him what sorts of protections are in place for the disabled in London. He responded:

> Many UK job adverts state that they aim to be an
> "equal opportunities employer" and "welcome appli-
> cations from ethnic minorities and people with dis-

abilities." It must be difficult for recruiters to uphold this though. They need to employ people who will work well within their team and someone with a stutter, for example, might have problems fitting in with an established and well running group. Patience is unfortunately rare in busy London commercial office environments. Most companies do have equal opportunity policies in place, but need enthusiastic staff who will fit in with their ethos. Someone who stutters probably has just as much chance to be successful in a job as anyone else, but I don't think employers see it this way. If more of them could see talent and potential, rather than just stuttering, the fate of so many would be much different. Another problem: Employers are worried that someone on their team would mock or laugh at the person who stutters. If someone did that, even accidentally, the procedures to deal with that scenario would potentially be complicated and costly (although I anticipate that not many people who stutter would have an issue with a few light hearted jokes) (Campbell, J., personal correspondence).

Oddly, it appears that laws designed to assure humane treatment of the disabled might actually backfire during the hiring process. Of course, that assumes that the employer in question is unable to train their staff to behave in a civilized manner.

Another counter-argument to concealing stuttering is that all it really accomplishes is to prolong the rejection. That is, the ignorant employer rejects the stuttering candidate after the interview rather than at the time the resume is received. On the other hand, job seekers who disclose early do not waste time with boorish managers like the one who laughed at Jaik. However, in my experience, most people who stutter do not seem to find this argument persuasive. They would still prefer the interview opportunity, as it allows them to make a positive face-to-face impression and show future co-workers that stuttering has nothing to do with competence.

Another potential concern with omitting any reference to stuttering is that it constitutes a deception. To this, I would argue that personal traits are not normally included on resumes. For example, no one states "right-handed" in the section on personal attributes. As long as stuttering has no bearing on the candidate's ability to do the job, it is just another trait.

Unfortunately, in Jaik's case, the difficulties occurred during the actual interviews. Still, open stuttering was the right way to go. Of course, he may have had no choice than to be overtly disfluent. Sometimes, stuttering is obvious from the first utterance. But there are other times that people can employ enough secondary behaviors to mask any noticeable stuttering. I would argue that these individuals would be better off visibly stuttering, self-disclosing with confidence, and making it clear that stuttering will not hold them back.

Stuttering and Employment

Needless to say, once a job has been obtained, communication pressures don't end. Daily conversations with colleagues, supervisors, and customers are made more challenging with a stutter (Bricker-Katz, Lincoln, & Cumming, 2013). Such challenges can lead to feeling different or excluded (Bricker-Katz, Lincoln, & Cumming, 2013; Klein & Hood, 2004) and possibly avoiding advancement opportunities (Bricker-Katz, Lincoln, & Cumming, 2013). In addition, there is the possibility of upward mobility being stifled by people uncomfortable with disfluent speech and/or who believe that stuttering individuals are too introverted and unsure of themselves to handle high level positions (Blumgart, Tran, & Craig, 2010; Klein & Hood, 2004; Palasik et al., 2012). Indeed, recent research (Logan & O'Connor, 2012) suggests that stuttering speakers are viewed as relatively less suitable for high speaking demand occupations in comparison to those with low speech expectations. This finding suggests the possibility that the perceived stereotype might force people who stutter into a relatively narrow set of occupations.

Although it is true that people who stutter can restrict their own advancement (see chapter 8), so too can others in the work place. Although it takes some time to reach the required level of desensitization, the best approach with co-workers is the same as with interviewers: be honest and open about stuttering (Bricker-Katz, Lincoln, & Cumming, 2013). As Jaik discovered, stuttering can actually be beneficial in the workplace. In fact, many of the benefits cited in chapter 10 apply to his story. For example, he noted that his stuttering helped him to stand out among the numerous comedians in London. Certainly, it is a difference that can make someone memorable for the right reasons. Again, it is a matter of how one presents him- or herself. If his stuttering had been viewed as a weakness, Jaik would only have been remembered as a comedian to avoid.

Determination, another stated advantage of having to deal with a stutter, was certainly evident in Jaik's search for stage time. It seems he was in almost constant contact with promoters, TV producers, and the like. It is true that 1) there is no way to know whether this determination resulted from a lifetime of stuttering and 2) he spent much of his day job writing scripts and sleeping in the company toilet, behaviors not exactly indicative of determination. On the latter point, however, it should be noted that his motivation to excel at structured employment was far less than it was for comedy.

The stutterer stereotype also offers a potential advantage to employment in service industries, such as those Jaik noted were all over London. To the extent that customers perceive the disfluent sales associate as timid and reserved and thus unlikely to give them the hard sell, they may be more apt to listen to him or her than to salespeople viewed as more aggressive. One salesman who stuttered pointed out to me that his public display of a perceived weakness made him interesting, worth listening to. In other words, stuttering allowed him a chance to be heard.

Personality and Stuttering

Of course, exhibiting one's stuttering requires a relatively high level of desensitization. The question becomes how realistic it is for a given client to achieve this level. At least some of that is dependent upon personality and, as mentioned in chapter 2, no real evidence exists that those who stutter possess characteristic personality traits that disallow boldness and self-assurance. There is, however, some research that supports a connection between temperament and stuttering (Alm & Risberg, 2007; Bleek et al, 2011, 2012; Eggers, DeNil, & Van den Bergh, 2010; Jones, Conture, & Walden, 2014; Kefalianos et al., 2014; Schwenk, Conture, & Walden, 2007), specifically that people who stutter present differing levels of anxiety, reactivity to stress, task persistence, and distractibility when compared to nonstutterers. Despite the fact that temperament is generally considered a characteristic that emerges in infancy and remains relatively stable over time (Anderson et al., 2003), these differences seem to be more a result of stuttering than a cause (Alm, 2014; Alm & Risberg, 2007). Furthermore, there are research findings indicative of no temperamental differences between children who do and do not stutter (Reilly et al., 2013). More to the point, one cannot assume such a difference with any specific client, given what an individualized disorder stuttering is.

Getting to know a client's personality traits is important because they can impact progress in therapy (Conture, 2001; Craig, Blumgart, & Tram, 2011) and, likely, their overall recovery. Someone who is cautious, sensitive to external stimuli, and afraid of making mistakes is going to have a harder time reaching the desensitization level of the aforementioned salesman who jumps into conversations feet first (see Brocklehurst, Drake, & Corley, 2015). It is also true that anxiety is correlated with the self-esteem of people who stutter (specifically, the greater the former, the lower the latter) (Blood et al., 2007). SLPs are wise to remember that some comfort zones expand more easily than others. In addition, some zones will require a lot of expansion before they include all of the client's communication wants and needs.

In this regard, Jaik's story offers hope to professionals. By his own account, he is naturally cautious and anxious. Despite such obvious obstacles to a comedy career, look what he accomplished. He excelled in a field most fluent people would not venture near. Moreover, in doing so, he learned to communicate effectively with a stutter.

One trait that did help him is intelligence. A former honor student, he made his living via an ability to cleverly phrase commonalities and offer unique observations, skills requiring high aptitude. This same intelligence eventually helped him to accept the reality of his stuttering and how to manage it. Clinicians should understand, however, that being smart can also hold stuttering clients back. It has been noted that gifted children are reticent to attempt new tasks because they will not excel at them (Silverman, 2003). They quickly see all of the ways that any risk can go wrong. In therapeutic terms, maybe the technique won't work or the listener will find it strange or something else will happen that makes the cost of failure too high. Given the importance to recovery of ideas such as risk-taking, adaptability, and expanding one's comfort zone (see chapter 8), it would seem that highly intelligent clients would be less likely to make progress in therapy. Yet, experience suggests that this is not always the case. Intelligence often has a way of winning out.

To draw a parallel, pretend someone asked you, intelligent reader, to tell your three best jokes at the London Comedy Store tonight. What is running through your head? Likely, it is everything that could possibly go wrong. You'll mess up the punch line or your voice will quiver or the audience won't like your delivery. Perhaps the jokes suddenly don't seem as funny as they used to. Or maybe it's another worry. After all, there are many paths to anxiety, fear, and perceived humiliation.

If you had a month or two to prepare your jokes, some level of anxiety would still be present, but you would at least have time to think through what you were being asked to do. You could make observations, seek advice, and decide on strategies that make sense for you. Similarly, most intelligent clients eventually discern the ins and outs of stuttering treatment. Their intellect helps them realize why techniques and activities fit their goals and also when to go against their instincts. Once the goals are understood, progress toward them becomes feasible.

In Jaik's case, for example, he was able to use a high stress situation to his advantage. Save for the occasional heckler, no one else was interrupting, talking over him, or finishing his sentences when he was performing. He was the only one speaking and could thus employ speech modifications without the usual conversational distracters. It was his choice to stutter openly, stutter easily, employ fluency enhancing techniques, or whatever he chose. For stuttering individuals, in fact, public speaking offers a rare opportunity for complete control over how speech is produced.

As a bonus, it provides a chance to disclose stuttering to a captive audience.

Discussing stuttering on stage turned out to be key to Jaik's process of acceptance. In fact, "I've got a slight stutter. Not a great start, especially when you've only got three minutes on live TV!" may be the best illustration of acceptance I have ever heard. Accepting a condition doesn't mean liking it. Jaik was saying that he recognizes that stuttering is part of his speech—part of his life, actually—but it can nevertheless be a considerable nuisance. That, in a nutshell, is acceptance.

All of the reasons to advertise mentioned in chapter 2 applied to Jaik in some way. Addressing his stutter helped the audience understand what they were hearing, thereby reducing potential confusion (and increasing the chances of an appropriate reaction). Mentioning the stutter also made it less tempting for Jaik to employ avoidance behaviors (as there was nothing to hide).

Self-disclosure gave him more control over his stuttering and even lessened its frequency.

In addition to Jaik's determination and intelligence, his well-developed sense of humor likely helped him mange his stuttering. Not only did it lead to personal satisfaction and recognition in the world of comedy, humor was also helpful to the process of recovery. There are lessons to be taken from his experiences.

Humor can help one to understand a deeply personal matter (Orben, 2001). This understanding leads to changed behaviors when the illogic of the old ways becomes apparent (Lyttle, 2002). Expanding chapter 8's proverbial comfort zone also becomes somewhat easier when one can have some fun doing it. It is empowering, for example, when the speaker can turn the tables and see the ridiculousness of listeners' reactions to stuttering (Lyttle, 2002; Martineau, 1972; Williams, G, & Campbell, 2015). There are examples of writers and filmmakers (e.g., G & D, 2012) making fun of the responses they get. That is, through humor, they create a therapeutic activity from situations usually associated with negativity.

Along with improved understanding, treating a personal subject with humor permits one to objectify it. In doing so, the individual distances him- or herself from the issue and makes it less personal, allowing new insights to emerge (Lyttle, 2002; Manning, 2001; Sultanoff, 1995). Jaik's example of stuttering with a suspicious police officer (in chapter 7) is a situation that would normally be associated with embarrassment, shame, and stress. When Jaik took a step back to view it, however, he found an aspect of the interaction that could be amusing. In such a case, one might even argue that he rose above the old negative feelings. Such perspective is valuable because it keeps the speakers from dwelling on mistakes or overrating achievements (Morreall, 1982), either of which could hinder the process of recovery.

As Jaik learned, humor can reduce not just the stress of the speaker, but that of the listeners as well (Lyttle, 2002; Orben, 2001). As soon as Jaik says, "…especially when you've only got three minutes of live TV," the audience understands where the humor lies with stuttering. They are now on Jaik's side and feel that they have permission to laugh along.

Of course, Jaik walks a fine line here. As noted in chapter 10, sometimes (OK, usually) stuttering is not funny. Being told you could never be hired because of your speech, for example, didn't evoke any laughter from Jaik. Humor is not necessarily the highest form of acceptance or a reflection of the best attitude one can have about stuttering. As outlined throughout this book, it is a disorder that different people handle in different ways. Some people learn to stutter confidently, almost daring listeners to respond negatively. Others stutter openly and simply ignore the reactions. Yes, humor can help some people. But they have to decide that it is what works for them.

Also worth pointing out is that with some listeners, a sense of humor will not be all that effective. Simply put, they won't get it. Another approach is needed. In chapter 10, arrogance, informally defined as assuming that what you have to say is more important than any squirming your listener feels the need to do, was mentioned as another means of dealing with listeners. Such a strategy places all of the speakers' focus on themselves and none on their listeners.

Jaik's experiences with his audiences might prove instructive here. Unlike arrogance in its purest form (*I talk, you listen; or don't listen, who cares?*), he had to strike a balance between "listening and reacting to their needs" and talking "the way I want to." As Jaik explained:

> *Listening and reacting to their needs is as much as part of the communication as my delivery. Yes, I talk the way I want to, even pausing for long periods of time to improve my timing...I am telling people my thoughts, and checking in with them now and then to see if they are still with me. The best comedians have a relationship with the audience and are very attentive to them. A speech flaw just means finding other ways to project my point of view.*

Although his approach appears far removed from arrogance, it actually falls in line with its therapeutic use. While courtesy to listeners is important, it is also true that desensitized clients place greater importance on their own speech content and less on how others might view its delivery.

In retrospect, what Jaik accomplished with his newfound arrogance was not superiority, but, rather, equality. He respected the needs of his listeners, without letting them determine how he spoke.

Speech Naturalness

The topic of consideration for listeners also encompasses speech naturalness. As noted in chapter 6, regardless of the treatment employed, the resulting speech will differ to some extent from that of the average non-stutterer. That is, it will include comparatively more disfluency, both tense and modified, and/or sound more controlled.

Research in the area of naturalness has focused on speech following fluency modification therapy. Quite consistently, listeners rated post-treatment speech as more unnatural sounding than the speech of fluent speakers (Ingham, Gow, & Costello, 1985; Ingham & Packman, 1978; Kalinowski et al., 1994). In fact, one study (Kalinowski et al., 1994) found that the pre-treatment speech of adult subjects was actually rated as more natural than their speech following treatment. Thus, it appears that treated speech not only sounds less natural than that which was never stuttered, but also when compared to speech that is.

Before placing too much importance on these results, it should be noted that naturalness research suffers from low reliability (Onslow, Adams, & Ingham, 1992). That is, individual judges are often inconsistent in their ratings. In addition, just because one speech sample is rated as less natural than another, that does not mean that the former sample is necessarily *un*natural. It might simply rank lower on the normal range.

Even if we determine that treated speech is unnatural, however, the importance of such a determination makes for useful discussion. From the speaker's perspective, it could be argued that naturalness is not a critical issue. The speaker, after all, is learning to express him- or herself openly and become desensitized to listener reactions. Still, if the main objective is effective communication, the less natural the speech, the further one drifts from this goal. Perhaps because of that reason, attempts have been made to improve the speech naturalness of people who stutter (Jayaram, 2014; Ratyńska, et al., 2012), although Jaik's therapy history (and likely, that of most people who stutter) did not include any such attempts.

Rehearsal

As a final note, let us briefly address the television show director's advice to Jaik to silently repeat his name over and over so that he would be able to produce it fluently on command. Helgadottir and colleagues (2014) called such rehearsal a "safety behavior," and argued that all it really accomplishes is to sustain speakers' social anxiety while forcing them to miss out on what is happening around them. Furthermore, as Jaik learned, it is a strategy unlikely to work. As noted in chapter 10, the complexity of human speech leaves it vulnerable to even minute situational changes. Thus, repeating a word off camera is not the same as saying it aloud into a microphone. There is no reason to assume that fluency in a relatively simple speaking situation would disallow the presence of stuttering in a difficult one.

Questions for Discussion

What would you tell a client who asked you whether to self-disclose his stuttering to a potential employer?

Do you agree that "someone who stutters probably has just as much chance to be successful in a job as anyone else?" Why or why not?

Your client wants to let his co-workers know that he stutters. What advice do you give him?

If you had a client wanting to try stand-up comedy, what would be your advice? How would you tell him or her to address stuttering?

How important is speech naturalness to stuttering therapy?

How would you teach desensitization to a client whose culture stressed subservience to authority figures?

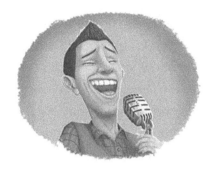

Chapter 13: The Edinburgh Fringe Festivals 2001-2008

The Edinburgh Festival Fringe is the largest arts festival on Earth, celebrating some of the best performers and entertainment from all over the planet. In 2014, a record-breaking 3,193 different shows staged 49,497 performances in 299 venues (The Fringe, 2014). Entertainers from various genres, backgrounds, countries, and nationalities rub shoulders and view each other's work, which spawns new ideas and future collaborations. As such, The Fringe is an unparalleled training ground, giving artists the opportunity to develop their productions, hone their skills, and network with producers, promoters, journalists, festival directors, and media professionals. It is an exciting place to be in August and the diversity of people and productions from all over the world is truly inspiring.

The Fringe began after World War II, as a small experimental arts festival and a maverick element of the main Edinburgh festival. Over the last 20 years it has become a huge marketplace for the comedy industry. It has launched the careers of many big stars, including Derek Jacobi, Rowan Atkinson, Stephen Fry, Hugh Laurie, Steve Coogan, Emma Thompson, and various members of the Monty Python team. A good Fringe review can rapidly boost a performer's reputation, improve his or her ability to get better paid work, and possibly land an agent (a bad review, on the other hand, can require a year or two recovery time). In one location, an unknown comic can put on a 55 minute show, get a collection of "5 star" reviews, win a comedy competition, and potentially become a household name. The hope of every performer is that a TV production company, a commissioning editor, or a radio producer will see his or her show, understand its potential, and offer a contract to transfer it to radio or TV. However, *hope* is a key word in Edinburgh, as numerous comedy shows get written, rehearsed, and performed there, and then sink into oblivion without a trace (except for the debt with which the performer is saddled).

Problems

There are many potential pitfalls with performing at the Edinburgh Fringe. A primary one is not having enough decent material for an entire show. Most time slots are 55 minutes long, featuring one comic or several. Either way, this length of time requires many, many jokes, and even if the script is sound, there is the matter of finding an audience. Because of the incredible number of acts, the Fringe Festival has an average audience of about seven people (The Fringe, 2014). Obtaining a top venue and evening show time can help draw people in, but competition for those is fierce, and venue mangers understandably need bankable, well-known acts.

Everything is also extra expensive in Edinburgh during The Fringe. Rents triple and venues can cost more than £2000. There must be enough posters and leaflets to last the whole month and, if the budget allows, paid "leaf letters" to hand them out. In addition to these necessary costs, there are the people asking for money. Publicists will contact acts insisting that without their help no one will hear about the show (which, of course, isn't true). Newspaper advertisers will e-mail offers to place adverts in their papers. There are even managers willing to find the act a venue and good time slot for the right (i.e., extravagant) price. This is for a show that they probably haven't read or seen. For all its renown, The Fringe is not a big money generator for the average artist.

It exists to help artists raise their 1) profile, 2) level of comedy, 3) lists of professional contacts, and 4) glasses in the many bars in and around the festival.

Benefits

Performing professionally at the Edinburgh Fringe requires self-discipline and practice, and not watching too many other shows and socializing. But it is a place people go to enjoy themselves, including the performers. Besides, viewing headliners in 2001-2 made me appreciate the level of quality the audience and press/critics were expecting to see. That was important because without press support, nobody would have known I existed. I had to learn what it took to persuade the press to read and publish my marketing releases.

Participating in Edinburgh not only improved my self-reliance as a performer, it also enhanced the confidence of promoters wanting to book me for a 20-minute spot after the Fringe had finished. In addition, the festival provided a benefit beyond professional utilities. By the time I did my first Edinburgh show, I had spoken about having a stutter so much, that I was well on my way to acceptance. The importance of effective communication (with or without stuttering) was magnified at The Fringe. Speaking to people on the street to persuade them to see my show, talking to the venue organisers and technicians, and, of course, performing shows night after night all required the ability to communicate well. Spending evenings getting my name out there to other acts and promoters obviously required that I identify myself. In fact, some of the more legendary Fringe parties required giving a name at the door to be let in, always a tricky proposition with a stutter (even when it was not my own name that I was trying to say).

Edinburgh 2001 - *So You Think You're Funny?*

Sometimes performers have to take risks before they are ready. In 2001, I was chosen to be in the semi-finals of *So You Think You're Funny* (SYTYF), one of the biggest comedy competitions at the Edinburgh Fringe. My material was limited but my audition was memorable, mainly because I was drunk on stage. I remember one of the judges telling me afterwards that it was my personality that got me through to the semi-finals (i.e. not my material), and she was probably right.

So I flew up to Edinburgh to do 7 to 8 minutes of stand-up in the semi-final. Using my annual leave, I stayed there for ten days, watching other shows, meeting comics, and frequenting too many bars. I bumped into an old acquaintance on the plane at Luton and this led to a very drunken first night. As a result, I wasn't in top form for the semi-final, as I didn't cope with the hangover very well. Some days before the gig, someone told me that the best comedians don't drink before getting on stage and I was watching my weight a bit at the time too, so on the night I performed I was sober and fairly self-conscious. Needless to say, I wasn't chosen for the final. At the time, I concluded that the lesson from this experience was to always make alcohol part of my preparation before going on stage. Clever me!

There were some silver linings to that first Fringe. I remember finding the whole experience very inspiring and educational, and feeling very much at home there. Also the artistic director of the *Gilded Balloon* venue, Karen Koren, came up to me after seeing my semi-final performance and told me that I "must keep doing comedy" because I "had talent." It was nice to hear, though her compliments did not result in any tangible benefits.

My return to London was somewhat gloomy, having not made the final of SYTYF, and having spent quite a few hundred pounds in the process. I reassured myself, however, that I didn't yet have enough decent material to cope with the better gigs that being in the final would have generated.

Edinburgh Fringe 2002 - *The Amused Moose Hot Starlets*

Following the Amused Moose semi-final in London (noted in chapter 11), I was chosen to be in their new acts show for the Edinburgh Fringe 2002. I was even in the main press release for the festival, which announced both my "debut" (apparently my 2001 performance didn't count) and my stuttering (Alberge, 2002).

I performed five shows in the The Amused Moose Hot Starlets. Part of the deal was to do two hours of "quality flyering" before each show. This was the first time I had regularly stood in front of the general public and spoken to random strangers. It definitely helped my confidence and made me feel less self-conscious about my speech. This was a fun week, mainly because I was in a show with friends, at least three of whom are now quite well known (Mark Watson, Nina Conti, and Rhod Gilbert). We did ten minutes each during the 55 minute show. One of the shows was attended by a well-respected comedian called Jerry Sadowitz, who told the promoter that I was destined to be "a big comedy star of the future" and that my stutter was "a comedy gold mine." So maybe I was moving in the right direction. The promoter's recommendation to me was to "use the stutter" as much as I could, but to "keep it controlled." This, of course, is not easy advice to carry out, given the realities of non-controlled stuttering.

In any case, *The Scotsman* gave me a good review, referring to me as one of a "strong line-up of comedians with disabilities" who was part of the "taboo-busting zeitgeist" willing to challenge the "attitude which cannot see past a disabled person's condition" (The Scotsman, 2002). The writer further noted that "the non-disabled punter's pity is at least as much a target for the humour as the performer's disability itself," which turns the tables on those with whom we interact (in my case, listeners) and thus "stimulates thought within the audience." It felt good to be part of a small movement pushing the boundaries, even though in reality I was simply trying to overcome my stutter.

After all of the excitement of The Fringe, I flew to the island of Gozo with two old school friends, which was good fun, though I remember thinking that I would rather be back in Edinburgh than lying on a beach. This longing was partly due to my love of comedy and also because I thought one of my friends (who was, unfortunately, later diagnosed with schizophrenia) threatened to kill me after a silly argument about our comparative driving skills. I spent that night sleeping on the beach, as I was too scared to stay in the flat.

2003 – *Birds*

In 2003, I was asked by comedian and friend Phil "Pigeonman" Zimmerman to perform in *Birds*, a show that ran the entirety of the festival. Performing at the Edinburgh Fringe in 2001 and 2002 taught me a great deal, but was not the same as doing a full run of three weeks. Having to be funny every day for 23 days in a row (15 to 20 minutes a day, plus a 5-minute sketch at the end) was a much greater challenge than the one week I had performed the previous year. More audiences meant greater diversity and I found myself trying to please drunken students, couples on dates, families with children, and even some very prudish and conservative elderly people, often simultaneously. Doing so required a kind of universally likeable and humble persona, and reasonably clean material, as an eight year-old was just as likely to be in the front row as an inebriated loudmouth.

Performing in *Birds* required us to work out a budget and I realised sponsorship was needed. Thankfully, the British Stammering Association stepped in, providing both a morale boost and financial rescue. They paid the printing costs for the posters and flyers, which was a huge help.

Our 40 word entry into The Fringe magazine read:

> *A journey into feathers and frustration starring Pigeonman Phil Zimmerman ('A genius' Omid Djalili), ITV's Stand-up-Britain finalist and stutterer-extraordinaire Jaik Campbell ('Big star of future' Jerry Sadowitz) and Welsh surrealist Steve Williams ('Simply enjoyable' Time Out.) Featuring Dolly Bird.*

The *frustration* part turned out to be prescient, in part because I hadn't focused enough time on my material and the time slot, 5.30pm – 6.30pm, was too early for me to get sufficiently tipsy. I still believed in the necessity of pre-show alcohol but, because that was our first Fringe show, getting a time slot more conducive to that sort of preparation (i.e., evening or later) wasn't realistic.

Other problems emerged as the weeks wore on. The room was too big for the audiences we attracted. One of the comedians constantly overran her time slot, which threw off the rest of the show. I also lived with three of my fellow performers for the month and secretly had a crush on one who didn't fancy me. This circumstance was a little difficult to accept and probably kept me from practising as much as I should have.

The last week of *Birds* was complicated because two of the comics were not able to perform and another wasn't feeling very well. That week is always the busiest, and so a few shows which were nearly sold out featured only Phil, the act's founder and headliner, and me. Hence, I had to open the show and hold the audience for 27 minutes before the Pigeonman flew out. It was a big challenge, requiring a great deal of lager and cigarettes, but the experience definitely sharpened my skills as a comedian. It also highlighted a dire need to have better, funnier material and so I focused more on writing when I returned to London.

Birds reviews

The reviews for *Birds* were mixed. Some were good, others representative of our general writing apathy, decreased commitment, lack of concentration, material shortages, unrequited love problems, hangovers, and overall despondency about the show's various setbacks. Kate Copstick, an important reviewer from the *Scotsman* newspaper, appeared when there were only six people in the audience and unfortunately that evening's show didn't go particularly well. She gave it one star, writing a particularly memorable review that still haunts me today:

> *The obvious reason for calling this show "Birds" is*
> *that when you play word association, the first word*

you get when you say "bird" is "s***." Cue a weak
Welshman, a nervous bloke with a stutter, and a guy
who had self-evidently decided to forego his medica-
tion for the night. I nearly bit out my own ovaries just
for light relief (Copstick, 2003).

To make matters worse, the review accidentally got printed twice on different days! Luckily, other critics viewed me differently. Ben Dowell of *The Stage* wrote, "Campbell's material is first rate but he needs to sharpen up his presentation and make stammering his comedic raison d'etre" (Dowell, 2003). An independent review-er (Styxx, 2003) wrote, "Jaik Campbell and his stammering ways were absolutely hilarious. I'd probably have been happy enough to pay the ticket price to see him only. New stuff, a different avenue of comedy, so very entertaining." Finally, a *Three Weeks* reviewer said, "Jaik Campbell was the only saving grace and a blessed re-lief" (JS, 2003). Comments such as these boosted my morale and inspired me to keep going with my stammering related material, as at least it was unique.

Back to London

The Fringe left me broke, both mentally and financially. Sorting out the venue bills, flat payments, and who was owed what from the ticket sales was basically a nightmare. After hours of emails it was all finally resolved (well, actually I'm still owed some money for the flat). I went back to Suffolk for a week or two, then returned to London, keeping myself busy with a mixture of stand-up gigs, extras work, and even a TV recording for a BBC2 sitcom review promoting the stuttering Arkwright character in the British sitcom *Open All Hours*. I also was filmed for a London Weekend Television programme in which people talked about funny occasions when they had been drunk. My story was related to the time I went to the toilet one night in my hall of residence and instead of walking back into my room afterwards, I accidently climbed into bed with a woman who's room was in the same corridor. There I stayed, too drunk to realise my mistake.

Between these London projects, I had two job interviews in Suffolk and, in both, mentioned being a comedian. Divulging this was probably my subconscious way of saying, "Please don't give me the job." If so, it worked.

2004

My move back to London in February 2004 (over my father's loud objections) was quite exciting. It featured a new job, a new flat in the borough of Enfield, and effectively a new life (for a while anyway). I liked living in Enfield, as it was part of London but felt like small market town, with its relatively relaxed atmosphere and pleasant parks. The setting contrasted the rest of my life, which was quite hectic. Not only were there new challenges at work, but before I left Suffolk I had applied for an "Arts Council East" grant to do a show at the Edinburgh Fringe 2004, and in March, just after I started my new job, I was informed that my application had been successful. From that point forward, I had difficulty organizing all of my new responsibilities. I was regularly late for work and, when I was there, I was tired and spent the first hour or so of every day replying to emails about the Edinburgh show. I actually got away with this schedule until I had to take the whole of August off to be in Edinburgh, which understandably didn't go down too well with the managers.

The idea was to do a "Three Man Wise Monkey" show, featuring comics who could not hear, see, and talk (I would be the latter). Unfortunately, the hearing impaired and partially blind comedians I had in mind both pulled out in April. So I had to find two new "monkeys."

330

I also had to write my material, handle all of the Arts Council and Fringe paperwork, and do a fairly complicated day job. I was busy from 8am to 11pm every day and there was little time for anything else. I did manage to work in an evening 30-minute jog, but still put quite a bit of weight on during this period.

Due to the nature of the Arts Council grant, I couldn't change the basic show concept. Luckily, I found Kevin Knite and Inkey Jones, two comedians who just about fitted the bill. We came up with the new title of *D-D-D-Don't Mention the Disability. I Did Once and it Took 15 Minutes,* or alternatively *The Good, The Blind and the Speechless.* This show was helped by having a good preview venue upstairs at the Round Table Pub, near Leicester Square in London, where we shaped our material. The Fringe program entry read:

> *Jaik Campbell brings you Kevin Knite, the world's only non-observational comedian, and Inkey Jones, Montenegro's official Steven Hawking's Tribute Band. The show that everyone¹s talking about, except Jaik.*

I tried to tell stories that were amusing and also educational, which I've always thought comedy should be. For example:

> *I've got what's known as the blocking type of stutter and the problem with blocking is that you force the word out so much that it comes out much louder than you had intended. Like I'm in a cinema on a date, and I want to whisper that I've got to go to the toilet, but I get stuck on the "t". So I say, "I've got to go to the (pause) TOILET!" Which leaves her thinking maybe a second date isn't such a good idea.*

331

Despite my efforts to keep the information humorous, one reviewer wrote, "Comedian or university lecturer on stuttering? He should decide" (Kay, 2004). Luckily, however, not all of my reviews were negative. For example, the words "Jaik Campbell" begin all of the following sentences:

- "...was endearing and enjoyable" (Healy, 2004).

- "...opened my eyes, unexpectedly, to what a useful tool a stammer can be in achieving perfect comic timing" (Disability Now, 2004).

- "...was the main act and...rightly so...not only did he keep the humour up but he also managed to educate the audience on the plight of those afflicted with stammering" (Ed-Fringe website, 2004).

Doing a show based on our own disabilities and shortcomings was a refreshing concept for The Fringe, which at the time lacked acts with that type of subject matter. The UK Arts Council likes shows that make "a contribution to peoples' lives" and increasing awareness of stuttering, poor sight, hearing, or other problems in a funny and positive way was a good way of achieving this. I believe that comedy should be thought provoking, and an honest and humorous view of life with disabilities is consistent with that belief. Our aim was to make the public treat disability in a more positive way, and help to change people's beliefs, perceptions, and judgements about it. In hindsight, we should have played it safe less often and pushed the boundaries more. Although saying the unsayable (not easy with a stutter) would have made a bigger impact, that's a relatively minor shortcoming in the grander scheme of things.

The show was kindly supported by the British Stammering Association and the Dominic Barker Trust, which helped alleviate some of the extra costs of what would otherwise have been an expensive month. Overall, we pulled off a reasonably professional comedy show, as most of the reviews reflected. We also obtained some good feedback from the audience. We were even asked to perform the show after The Fringe at the Queen Margaret University in Edinburgh in October, The Cut theatre in Halesworth, Suffolk, in November, and the Ipswich Arts Festival in July 2005. All of these performances were well received.

My return to Enfield was a self-imposed fairly solitary experience. I lived there from February 2004 to March 2007 and during that time I never saw one family member or friend in Enfield (not that I ever invited them, or even wanted anyone there). My time was spent working, gigging, jogging, reading, and writing at Enfield library, and religiously studying the *Timeout* magazine comedy listings. Becoming a better comedian was all that I was really concerned about. Once I lost my proper job in November 2004, I primarily focused on comedy and 2005 was spent preparing for a one man show.

2005

In January 2005, Griff Griffiths, a friend and fellow comedian, and I had a meeting with a producer from London Weekend Television to show him some sketches we had filmed for a program called *The Morning After Show*, a live Sunday morning offering on Channel 4. The next day I flew to Gran Canaria with my comedian friend, Alan Wilde, to film some more sketches for potential TV use. This trip proved to be creatively very productive and possibly one of the funniest weeks of my life.

Upon returning, I had an audition for a Channel 4 show called *FAQ U*, which went badly (mainly because I was sober). I was still living in the Enfield flat, but my roommate was about to leave and so I had the choice of finding either a new person to move in or a new place. In March, I found the latter. For the next six months I focused on preparing, organizing, structuring, and publicizing my 2005 Edinburgh show.

In hindsight, I should have waited a year or two before doing my own Edinburgh show, especially in a proper venue. My decision to do the 2005 Edinburgh show was rushed because I didn't know how long my time in London was going to last and because I realised that making a name for myself at the Fringe was going to take a long time. My mother was also keen for me to get all this "comedy stuff" out of my system as quickly as possible, and encouraged me to do it. Besides, I had wanted to perform a 1-man Edinburgh show ever since I had watched one in August 1996. On top of all that, I felt that doing a show about stuttering was a good idea whilst the material, media interest, and concept were still fresh. However, I did not give myself enough time to write the necessary amount of quality material and I probably spent too much money on the venue hire, as there was no *Free Fringe* in 2005.

By July, I was doing my first 55-minute preview of the show (which I had not finished writing) at the Etcetera Theatre in Camden, London. An experienced theatre director was in the audience and told me afterwards to make the show "autobiographical with a time line" so it would flow logically and be easier to learn. I thought this was good advice, but it meant spending the rest of July frantically trying to restructure, rewrite, and relearn the show, not to mention publicize it.

I felt that stuttering was a good angle to focus on and a good hook for audiences and the media, and this idea generated quite a few press stories published in local and national newspapers. In fact, my speech was so much of a focus that I called the show *I've Stuttered So I'll F-F-Finish.* My 40 words for The Fringe program read:

> *Campbell's award-winning, unique insight into love, life and stuttering. The show everyone's talking about, except Jaik. 'Genuine pathos' Scotsman. 'Sharp wit' Evening Standard. 'Satisfying comedy' Three Weeks. 'Endearing and enjoyable' List.*

2005 - I've Stuttered So I'll F-F-Finish

At Edinburgh 2005, I had a good timeslot (8.20pm) at a respectable venue (Cvenues, "Electric"). Before my first show, I had performed four previews in London. Nevertheless, the show wasn't in a perfect state when I got to The Fringe, and on the opening night, reviewers from two important publications, *The List* and *Three Weeks*, came to watch. Even for experienced comedians, having a critic sit there and take notes or peck away on a laptop on the first night is a fairly daunting prospect. I also had to quickly find an audience to contribute some laughter to the event. Whilst out flyering, I happened to meet two young women who both agreed to flyer for me over the next three weeks (I'm still friends with them today). I was allowed to "paper" the show a bit too, a process in which the production company (me) is allowed to give away free tickets reluctantly provided by the venue, because they realise that a good review, helped by a big audience, increases future ticket sales. Fortunately, both reviewers enjoyed the show, gave me three stars out of five, and praised the show.

I've Stuttered So I'll F-F-Finish was a one man show, 55-minutes long, sometimes going on longer as there was no show in the slot after me and the venue managers did not seem to mind me over-running. However, it was probably a mistake in terms of maintaining quality. I performed it for 26 of the 27 nights of the festival. The show was an egotistical journey: Short anecdotes about how the stutter had affected growing up, school, university, and jobs. Examples included:

> *Yes, I have got a slight stutter. I'm not actually a rap artist. It's not a glitch in the matrix.*

> *I come from SSSSSSSuffolk. That's Suffolk.*

> *It's a good thing I don't come from Cincinnati, otherwise we could be here all night.*

> *My father has a stutter, my grandfather has a stutter, and I have a stutter. Us three in a restaurant lasts forever.*

> *One of us says to the waiter: "I'm having what he's having."*

> *And then we realise no one has actually said anything yet.*

> *People at university didn't know how to react to the stutter.*

> *They'd say, "Sorry, have you got some kind of stutter?"*

> *I'd say, "No I just like making stupid facial expressions. It helps me get through the day."*

> *My first three panel job interview, I simply couldn't speak.*

336

I said "d- d- d- d- d- d- d- d- d- d- d- d- d- d- "

He said, 'Shall we turn the central heating up?'

I replied "D-D-D-D-   D-D-D-D-   D-D-D-D-"

He said, "I'm sorry we don't know Morse code."

Greene King IPA, a British beer company I had contacted a month earlier, offered to sponsor the show. They kindly couriered 192 cans of their product free of charge, which I divided up and left out on the seats for the audience before each show started.

As the days rolled by, I noticed that my speech improved, which led to greater self-confidence. I wondered about that link and, in a more general sense, how to become more confident and the different types and levels of confidence that people have. Why aren't we all just born with self-assurance? How much should we have? In an increasingly competitive society, confidence is useful, but too much leaves one arrogant and unable to see his or her own faults. I hated not feeling very confident, and felt my shyness was holding me back, both professionally and in my friendships.

I've been embarrassed so many times by my stutter that failures occurring on stage or in front of a camera were never that worrisome to me, no matter the size of the audience. But *I've Stuttered So I'll F-F-Finish* was the first time I felt that I might be doing more than I could handle. Performing for 55 minutes a day in front of a paying audience pushed me completely out of my comfort zone. Still, I trusted myself to do the show in spite of my fears, and this trust gradually morphed into confidence. If I had waited until my fear had disappeared, I would still be waiting.

Tickets were priced between £7.50- £8.50, so the performances had to be worthy of this. I needed to focus on everything that was going on around me and ignore any doubts inside my head. To accomplish this, I once again turned to my old friend, Mr. Alcohol. Looking back, I sometimes had to force myself to drink in order to be funny which regrettably has made me hate the taste of lager now. Given that I was performing every day, I had to be disciplined to make sure the alcohol intake was at least somewhat restrained.

My days were spent waking up at about nine, doing some exercise, having a leisurely sugar-filled breakfast, walking over to the venue to check ticket sales and note which reviewers were coming in that day, and then going on a long run, which doubled as rehearsal time. The jogging prepared me for the next onslaught of alcohol and the mental stress of trying to remember the material. I gave myself at least an hour before I went on stage to eat, go over the script, drink lager, and try to relax. The afternoon was spent flyering for at least two hours and speaking to people to encourage them to watch my show. Fortunately, it worked. Attendance was normally good. When the act personally leaflets his or her own show, ticket sales multiply radically. Thus, it was no time to be shy.

At 8.20 every night, I walked onto the stage as relaxed and confident as I could be. I was in a proper venue and couldn't show any nerves. I performed the show and then returned to my room, had a good meal, sobered up as much as I could, and normally listened to a recording of that night's show (so I could hear which parts of the routine worked and which might need to be changed). I tried not to go out too much, so the days were quite solitary.

Sticking to this schedule, I was able to produce quality shows by all accounts except one: *The Scotsman* gave me one star, calling the show "painful" with "weak material" (Cox, 2005). That description would have bothered me more, but the same evening I met an Italian woman who told me that most Scotsman reviewers 1) are 50-60 years old and 2) spend their time outside of August writing travel or business features and thus lack any understanding of modern comedy (her words, not mine).

My show improved as time went by. I became more familiar with the script and I felt more comfortable with the venue and with the types of audiences that turned up each night.

Staying committed to the material every day was a challenge and I didn't watch many other shows because I found doing so normally affected that commitment. However, it was sometimes useful to watch the bigger names to see how other one-person shows were put together. One of the most successful shows of Edinburgh 2005 was Demetri Martin's *These Are Jokes*. He stood on the stage, sometimes with a guitar, and simply told funny, concise, and original jokes, e.g.:

I think it's interesting that cologne, rhythms with alone.

It was a very cleverly written, well-structured, and critically well received show. It made me want to write some quality, pathos driven, rueful, honest, and original material. Except for the most brilliant story-tellers, character comedians, or ventriloquists, quality performances need a lot of punchlines. Otherwise the show should go in the drama section.

By the end of the run, I slowly learnt the complexities of holding an audience for an hour, but definitely needed new material. I wanted something uplifting and positive, not just some bloke going on about how depressing his life has been.

Life affords stressful and dismal times for all of us, and people watch live comedy to escape from the reality of life.

Overall, I'm pleased that I took the risk and tried the solo performance. It helped my stage presence and made me a better comedian. Acceptance of and even pride in having a stutter were additional benefits from this experience. I no longer viewed it as a negative thing. All told, the gains were worth the £2,300 I spent on venue rental, accommodations, travel, and marketing.

I also realized that organizing a show, writing it, and learning all the lines, as well as staying physically and mentally fit, required a great deal of organisation and/or a complete lack of any social life. Fortunately (sort of), I didn't have a personal life at the time, having lost contact with most of my friends due to my self-imposed hectic schedule.

After The Fringe, September and October 2005 were spent mentally recovering. My mental tiredness and frustration again weren't conducive to having a relationship. Indeed, one female comedian I met at The Fringe promptly declined to go on a date with me after she said I sounded too angry on the phone. I was also doing the odd bit of extras work, as well as gigs here and there. One of them was a performance for the Dom's Fund Charity Evening in Suffolk, in memory of Dominic Barker. Mr. Barker was a man who shot himself because of his stammer.

My act at this point started to go off in two directions. One was doing a series of one-liners, such as Jimmy Carr, Milton Jones, or Tim Vine do, and the other was exploring the humour of being in a minority group (i.e., as a stutterer). I decided to continue writing about the stutter as there were just too many comics aiming at the sharp gag route. I felt that stuttering was a unique selling point. I also enjoyed the self-deprecation of doing stuttering-related material as it was easier to make the audience warm to my act.

2006

I didn't do an Edinburgh 2006 because my performance scripts needed improving and because I couldn't afford to perform again at a proper venue. I also increasingly felt obliged to help with a few routine family business matters back in Suffolk, as well as fit in a wonderful (and solitary) 2-week holiday in Gran Canaria.

I did do two shows at the 2006 Camden Fringe called *Leastwanted-UK*. The name was born of a realization that there weren't many moments in my life when I felt particularly wanted, either by my parents, my siblings, or my friends. I think that was my fault a bit. I was never a big fan of people in general and it was difficult to let people love me when I hadn't learnt to love myself. I also let my need for behavioural confidence (i.e., being professionally successful) override my need for emotional confidence (i.e. my need to be in a good relationship). If I had been less worried about trying to make it as a comedian and simply enjoyed my one and only life, I would have probably liked myself more. I had gone from letting my parents have too much control over me to allowing my ambition to do the same.

My stutter, hair loss, and general insecurities gave me a few personal issues to deal with. Regular exercise seemed to help my self-esteem, as did becoming less daunted by women. Also, borrowing from other peoples' confidence worked. I watched how actors stood, held themselves, breathed, walked, and smiled and tried to transfer these mannerisms to my own life.

Life's issues added up but, luckily, I could find humour in them. This process would become the inspiration for my next Edinburgh fringe show.

Edinburgh 2007

In May 2007, I spent three pleasant weeks in Croatia, primarily to attend the World Conference for People who Stammer. I found this experience very enlightening. I met many different people from all over the world who were all united by their stammers. Some of the notable individuals I met included a Croatian film director, a singer, and even a Croatian politician. None had let their stammers get in the way of success. Many people at the conference seemed impressed that I was doing stand-up comedy, and I gave a routine at the end of the gala dinner, and a workshop on, of all things, improving confidence. One of the things I recommended to the audience was to run naked along a Croatian beach to increase self-confidence and reduce self-consciousness. This raised an eyebrow with the aforementioned politician, who was sitting in the front row.

I came back to Edinburgh in 2007 with another stammering-based show at a free venue run by the Laughing Horse promoters with whom I got on well. My aim was to make the first 30 minutes gag after gag of funny punchlines, but the theme was less positive than the 2005 show. The 2007 offering was primarily an act about my life, loss, and overall despair. I called it *Jaik Campbell: L-L-Lost for Words - My Life with a Stutter – Free*. In The Fringe magazine it stated:

> *Winner of the BSA writing award and ITV's Stand-Up-Britain finalist, Jaik explores his life and stutter. 'Genuine pathos' Scotsman. 'Sharp wit. Smart one-liners' Evening Standard. 'Original gags' List.*

342

The show was originally going to be called *Least Wanted UK* but I had a girlfriend when I named it, so I went with my second choice. Shortly thereafter, of course, she dumped me, claiming that she wasn't the right girl for me. Then I thought a more apt title would have been *Jaik Campbell: I'd happily dance over my own grave.* I was in a black mood!

The time slot I was given wasn't good (4 to 5pm) but I didn't negotiate very well or want to cause a fuss, and so decided to go ahead with it anyway. My objective was to simply enjoy it this time, rather than worrying about every little detail. This resulted in a better, more relaxed, and laid back show, notwithstanding the less-than-ideal slot.

Despite being a free venue, I normally had a fairly full room of people who were quite generous about putting money in the bucket at the end of the show. That was a nice bonus. As noted earlier, performers are not necessarily at The Fringe for the money. They're basically there so people go from saying, "Who in the world is that?" to "Oh yeah, it's that guy."

In 2007, I worked a little with the comedy writer Nick Thomas, who thought the stuttering gags were unique and original enough to be the show focus. The logic was simple. There were many white, middle class comedians doing jokes about how they can't get girlfriends. But few can talk perceptively about stuttering. The material this time was a bit darker than the 2005 show, and still fairly self-deprecating, as the following examples show:

> *I was a bit of a reclusive, shy child. At school instead of writing an essay on "what I did in my summer holidays," I wrote an essay on the places I hid in my summer holidays.*

I live in Brixton, London, which is quite a scary place to be honest. I don't really like things that generate constant terror and stress. Having said that, I am thinking of getting married next year.

There's no easy cure for a stutter. There's no drug you can take, although the drug "speed" is useful.

There's something called a speech therapy CD you can buy, which plays speaking exercises through the night to help someone get over their stutter.

I bought the CD, put it on, and went to sleep, hoping to be cured.

It got stuck. I woke up in the morning, I couldn't speak at all.

I used to think that nobody cared if I was dead or alive in London, which luckily wasn't true.

Nobody cared if I was dead or alive anywhere.

I went to the World Congress for people who stutter a few months ago. All the other stutterers were there to learn about their stutter. And I was there just to get material.

And because the girls couldn't say no.

Although they could still write "no".

The queue to the bar was a nightmare.

Again I did quite a bit of flyering before the show and made a point of speaking to as many people as I could to encourage them to attend. Persuading people to watch the show was easier than in 2005, as "free" is a good selling point. I decided that if I was having a good time on and off stage, so would the audience. This decision led, for the first time in my life, to a surprising bit of female attention. My timeslot meant that I was fairly drunk each day at 5pm, leading to a few early evening flirting antics. These exploits backfired on me badly when my girlfriend heard that a friend of her flatmate had been chatted up by a stuttering comedian. That description was difficult for me to deny.

Based on at least one review, the show was moderately successful. *The Stage* (Wilson, 2007) noted my alleged "charm," "warmth of character," and "first-rate gags," but saw a "faltering performance" that was short on "confidence (and) structure." I returned home feeling definitely more self-assured and enriched by the Edinburgh experience.

2008

I started 2008 with a new job. Going to Edinburgh every year costs money, after all. Unfortunately, the role—digitising satellite images for the Ministry of Defence—was seriously tedious, requiring me to practice a great deal of patience, which nearly drove me insane. In fact, someone who had previously worked at the same place on a longer shift pattern actually did end up in a mental institute. Some of the people I worked with told me that the two occurrences were possibly connected, and after a few months working there, I could see why.

Difficulties started early when someone told my boss about my comedy side-line. He called me aside one day and said, "Tell me I haven't just hired a comedian."

I said, "No, to be honest I'm not very funny. *The Scotsman* newspaper once only gave me one star." He unfortunately wasn't laughing and kept a close eye on my daily output from that day forward, sternly telling me "not to let comedy interfere with my work."

All told, my time there was a dreadful, soul destroying experience and the job basically involved working with the living dead. In all the months I was there, no co-worker ever asked me a question about the work, or even how I was. From my experience there and my life in general at that point, I was inspired to write a new show called *The Audacity of Hopelessness*. I originally wanted to call the show *Jaik Campbell: C-C-Confidence*, but somewhat ironically ran out of the confidence to do so.

The Fringe programme description read:

> *Fringe regular and ITV's 'Stand-Up-Britain' finalist, Jaik Campbell, speaks from the heart to explore hopelessness, confidence and finding happiness in today's society. 'Brutal honesty' (Three Weeks); 'Gifted' (Stage); 'Terrific. Smart one-liners' (Evening Standard).*

My press release elaborated:

> *"The Audacity of Hopelessness" is the 3rd one-man show from Fringe regular and ITV's 'Stand-Up-Britain' finalist, Jaik Campbell, who speaks from the heart to explore hopelessness, confidence and finding happiness in today's society. Natural disasters, wars, failing economies, global warming, getting older, failed relationships: it's easy to feel lost and hopeless sometimes and unable to change things*

and most of the time, the sad fact is you can't. Fol-
lowing on from then-US Senator Barack Obama's
book, "The Audacity of Hope", Jaik comedically ex-
amines various subjects and concludes how essen-
tially nothing can be changed, but avoiding fear and
getting more confident are useful.

Jaik says: 'Without wanting to sound too depressive
or political, the fact is the World is going through a
fairly hopeless period. Indeed, surely hopelessness
is better than hope? When you're hopeless you don't
care, and when you don't care, the world is an easier
place to live in. It's only when you start caring that
you have hope, which can lead to frustration and
despair, so perhaps it's best just not to care at the
start. So maybe hopelessness is the key to life. It's
certainly my only hope.

Edinburgh 2008

I performed for ten shows at Edinburgh 2008. What is sad is that
I had a good venue and a great time slot (*Laughing House Espio-*
nage, at 10.20pm- 11.15pm), but due to the demands of my job,
I couldn't take more than ten days off. I was too scared to ask for
more time, thinking I would be fired. This seems silly looking back,
given that I hated the job so much.

I think there was also a part of me that wondered whether doing any
more Edinburgh shows was really worth the hassle. Given the mental and financial stresses, lack of decent material, negative effects
on my health, and constant offers to part me from my money, the
experience was a fairly costly one. In addition, I remember feeling
that the public is constantly bombarded with information about new

fads, pieces of technology, or TV shows. They have the internet, cable TV, mobiles, and many other sources of entertainment at their fingertips. To get people to pay for a live show is not easy.

Eventually I would conclude that entertaining, writing jokes, and performing a show I could be proud of were very important to me. Much of that goes back to having a stutter and growing up with a workaholic father who didn't like me. Part of my inferiority complex was a need to show the world that I'm not just an idiot who can't speak. Also, I believed I had a talent for writing, learning, and performing comedy. It was something I felt very passionate about and I needed to fulfil that passion.

Some of the most successful acts of recent years in the UK have been based on material about belonging to unique groups. They enlarged upon their distinctiveness, and clever gags emerged. The comics established characters that audiences tuned in to see. An example is Omid Djalili, who talks about being Iranian. He uses his accent to great advantage. In terms of both style and content, I was doing much the same with my stutter. Writing comedy is a fairly organic process, somewhat like a flower on a plant. It takes time to grow (although alcohol is sometimes the water), but when it does eventually flourish, it can look quite good!

My 2008 act was half comedy show and half self-help, the latter because I felt that my life contained too many compromises. It was an expression about not living up to my full potential and the difficulty of finding the right partner. My soulless job and lack of girlfriend were once again affecting me! It was a show that was honest, mainly because I wanted to avoid meaningless jokes and talking about nonsense for an hour. My theme was that I could stop being a pawn in the game of life and take more control. As such, the show covered love, confidence, and both hope and hopelessness.

I went on a confidence course. To pay for it I sold my car and my laptop. At the end of the course they said. "You'd be more confident with a car and a laptop."

I've just finished a confidence course to help with my dating. Now I have the confidence to handle the rejection from three women instead of two.

I once said to my mother that my stutter sometimes makes me feel like the whole world is against me. She said "That's not true. Some countries, like Switzerland, are neutral."

My stutter has given me quite low self-esteem. I ran up to a garbage truck a few weeks ago.

I said, "Am I too late for the rubbish?"

He said, "No, mate."

So I jumped in the back.

I was never very good at meeting women. In fact, my love life now is like a fun fair.

It's not fun. It's not fair.

Despite the darkness of the material, those ten days in Edinburgh 2008 were a good time. A number of factors came together in my favor. The favorable time slot meant I had all day to prepare, exercise, and focus on doing a good show. The audiences were also more relaxed and therefore up for more fun and laughs (certainly a contrast from the 4pm audiences of 2007). I also liked the venue, as it was part of a large nightclub called *Espionage*, with great bars, a good sound system, and at last some decent toilets! Once the show was finished at about 11.15pm, there was a two to three hour calm down period, spent in the nightclub chatting to audience members, watching other acts, dancing, drinking, and basically enjoying myself.

Dare I say it, but as a single man, to have several hours each night being surrounded by a largely female audience I had just made laugh, with my posters on the wall, was quite an ego boost. I enjoyed the attention and chat. My accommodation for those ten days was in a nearby student hall of residence, so there wasn't a long walk back at 2am either, which was quite handy. The show was also the funniest I had written, with stronger punch lines and higher quality material that generated big laughs. My only regrets were the free venue status and not doing a full festival run. Unfortunately, these factors kept me from being reviewed, but I took solace in the (mostly) positive audience comments on the EdFringe website.

The 2008 Edinburgh Fringe was a necessary escape from the pressures of reality, especially having been stuck behind a desk for many months. It was also a chance to catch up and have a laugh with some old friends who valued my company far more than the people in the digitizing office did. I was at a time of my life when I had no commitments, having split up with my girlfriend in July, and I was enjoying being free and single again. And because of my job, I at last had some money at Edinburgh, which didn't hurt.

The reality of the job gave me a sense that this might be my last Edinburgh Fringe. That kind of lifestyle with responsibilities is difficult. Someday adding a wife and children would make it impossible. But that festival provided me with some good memories and a different identity. For the first time in my life, I didn't wear a jacket on stage, partly because it was hot but also because I wanted to look more relaxed and laid back. I usually held a pint of lager or had one on a nearby table. It was intended to be a security blanket, but ended up serving mostly as a prop, reminding me to enjoy being on stage and savor the moment as much as possible.

The audience was much younger (normally in their twenties/early thirties) than the 2007 show. I was worried that they wouldn't want to hear about my inabilities to find a girlfriend and a good job. But the usual material comedians use for such audiences—the difference between men and women, sex related gags, relationships, airport security, flying, society's absurdities—is quite difficult to make original, as so much has been written about these areas already. The moment a comedian starts in on such standard comedy topics, it can sound plagiarized.

Despite the overall positive response, a few audience members told me after the show that they thought that the title was too negative and the act a little depressing in places. They had a point, though in my own defense, I had just split up with my girlfriend and had a job I hated. Besides, the show ended with me singing an upbeat karaoke version of Frank Sinatra's *New York, New York*, with lyrical changes to make it about Edinburgh. The audience seemed to like that and, as a bonus, I don't stutter when I sing!

As an aside, returning to the office and digitizing lines onto maps after such a successful two weeks had to be one of the most depressing come downs of my life.

Conclusion

Edinburgh taught me pathos, humility, charm, patience, and emotional empathy. In a way, my father had already honed these skills by his criticism and showing me the negative effect he had on people. So I lived my life trying to do the opposite.

In the same way, I hope to bring my children up in a more patient and understanding manner, although I appreciate that this is not always easy.

The Fringe had other lessons to teach me as well. Performing comedy at Edinburgh takes a great deal of time, effort and preparation. The London circuit was a useful foundation course, but The Fringe was advanced training. Learning to perform for the audience rather than for myself took a while, but it was an important lesson. Figuring out how to engage with them took time too. The first five to ten minutes therefore normally involved speaking to the audience and having some fun with them. For example, I might ask, "What do you do for a living sir?"

"I'm a builder"

"How long have you done that for?"

"Ten years."

"What is that—an estimate?"

There's a skill to poking fun and being "nice" at the same time. I was careful to avoid alienating or demeaning anyone in the audience. Interestingly, because of my laid back, stuttering "nice guy at a party" persona, I could get away with being ruder than perhaps the average male comic.

Looking back, I should have put more effort into writing material that pushed the boundaries. To please a critic from a broadsheet newspaper is a serious challenge and takes writing to a new level of consciousness and originality, something I wasn't prepared to put the time into, given that I normally had to work real jobs to pay real bills. Edinburgh was a good platform to challenge concepts such as prejudice toward the disabled. The best Edinburgh shows take the audience on an emotional ride of highs and lows, and makes them think about the world in different ways, something I could achieve only through comedy. My priorities were my stutter and self-confidence issues, rather than writing excellently crafted jokes.

Although I went to Edinburgh to stutter, I often felt, strangely, that there wasn't time to stutter there, especially during the last week which was always the busiest. I had to be a performer, as well as a salesman, persuader, and technology geek, all at the same time. Like the London comedy circuit, The Fringe was desensitizing. I could potentially spend many hours a day talking about my stutter in radio and newspaper interviews to promote the shows, whist out flyering, on stage, and even perhaps in the bars afterwards, especially if someone who stutters was in the audience, which quite often happened.

Performing in front of an audience for 55 minutes every day for nearly a month allowed me to accept my stutter. In fact, my speech was a unique selling point and therefore a useful "hook" when speaking to newspaper journalists. But I had to marry it to a friendly, non-threatening, non-depressed image (not easy on a daily basis).

When I was feeling confident, I tried to generalize that feeling to every aspect of my life and control more everyday situations. For example, I tried to smile at the newsagent when I bought a paper or sound more relaxed when answering the phone. I tried to believe in myself more as a person. When I started to feel independent and more in control of my life, the better my speech became (though not necessarily my bank balance).

If money is your God, the Edinburgh Fringe probably seems a fairly pointless exercise. Still, I learnt about entrepreneurship there because putting on a show felt like a small business start-up: a product, advertising, sales, and constant evaluation. Its success or failure was based on whether the customers (i.e. the audience and critics) liked the product (i.e. the material and performance). In addition, it provided a platform for experimentation. I could try out new, unusual, and edgy material and personas at relatively low cost and risk, and get instant reaction and feedback. It was a reasonably safe place to fail. A few bad reviews one year meant that I could return the next and try again with a different approach. Through this type of trial and error, I learnt what worked for audiences and what did not, a process that stimulated my own innovation. Other types of start-ups need a similar way to learn from mistakes. Perhaps if we want more entrepreneurs and more new businesses, then the Edinburgh Fringe might be a useful model to follow. We need safe places for creative entrepreneurs to try out their ideas.

A friend once said to me, "The thing is Jaik, I'm not being harsh, but I think you are capable of so much more than comedy."

I answered, "Well the thing is, I think comedy is capable of so much more than comedy. That's why I keep doing it."

I have often considered comedy to be one of the most important of the unimportant things in life. We're not saving lives but we can effect small change.

I honestly believe that comedy has the potential to break down barriers between people (for example, seeing that stuttering does not have to be an insurmountable obstacle to public speaking opportunities).

On a personal level, the Edinburgh Fringe was a therapeutic process. Making jokes about the past and turning negatives into positives was healing. I learnt about myself and how the past is simply that and I must try to move forward positively. Life in many respects is out of our control, so there's little point becoming too upset. Comedy was a way of making sense of experiences such as growing up with a stutter, time at university, and a bullying father. It is amazing how such negatives from the past lingered. It was do the Edinburgh Fringe, see a therapist, or take drugs. Despite the hundreds of hours of writing, performing, and analysing, I have not achieved full resolution of all my life's issues, but then maybe no one ever really does.

If I ever go back, it will be a more upbeat show, called something like *Positive Life Lessons* or *Smile—You Know You Want To*. In contrast to my last appearance, I could talk about positive life lessons, namely the joys of being in a stable relationship, settling down, and having children. The trouble with that, however, is the difficulty of writing funny material when everything is positive. Comedy is, after all, about conflict. When people laugh, the joke is on someone. For me, that someone was usually myself.

> *If I'm in a nightclub, I try and tell the girl at the start that I have a stutter. But I usually get stuck.*
>
> *I say, "Hi. I'm a st- I'm a st- I'm a st- I'm a st- "*
>
> *And my friend says, "He's a stalker."*
>
> *She then asks, "So what do you do for a living?"*
>
> *I say, "I'm a comedian."*

And she says, "A comedian with a stutter?"

I say, "Yes it's my way of getting more stage time."

Questions for Discussion

Would all people who stutter benefit from a festival-like experience of constantly talking to people about stuttering? Why or why not?

To promote his shows, Jaik had to talk to random people attending the festival? Was that good for him? Explain your answer.

Why do you think an established comedian referred to Jaik's stuttering as "a comedy gold mine?"

A promoter recommended to "use the stutter," but "keep it controlled." Why would someone believe such a balance was possible?

It appears that Jaik got mostly positive reviews, yet is haunted by the few negative ones. Do you believe such sensitivity is human nature, or somehow related to growing up with a stutter?

Another reviewer wrote that Jaik should "make stammering his comedic raison d'etre." How would that be accomplished?

Did Jaik's humor about stuttering change across his many Fringe appearances? If so, how?

Can humor help the plight of people who stutter? If so, how?

Stuttering is a theme in every new show. Can an entire comedy show be based on a disability? How much time is the right amount to talk about stuttering?

Does the 2008 theme of "stop being a pawn in the game of life and take more control" reflect the stuttering journey? Explain your answer.

Jaik discusses comedy that pushes the boundaries. How would that be accomplished with the topic of stuttering?

If one of Jaik's priorities for performing at Edinburgh was to help his stutter, was he successful? Why or why not?

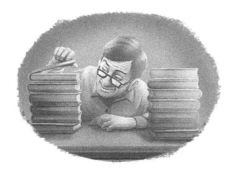

Chapter 14: Recovery, Correlates, and Suicide

Once again, Jaik writes of the relationship between confidence and fluency. In his early Edinburgh Fringe appearances, he longed for improvements in both in order to better speak to venue organizers, technicians, colleagues, partygoers, producers, directors, passers-by, and, of course, his audiences. Although he described his then-self as low on confidence and terribly self-conscious, performing at a major international festival, with all of the associated speech demands, requires not only courage, but a level of confidence that is well above that for which he credits himself. In fact, if a client told me he wanted to work on confidence, but could not begin until after he staged three weeks of stand-up comedy at Edinburgh, part of me would wonder if there was anything I could really do for him.

As noted (see chapter 4), the research on fluency and confidence is sparse and seems to indicate a relationship that stems from the former (or, more precisely, that disfluency can lead to reduced confidence). In previous chapters (and parts of chapter 13 as well), Jaik did view confidence as an attribute that rises and falls in direct proportion to fluency, but to him, the two features influenced one another. That is, not only could fluency improve confidence, but a confident speaker would necessarily be more fluent. From this perspective, confidence is easy to track—it is there when speech is good, missing when it is not.

Jaik is referring the *state confidence*, which is situation-specific and notoriously changeable (Harrison, 2013). Given that description, it makes sense that it can be directly proportional to fluency, just as it seemingly is to audience feedback. Contrast that with *trait confidence*, a more innate and stable attribute (Harrison, 2013). Trait confidence is what keeps getting Jaik back on stage after disfluent or poorly received shows. He has an inherent belief in his ability to succeed.

Later in chapter 13, Jaik began to consider the idea that confidence is actually a complex concept. Yes, some people are more confident than others, but everyone has situations in which he or she is comparatively more (or less) self-assured. And although added confidence feels good, it is not really true that the more one possesses, the better life will be. We can all think of examples of individuals whose excessive confidence makes them, as Jaik put it, "arrogant and unable to see his or her own faults." What Jaik longs for is an ability to handle every situation appropriately, always saying the right thing, projecting an assured attitude, and having no regrets afterward. Given that most nonstutterers desire this ability as well, its absence may not be associated with stuttering to any large degree. And if fluency does not necessarily lead to confidence, could it also be said that confidence doesn't require fluency? Jaik does not answer this question outright, but his journey toward acceptance seems to suggest that he will do his best to find out.

Recovery

Over time, the communication experiences associated with The Fringe (and with comedy in general) and Jaik's gradual acceptance of his stuttering seemed to shift his priority from fluent speech to effective communication. Without this transition, I would argue, he could not have accomplished all that he did. To someone who stutters and makes a living with his voice, talking only when fluent is next to impossible. Doing so would require both constant and successful use of fluency-enhancing techniques, an approach he has already rejected as unsuitable (see chapters 5 and 6), or spontaneous recovery, which is also improbable.

This is not to say that people never stop stuttering during adulthood. Some do, often for no clear reason (Cooper, 1972; Finn, 1996, 2005; Wingate 1964). Their number is clearly small, but exactly how small is difficult to estimate. For one thing, some who claim to have recovered probably never stuttered in the first place (Lankford & Cooper, 1974). Confusion also stems from the likelihood that "recovered" is sometimes defined as greatly diminished (but not terminated) stuttering. Perhaps more important than determining the prevalence of late recovery, however, is the evidence that there are some people who recover from stuttering as adults and others for whom the severity is greatly reduced.

One question raised by such evidence is: *Why* do some people experience late recovery from stuttering? In separate summaries of the data, Logan (2014) and Finn (2004) identified some of the subjects' self-professed reasons for it:

- Practice and eventual habituation of speech modifications (e.g., Finn, 1996; 1997),

- Motivation to change (Finn, 1996; Quarrington, 1977).

- Improved maturity (Johnson, 1950),

- Increased confidence (Johnson, 1950),

- Greater awareness of problem(s) (Shearer & Williams, 1965),

- Relaxation (Shearer & Williams, 1965),

- Change in attitude (either general or speech-associated) (Quarrington, 1977; Wingate, 1964), and

- Making a conscious decision to change (Anderson & Felsenfeld, 2003).

Of course, Jaik could not sit around and wait for an event as unlikely as spontaneous recovery. He had a life to lead and, with it, a limited opportunity to climb the ladder of comedy success. For him (and indeed for most people who stutter), acceptance offered a better way to proceed toward his goals.

Jaik mentioned acceptance several times, always with respect to how performing stand-up allowed for its occurrence. Equally interesting, however, are the indirect references to this process. For example, he stated, "I've been embarrassed so many times by my stutter that failures occurring on stage or in front of a camera were never that worrisome to me, no matter the size of the audience." I find this to be a very provocative statement. It reminded me of a story about a professional baseball team that lost a 5-run lead in the bottom of the ninth inning of an important game.

The question that emerged subsequently was, "How can they possibly recover from such a crushing loss?"

Commentators agreed that they could not. When former and current professional athletes were interviewed, however, the answer was much different. The losing team would simply accept the reality of a bitter defeat and move on. The logic was that because of the large number of games each of their players had endured—from T-ball to professional ranks—they had all repeatedly suffered every type of baseball-related disappointment imaginable. Given that they kept playing anyway, it follows that, like Jaik, they possessed the ability to put failure behind them.

That raises the question of why everyone who stutters is not able to shrug off embarrassment. After all, they have all had plenty of experience with it. So why is acceptance of stuttering so difficult? There are two ideas to keep in mind regarding this question. One: failures performing a basic function such as speech are more shameful and less acceptable than losing a baseball game. Thus, moving past them will surely prove to be more difficult. Secondly, the example given does not refer to all athletes. Rather, it references only those who were able to accept disappointment well enough to reach the highest level of their profession.

Also interesting is how others accepted Jaik's stuttering. Once it was established that he was going to stutter on stage, promoters and others contemplated how to take advantage of it. Stuttering became an angle, a means of showcasing their star. One promoter recommended that he "use the stutter" as much as possible, but warned Jaik to "keep it controlled," as if stuttering is a faucet that can be adjusted for flow. It is not quite the same as "slow down" or "think before you speak" or some of the other common pieces of advice received by stuttering individuals. Those are designed to induce fluency. Recommendations to manipulate the stuttering to proper effect seems to suggest that somehow the amount and severity of disfluency is under conscious control, even if its presence is not.

Stuttering as a Learned Behavior

It is instructive that the notion of stuttering as a voluntary act is still present in the general population. It is an idea that was prevalent in early learning theories of the disorder, the most well-known of which are more than a half century old:

- In the *anticipatory struggle hypothesis*, Bloodstein (1958) theorized that stuttering arises because children become convinced that speech is difficult but must be done well. The results of these beliefs are tension and struggle when attempting to execute perfectly fluent speech movements. In this way, the anticipation of stuttering is also its cause.

- Sheehan (1958) wrote of stuttering as an *approach-avoidance conflict*, whereby individuals struggle with desires to both speak and not speak (leading to ill-timed starts and stops that are manifested as disfluencies).

- In perhaps the most famous learning theory, Johnson (e.g., Johnson, 1942) hypothesized that a child's normal speech breakdowns are mislabeled (by parents) as stuttering and, consequently, the child is instructed to change how he or she talks. By definition then, the child has moved from normal to abnormal speech patterns, which over time emerge as stuttering. This model has been called both the *diagnosogenic theory* (as the diagnosis of stuttering causes it) and the *semantogenic theory* (because the word *stuttering*, applied incorrectly to some children, carries enough power to permanently disrupt speech).

More recent research has contraindicated such theories, as well as the general notion that stuttering is voluntary. For example:

- Stuttering children are *not* normally speaking individuals who just happen to present ill-timed speech breakdowns. As noted in chapter 2, the disfluencies of incipient stuttering children are qualitatively different from their non-stuttering peers; they present significantly more part-word repetitions, prolongations, and hesitations. This finding makes it more difficult to explain how mislabeling normal disfluency leads to stuttering.

- Parents of children who stutter interact with their children in basically the same ways that parents of non-stuttering children do (Cox, Seider, & Kidd, 1984; Meyers & Freeman, 1985). There are no differences in how they identify disfluencies (Zebrowski & Conture, 1989) or with their parent-to-child verbalizations (Miles & Bernstein Ratner, 2001), calling into question the supposition that perfectionistic parents are the cause.

- Direct therapy methods, designed to teach and reinforce novel speech techniques (i.e., to focus on the child's speaking), are reportedly effective with many preschool clients (see chapter 6). Such success counters the belief that there is harm in calling attention to stuttering.

- When the diagnosogenic theory was tested empirically (Tudor, 1939), no basis was found for the conclusion that badgering children about their speech can make them stutter.

Stuttering as a Physiological Disorder

On the surface, physiologic differences between people who do and do not stutter during speech is also contradictory to the notion that stuttering is a learned behavior. That is, such research findings seem to indicate underlying system differences associated with stuttering.

During production of fluent speech, functional variations have been found in the respiratory (Baken, McManus, & Cavallo, 1983; Williams & Brutten, 1994), phonatory (Bakker & Brutten, 1989; Tsiamtsiouris & Cairns, 2013), and articulatory systems (Hulstijn, Van Lieshout, & Peters, 1991; Janssen, Wieneke, & Vaane, 1983; McClean & Runyan, 2000) of adults who stutter when compared to non-stuttering samples. Furthermore, group differences were found when coordination *between* these systems was examined (e.g., coordination of respiration with phonation or articulation) (Perkins et al., 1976; Williams & Brutten, 1994). These sorts of differences have led theorists to speculate that people who stutter have difficulty making quick and necessary motor adjustments when speaking (Max et al., 2004; Neilson & Neilson, 1987). It should be noted, however, that some researchers did not find such differences (Bakker & Brutten, 1987; Cross & Olson, 1987). In addition, the differences found were based on group data. That is, they are not true of all people who stutter. More to the issue of this chapter, speech system variances do not necessarily reflect organic differences. It is not unreasonable to assume that one's communicative history could, over time, change motor speech patterns. Stated differently, experiencing difficulties with speaking could result in alterations within and between the responsible biological systems. Indeed, McClean, Kroll, & Loftus (1990) found group differences in articulatory movements, but only between non-stutterers and the stuttering subjects who had recently received therapy. The no-treatment stuttering sample, that is, the ones who presumably did not receive training related to speaking movements, were not significantly different from the control group.

Stuttering as a Neurological Disorder

In addition to physiologic differences, researchers have examined neurologic components. The idea is not necessarily to discover the precise site of lesion that causes stuttering. At this point in time, the proverbial haystack needle would be easier to find. Given that we do not typically observe comparable motor deficits in people who stutter (e.g., prolonged or repeated limb movements), it is probable that any key neural deficit would have to be microscopic. And in addition to the problem of size, there is the matter of location. As noted in chapter 10, human brains house numerous neural sites and generators that can be involved in speech at any given time. Moreover, the extent to which any one is activated depends on variables such as language level, feelings, environment, and countless others (Webster, 1999). Taking into account these limitations, finding the responsible brain area would literally be more difficult that finding the needle in a haystack, because at least the needle is there whenever someone is looking. When I first entered the field, I heard of microscopic brain damage being compared to finding one's house on a globe. First we need a workable map of the correct country, then the region, city, and neighborhood. Advances in technology since then have probably moved us beyond the globe level, but we cannot yet claim to be in the neighborhood.

All of that is not to imply that neurobiological research on stuttering is valueless, however. In fact, much the opposite is true. Research has established some important neuroanatomical and neurobehavioral characteristics that vary between people who do and do not stutter. For example:

- Neuroimaging studies have indicated atypical patterns of cortical, subcortical, and cerebellar neural activation in stuttering subjects during perception, planning, and production of speech (Brown et al., 2005; Chang et al., 2009, 2011; Fox et al., 1996; Watkins et al., 2008). A key observation was anomalous right hemisphere dominance. These results are consistent with a decades-old theory that suggests stuttering results from a lack of cerebral dominance for speech (e.g., Travis, 1978). That is, midline speaking structures receive neural input from both hemispheres; a dominant hemisphere is needed In order to coordinate the signals. When this coordination is absent (according to the theory), stuttering can result.

- DeNil and colleagues (e.g., DeNil et al., 2004) used positron emission tomography (PET) to uncover right biased motor cortex and cerebellar activation with untreated stuttering subjects during silent reading, a task which resulted in *left* biased activation in the nonstuttering speakers.

- Dichotic listening studies, in which auditory stimuli are presented simultaneously to each ear and the subject identifies which one was perceived (i.e., a word is presented to the left ear, a different word to the right, and the listener tells which he or she heard) have indicated that adults who stutter most often show a left ear preference (e.g., Sommers, Brady, & Moore, 1975). This is in contrast to the general population, for which a right ear preference most commonly occurs, indicating that language is being processed in the left hemisphere (because that is where information into the right ear goes most efficiently).

- Similarly, when visual material is presented concurrently to each eye in tachistoscopic studies, subjects who stutter more often show a left visual field (or right hemisphere) advantage when compared to normally fluent subjects (Hand & Haynes, 1983; Moore, 1976).

- Electroencephalography (EEG) findings indicate differences between stuttering and nonstuttering subjects (e.g., Weber-Fox, Wray, & Arnold, 2013), including atypical right hemisphere alpha wave suppression patterns (Moore, 1984) during language processing. This suppression indicates active involvement of a particular brain area, in this case the right hemisphere. Thus, EEG provides evidence of processing differences associated with stuttering.

- Foundas and cohorts (2003) found that nonstuttering adults presented greater right prefrontal lobe volume in comparison to the left prefrontal lobe. In contrast, stuttering subjects were unlikely to show such a pattern. This could well be an important distinction because, as the authors point out, "atypical asymmetry patterns have been found to be associated with anomalous functional cerebral laterality" (Foundas et al., 2003).

- PET scans reported by Wu and colleagues (1997) indicated increased dopamine activity associated with stuttering. Dopamine is a neurotransmitter that has been linked with other conditions for which speech is unique. For example, Parkinson's disease is associated with imprecise articulation, reduced pitch inflection, and monotone (Ramig, Fox, & Sapir, 2004), as well as decreased dopamine levels. On the other hand, an overactive dopamine system occurs with schizophrenia, a condition marked by, among other features, pauses, and unusual intonation (Alpert, Kotsaftis, & Pouget, 1997; Stein, 1993).

- In comparison to nonstutterers, reduced white matter integrity has been observed in cortexes of both children and adults who stutter (Cykowski et al., 2010; Sommer et al., 2002; Watkins et al., 2008), perhaps indicating disconnection between speech motor planning and production centers of the brain.

As noted earlier with the physiologic differences, these results are based on group differences and do not apply to ever individual who stutters (Foundas et al., 2001; 2003). Another similarity between the two lines of research is the chicken-and-egg type of quandary with functional differences. In the case of neurologic findings, do brain variances result in stuttering behaviors or could a lifetime of disordered actions alter neural organization? Addressing this issue, Watkins et al. (2008) note that differences found in children suggests the former sequence. If so, it might help to explain the high relapse after stuttering therapy. That is, perhaps the innate patterns are strong enough to eventually usurp any new behaviors learned in therapy (see DeNil, 1998). Without constant updates, the operating system defaults to factory settings.

Stuttering as a Genetic Disorder

In comparison to the research addressed in the chapter to this point, investigations of heredity and genetics more strongly move hypotheses of stuttering etiology away from strictly learning. Some key findings include:

- Susceptibility to stuttering runs in families in patterns consistent with genetic transmission (Kidd, 1984; Records, Kidd, & Kidd, 1976). Interestingly, neither severity nor recovery appear to follow any predictable transmission patterns (Kidd, 1980).

- Based on longitudinal research, it appears that more than two thirds of stuttering preschoolers present positive family histories of stuttering (Yairi & Ambrose, 2005). When isolating the persistent cases (i.e., the preschoolers who did not recover), the chance of a stuttering relative jumps to 88% (Yairi & Ambrose, 2005).

- Studies of twins (Andrews et al., 1991; Felsenfeld et al., 2000; Howie, 1981; Rautakoski et al., 2012) indicated that far more monozygotic (identical) twin pairs are concordant for stuttering in comparison to dizygotic (fraternal) twin sets. That is, when the shared genetic material is closer to being identical, the chances of both twins stuttering increases rather dramatically. This appears to strongly implicate heredity as a causal factor of stuttering. As documented in chapter 4, however, it is often difficult to separate nature and nurture. To this point, Starkweather (1987) noted that monozygotic twins react to their environment similarly, so their resemblances do not necessarily exclude environmental factors. This would seem to be supported by the less than 100% concordance (i.e., some identical twins are *dis*cordant for stuttering, suggesting that something other than heredity is at work here). To this supposition, however, it must be noted that monozygotic twins are not completely identical in terms of genetic makeup (Bruder et al., 2008); genetic divergence can occur at various points in the genome during imprinting. Also, twins are more susceptible to perinatal distress (Stromswold, 2006), which could also make them less than identical.

- In gene marking studies, linkages have been found between stuttering and specific chromosomes (e.g., Dominques et al., 2014; Raza et al., 2013). More precisely, chromosomes that predispose individuals to stutter have been isolated within specific families. As Logan (2014) pointed out, however, the chromosomes identified vary across the families studied, allowing few conclusions to be drawn regarding which genes are linked to stuttering.

Given the aforementioned findings, it is now fair to state that the genetic contribution to stuttering is not really in doubt. The question is how big a contribution it is. Based on their investigations of twins, both concordant and discordant, Rautakoski and colleagues (2012) used structural equation modeling to determine that 82% of the variance in liability (i.e., the amount that can be explained by heritability) to childhood stuttering was attributable to genetic effects, with the remaining 18% due to environment. This is a greater discrepancy than determined by others (Andrews et al., 1991; Felsenfeld et al., 2000) and is unlikely to be the last word on the subject.

Stuttering as a Psychological Disorder

Although the idea of clinically abnormal disfluency being as manageable as Jaik's promoters would like is at odds with much of the research cited in this chapter, it does fit the misconception that stuttering is a psychological condition. This myth likely originated with repressed needs theories, a collection of hypotheses in which stuttering is viewed as the voluntary consequence of neuroses. According to such theories, people are disfluent because communication results in divulging thoughts and feelings that are shameful and/or frightening (Travis, 1957). The stuttering child both desires and fears speaking, resulting in speech that is disjointed and broken. What is bothering the child could be unresolved oral-erotic needs of childhood (Coriat, 1928), anal-sadistic level fixations (Fenichel, 1945), or something simpler, such as anger. Repressed needs theories are unsupported (Bloodstein, 1993; Manning & Beck, 2013) and not widely believed within the field. Still, SLPs should be wary, as these sorts of hypotheses do arise from time to time. Parents might believe (or, more correctly, have been told) that they have instilled deviant fears in their child, for example. Worse, the client may perceive stuttering as an emotional disorder, cured by greater understanding of self or fulfillment of basic needs. It is worth noting that attempts to eliminate stuttering via emotional counseling have not been particularly effective (Bloodstein, 1981).

Related to repressed needs theories is the idea that stuttering results from some emotional occurrence in childhood. As noted in chapter 2, there is no evidence to support this notion. Children are exposed to environmental stressors quite regularly. Thus, even if it could somehow be determined that a child's stuttering began right after his best friend moved away, this does not place the blame squarely on the move. If the child was genetically predisposed enough that one event could trigger the stuttering, it is almost a certainty that if the move had not happened, another equally effective spark would have soon lit the same fire. Clinicians are warned that the lack of evidence for sudden onset in response to emotional trauma will not stop people from asking an individual what caused his or her stuttering. Of course, the answer to this question is far more complex than they believe.

Stuttering and Suicide

Although emotional trauma does not cause stuttering, they can, of course, exist concurrently. In some cases, the results are devastating. Jaik writes of the sad case of Dominic Barker, a young man who stuttered and took his own life at the age of 26 (BBC News, 2006).

Any discussion about stuttering and suicide should begin with the point that most people who stutter are not at-risk (Donaher & Scott, 2014). Common warning signs, however—such as anxiety, anger, withdrawal, feeling trapped, fear of embarrassment or humiliation (National Alliance on Mental Illness, 2012) — are certainly not foreign emotions to many who stutter. Moreover, bullying, experienced by so many stuttering individuals (see chapter 4), increases the risk of suicide-related behaviors (Suicide Prevention Resource Center & Rodgers, 2011). Bullying can lead to depression, anxiety, and substance abuse on the part of the victims (Centers for Disease Control and Prevention, 2010), all of which are considered suicide risk factors (Suicide Prevention Resource Center & Rodgers, 2011).

Determining an individual's risk for suicide is outside the scope of practice for SLPs. Still, awareness of risk factors, and a means of making referrals to the appropriate mental health professionals can be beneficial (Donaher & Scott, 2014). After all, few professionals have as many opportunities to listen to individuals who stutter. Such referrals can save a life, a point made clear by Palasik (2013) who places an SLP and some communication disorders graduate students in the small group that rescued him from suicide.

Conclusion

Jaik concluded chapter 13 with some lessons learned at Edinburgh. Quite appropriately, he discusses acceptance, specifically how stuttering openly in performances and interviews resulted in his disorder becoming a regular and even necessary part of everyday life. What his story does not specifically say, but clearly demonstrates, is that stuttering was often secondary to such festival details as learning his lines, creating a suitable image, promoting his shows, checking ticket sales, and pleasing critics. Speech, forever his main worry in life, was relegated to the background. Although this may not fit everybody's definition of acceptance, it does show that stuttering's power over him was diminishing. In fact, given how his speech became a "hook" to draw attention to his work, one could even argue that stuttering went from handicap to benefit.

Acceptance was further demonstrated by Jaik's comedy, in which his targets were less himself and other people who stutter, and more those with whom they must communicate on a regular basis. As evidence, I present Jaik's report of an Edinburgh review (The Scotsman, 2002):

> "…the non-disabled punter's pity is at least as much a target for the humour as the performer's disability itself," which turns the tables on those with whom we interact (in my case, listeners) and thus "stimulates thought within the audience."

This is a common theme with stuttering comedians. As noted in chapter 10, many report transitioning from poking fun at themselves to the more fruitful area of comedy, listener reactions (Williams, G, & Campbell, 2015).

In a sense, they are saying that they are not the ones at fault for problems that arise within the stuttering communication dynamic.

Perhaps the distance he put between himself and stuttering was what Jaik was referring to with the statement, "When I started to feel independent and more in control of my life, the better my speech became..." If he is referring to independence from the negative emotions of stuttering and defining *better* speech as effective communication, I agree. His examples of confidence displays—increased control of everyday situations and greater belief in himself—illustrate that the concept of effective communication is not necessarily expressing profound thoughts without missing a detail. It can also involve simply interacting with newsagents minus the former apprehension or shame.

Finally, prior to Jaik's concluding thoughts, there was another statement deserving of reaction. He quoted the following line from a review (Kay, 2004): "...comedian or university lecturer on stuttering? He should decide."

Can't university lecturers be funny?

Questions for Discussion

Can you think of an example of a skill for which trait and state confidence were not aligned, that is, confidence seemed lacking at times, but you stayed with it because of your innate belief in your ability? How about a skill in which a lack of confidence led you to quit? What was the difference between the two examples?

A client says, "Some people recover as adults. Why can't I?" How do you respond?

What are the potential harmful effects of viewing stuttering as a wholly learned behaviour?

Do you think a stuttering client would feel empowered by the idea of stuttering being a neurological disorder? Why or why not?

Research suggests hemispheric differences between people who and do not stutter for variables related to silent reading, language processing, and prefrontal lobe volume. Do you believe that any of these findings are related to the old theory that stuttering results from a lack of cerebral dominance for speech?

There has been much research on genetic contributions to stuttering. How do you explain new cases (i.e., people who stutter with no family history of the disorder)?

A client says, "I can talk fluently by myself, to my dog, and when talking to babies. If I can do it then, I can do it any time. That proves that stuttering is psychological." How do you respond?

How would you set up a referral system for potentially suicidal clients?

Acceptance of stuttering is another theme of the last two chapters. How do you define such acceptance?

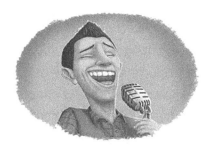

Chapter 15: Was It Worth It/ Any Regrets?
Moving On. What Next?

It's interesting to consider the different routes we all take once we leave school. Some people are happy staying at home with their parents, others want to travel; some can't wait to start flash corporate careers in the city while others stay in educational institutions; some go wild and others want to marry their high school sweethearts, settle down, and have children as soon as possible. There are those who desire riches and fame and those happy to take whatever they need to get by. There are no right or wrong answers regarding how we live our lives. In my case, I never quite knew exactly what I wanted, but losing my stutter and making a bit of money were on the list.

If we take the view that there is no afterlife and that the sun will extinguish its source of hydrogen in four billion years' time, thereby making all creative work meaningless, then maybe we should simply try to enjoy our short ride on this amazing planet. From that perspective, comedy is potentially a poor use of time. With or without a stutter, it can be a stressful and terribly frustrating activity. It would not be difficult to think of better experiences.

Many life choices are influenced by our parents and childhoods, no matter how much we resist that idea. In terms of proving anything to my father, stand-up didn't work. His view of me remained unchanged. He never said, "Well done getting as far as you have with the comedy." He never saw me perform a live show or commented on (or laughed at) any of the material I wrote. As chapter 7 revealed, I did comedy in large part because of his influences. But to expect any equilibrium or justice from a man like that is always going to be difficult; in fact, it's probably impossible.

By the time I performed my last Edinburgh Fringe Festival, I was living in Suffolk. As I mentioned, I had never really been comfortable in the big city. Reducing my comedy schedule and ending some of my London friendships had been mildly traumatic, as was moving closer to my father. But this time life had a pleasant surprise for me.

In early 2009, a friend set me up with Jennifer Humphreys, a popular, outgoing, and successful woman who I liked from the start. Naturally, and in true self-deprecating style, I convinced myself that she didn't much care for me. I even told her that at the end of the third date. Luckily, it wasn't true. To this day, I'm still quite surprised that we even made it to a *second* date. Jenn is very sensible and level-headed and, as previous chapters have shown, I am often the reverse. But we did have much in common. We had both been brought up by busy, self-employed, entrepreneurial-type parents. We attended the same primary and secondary schools (though she was three years behind me) and similar universities. In fact, I knew her older sister Suzannah at school (she apparently had the crush on me!). Jenn and I had both moved back to Suffolk after working in cities. More importantly, we both enjoyed comedy, travelling, music, films, beaches, good food, country walks, and jam and chutney making!

One difference between us is that Jenn is extroverted whereas I would hide away on my own for weeks on end if I could. This disparity can make family get-togethers awkward and I didn't really bond well with Jenn's late father. In addition to being outgoing, Jenn is self-disciplined, organized, well balanced, and has a professional career. Even so, she is very patient with my addictive personality traits, obsessive compulsive tendencies, moodiness, and dislike of authority.

Fortunately, our similarities outweighed our differences and we saw a great deal of each other that year. In August, we took our first holiday together, to Egypt. Jenn became quite ill with food poisoning. I did my best to help her feel as comfortable as I could and realised that it felt natural to care for her. From that point on, I recognized what a good partnership we are.

Being practical, Jenn researched me before our first date and knew that I had a stutter. From the start, however, she handled it with intelligence, patience, and understanding. It has never been a barrier to our relationship or even fazed Jenn in any way. As a result, I rarely stutter in front of her unless I'm very tired or stressed.

The Birth of Angus

When the time came to discuss having children, Jenn was more sure about the idea than I was. Being responsible for new lives who would depend on me for the next 18 years (and probably beyond) was a scary proposition. I had always imagined myself taking on this responsibility at some point in my life. However, I realise children tend to duplicate how their parents speak and act and I certainly didn't want them to copy my stutter. A moral responsibility rattled in my head.

My own childhood was also a consideration. When children are bullied at home and don't learn ways to resolve conflicts peacefully, they are more likely to react aggressively when events spiral out of control with their own children. I didn't want to be a bullying parent.

On the other hand, any children we had would have an extraordinary mother. And I had a partner able to soothe my worries. In the end, her certainty about starting a family won out.

My son, Angus, was born on 28th December 2011. One lesson learnt from the experience was that when it comes to having children, living 30 miles away from the nearest hospital is not ideal. The birth was induced, a process that the nurse informed me would take many hours. Receiving a promise that someone would call me when the contractions started, I calmly drove home, cooked myself a meal, and went to sleep, making sure my mobile phone was charged and next to my bed. At 7:30am it rang and panic ensued. I quickly got dressed, ate some breakfast, and checked that the oven was off, cat was fed, and house was locked before driving to the hospital. I arrived about 9:30am and Angus was born 90 minutes later.

Another lesson from that day is that there isn't really much a father can do during the birth of a child apart from look calm and reassure the mother that she's doing a great job. Unfortunately, it turned out that looking calm whilst my partner was in obvious agony was not in my skill set. Her pain instantly became my pain and I began to wonder if having me in the room with her was actually a help! Luckily it all went fairly smoothly; I even cut the umbilical cord. The relief that it was over reminded me of walking off stage after the Stand-Up Britain final.

The Birth of Emma

After some gentle persuasion about how Angus needed "some company" and that the house "had the space," I agreed to try for another baby. On August 13th 2014, our second child Emma was born, a birth more traumatic than her brother's.

The morning before the birth we were very relaxed, making marmalade, doing a bit of shopping in the local town, and playing with Angus in the playground. In one of the shops I met an old friend. Suddenly the first contractions started, but I was carried away talking. The seriousness of the moment was soon made clear to me, however, and we drove home. I attached Jenn's back up to a TENS (transcutaneous electrical nerve stimulation) machine to relieve the pain during the contractions, by then more regular. I rang up the hospital and nervously explained that the contractions were about seven minutes apart.

The woman on the phone asked, "Is this her first born?"

"N- N- N- No," I answered, "this is her husband."

She told me to drive to the hospital straight away.

At that point, I repeatedly checked the oven to make certain it was off and the door, to assure it was locked. Taking care of the little things while worrying about the birth was overwhelming. At least in comedy I could prepare for the scary moments. The birth of a baby allows little in the way of rehearsal. Mother Nature is firmly in control, but the costs of errors on my part were potentially great.

I drove as fast as I could to the hospital, ignoring a red traffic light just before the entrance. The contractions were getting stronger and by the pitch of the screaming, I could tell that the time was near. I parked outside the reception area and helped Jenn inside and onto the lift. We were escorted into a white and warm delivery room, Jenn in serious distress.

I turned to the nurse and said, "Have I got time to move the car? I didn't buy a ticket."

"No! You're about to have the baby!" she answered.

Sure enough, Emma was born about 2 or 3 minutes later. I cut the umbilical cord, and held my new child.

"What is it?" asked the nurse.

"It's a baby," I said.

"No. What sex is it?"

"I think it's a girl."

"You ought to know the difference by now," observed the nurse.

"I don't get out much," I admitted.

From that day on, I have had two beautiful women in my life.

Children

A family means I can't be a loner anymore. Social anxiety is no longer an option, as there are children's parties and school meetings to attend. Having an increasingly frail mother and a father who has limited patience with children puts more pressure on me to be an involved father, as I have to help quite a bit with the child care.

I can't simply hand my children over to my parents to watch.

Angus, now four years-old, is, unsurprisingly, more verbal than his baby sister. When we have friends over for dinner, he always wants to join in the conversation. All he is likely to add is a non sequitur about his love of trains, but I don't tell him to be quiet (well OK, maybe if he carries on too long). I certainly don't shout at him, as I know what it was like being a child looking for a little bit of positive guidance and support and instead receiving only criticism and negativity.

Writing this book has shown me the control parents can have on a child. I will no doubt face dilemmas with my own children in that regard. One of the big ones will be whether to let them head off into the world, or persuade them to stay nearby. Jenn has already told me that they are free to do as they please, so maybe the decision won't be so difficult after all. "If you love someone set them free" as the saying goes.

The four of us live in a house less than 600 yards away from my parents. That fact alone should serve as proof that priorities change with the arrival of children. Why did I move so close to stark reminders of childhood disapproval? Because we found a beautiful farmhouse that I know my children will enjoy growing up in. That's what's important.

I sometimes wonder whether passing my genes onto other human beings was sensible, what with my stutter, obsessions, depression, and the like. But then I look at my two children and find nothing wrong with them (yet!). My daughter Emma can only say a few words such as "Daddy" or "Duck," but luckily not "D-D-D-Duck." Angus likewise shows no sign of having a stutter. His speech is clear and he has a wide vocabulary. He doesn't display any negative emotions or behavioural problems, apart from the usual naughtiness that comes with being a child. In fact, he is very confident, already showing signs of leadership in his nursery.

Of course, I still have concerns that either or both of my children might show signs of stuttering in the future, but what I observe now makes me think about the whole "nature-nurture" balance. What if I had been less criticised growing up? What if I had been listened to and not constantly interrupted by my father? What if I had been allowed to have a year off before going to university, or had some support for the jobs I wanted to do? What if my father had instilled confidence in me rather than constantly overruling my thoughts and ideas?

My father views his cattle feed business like a special child. He put thousands and thousands of hours into it, but at what cost? He has high blood pressure, shouting fits, no proper holidays in which to relax and unwind, and three children who have never been able to spend any quality time with him. I would be mortified if my children grow up to feel the same way about me.

Genetically there is a high chance that one of my children will stutter, but by giving them time to speak, instilling confidence in them, and using early intervention techniques, I will try to keep it from ever starting (if I can). There is no doubt that my stutter seriously affected my life, and I would feel very guilty if their lives were tarnished in the same ways.

Reflections on Comedy

As my priorities shift and I look back over the years, sometimes I wonder whether I was really cut out for comedy. Ideas flow when I write this book, but an original joke with a hilarious punchline is agony to create. I have learnt the persona to help deliver a good line and may have even picked up a degree of acting ability in the process, but the costs were high.

My old friend, Jamie Bushman, emailed me in 2006 and advised me to stop doing comedy as he felt that I had gained enough through it and it was "having a warping effect on me." He may have been right. Except for the super talented writers and performers, the rewards from being on stage are limited. There came a point when I started thinking, "OK, it's time to stop doing this nonsense." Life is short, after all. If there were an afterlife where we can continue making people laugh, then having that "killer routine" would actually be worth perfecting. But that doesn't seem like a proper likelihood on which to base life decisions. Here on earth, our capitalist western societies tell us that cash flow is king and competition and money making are the ideals we must confront. Few of us can be "lilies of the field," existing in splendour while awaiting our dream opportunities.

Most men decide in their twenties or thirties whether to marry, which potentially forces them into a conventional, structured, and more disciplined existence, especially if children are added to the scenario. Deciding instead to go it alone allows for more maverick activities. Governments fear the lone man. They don't worry about the one married with children. If I had married my first or second girlfriend, I don't think either would have appreciated me suddenly announcing, "I want to be a comedian!" The need to earn money and learn a proper profession would have outweighed any show business dreams. So although I went through significant pain and heartbreak from not seeing either of those two women again, it opened the door to many interesting and nonconformist years, for which I am grateful.

President John F. Kennedy said "There are risks and costs to action. But they are far less than the long range risks of comfortable inaction." With this perhaps in mind, sitting on the comfy sofa in the evenings was certainly not an option for me as a young adult. With comedy, at least I was doing *something*. But like most things in life, there were pros and cons to this decision.

Pros of Doing Stand-up

I will start with some of the benefits derived from comedy.

1. Making people laugh was a good feeling and an empowering high

The high I obtain from doing a good gig is something I rarely experience any place else. The feeling of stepping onto a stage and having the audience in the palm of my hand for 10 or 20 minutes is simply empowering. Not even a heckler can ruin it. For those brief few moments on stage, the world is my oyster and I am untouchable. I'm not worried about doing the washing or even keeping my family happy. I'm doing it for me and I can feel nearly invincible.

The sad bit was, from being "the man" on stage, the next morning I would normally wake up and revert back to the same old insecure little boy, Jaik Campbell.

2. Good practice for work presentations, commercial life or even politics

My time as a stand-up comedian taught me various skills transferable to everyday life. For example, I learnt to deal with the pressure of being watched on stage and off, and hence have no problems being observed by a manager or assessed in an audit. I also am less worried than I used to be about asking a question in a meeting or giving a presentation.

For a time, I was interested in politics, and felt that in 20 years' time the Prime Minister of the UK would probably be an actor or comedian (a bit like Ronald Reagan was in the US). I was not training for that role particularly, but stand-up gave me the ability to practice the public speaking I would need if I ever decided to pursue politics. Today that seems unlikely, as I'm much less motivated about being a politician now than I was in the past.

On the other hand, comedy may have taught me to be too genuine for politics. Most high ranking politicians have been coached on how to make certain issues more dramatic and to emphasise particular parts of their rhetoric, but such histrionics are not always authentic. As a comedian, I have to make the audience believe that I experienced the personal events mentioned in my routine. I had to learn to connect emotionally to myself and my audience, to immerse myself deeply in the material in order to convey it as realistically as possible. When I trundled out lines that were over-rehearsed but devoid of any heart, the audience immediately saw through me. I realized why great actors are great actors. They don't just repeat lines; they move the audience at a deep level. With a few exceptions, politicians fail to deliver such convincing and authentic personas.

1. It (usually) cheered people up

Success is not necessarily about money or attention. It can be about giving the gift of laughter to even one person. Normally after a good performance, someone would come up to me and say something like, "Thanks, you really brightened up my week." At an Edinburgh show, an audience member once explained that he had been serving on a submarine for 40 days, only to be told by the Navy upon his return home that his mother had died (apparently it is not Navy policy to inform crew members of family tragedies whilst on board). He had missed the funeral as well as the death announcement, and was understandably in a very depressed state. Apparently watching my show had cheered him up and improved his mood. Upon hearing that, how can I argue that comedy wasn't worth it?

The emotional connection between a stand-up comedian and the audience can be something quite profound. According to Dr. Tim Miles (2014), there is "a complex symbiotic relationship between the stand-up comedian and their audience…a relationship that is, in some ways, similar to a doctor and patient." Indeed, some of the comedians in Dr. Miles' study stated that they offered a "therapeutic service" or some sort of "drug;" references to comedy as medicine, therapy, and a device for "feeling better" were made by audience members too (Miles, 2014).

If stand-up is done correctly, there is also a bond among audience members. Indeed, research exists to support the idea that laughter brings people together; we laugh "not so much because something is objectively funny, but because we want people to like us, or we want to feel part of a group that's laughing" (Miles, as cited in McNamee, 2014). As such, live stand-up comedy fulfils a need for feelings of truth, trust, empathy, and intimacy between strangers in a society where many experience different types of isolation.

3. It helped my stutter, self-confidence, shyness, self-consciousness

As discussed in chapter 9, the application of comedy to stammering is complicated. Stuttering is, after all, a sensitive subject, one in which laughter is usually equated with mockery. But like any problem, laughing at it is also a step in defeating it. The tricks are finding the funny side to stammering and using the humour to help people empathise with the battle.

In terms of reducing my stutter, stand-up comedy was mainly worth it. I still have a stutter, of course, but it is more controllable than when I was in my twenties or thirties. I guess it might have improved regardless of my chosen career, but I believe that public speaking week after week definitely helped. And I couldn't think of many better ways to improve my confidence or self-esteem. Stand-up gave me the ability to command a room or situation with empathy, respect, compassion, and charm. Comedy teaches situational control of communication environments: the ability to walk up to any human being and speak in a calm, respectful, and persuasive manner; the skill to handle a job interview and know that it will go well; the capacity to go on a date and know that the girl will not attempt to escape out of the toilet window.

There are few people I've met in my time who have perfect or even natural leadership skills. Most would rather follow others. Leaders have to learn how to lead, which involves pushing their comfort zones. Comedy forced me to do that, given that there is nothing comfortable about stuttering on stage. It also taught me more about (and therefore to be less scared of) women, though more learning is needed in that area.

I think one of the problems of having a stutter is that it can erode self-esteem. I found myself believing that negative inner voice that says, "You can't do this, you're not good enough." Over time, I became accustomed to not liking myself and addicted to the easy surrender that came with convincing myself that I wasn't very confident. I was gradually becoming an expert at suffering.

If stuttering leads to self-loathing, there then is a reasonably good chance of disliking other people as well. I might, for example, question whether a girlfriend really likes me or has other motives. What's her angle? Is she cheating on me? Predictably, the relationships break apart, leading to the downward spiral of more self-doubt and isolation. The world of stand-up comedy served to silence the negative inner voice. I learnt to accept and make light of my shortcomings and become stronger and more independent. In time, I saw myself as deserving of love.

I don't want my children to have the same confidence issues that I had. I regularly tell them that they are beautiful and clever, and I try to be kind and patient with them (most of the time). As a parent trying to pay the ever-increasing bills, I worry that there simply isn't time to instil self-belief and self-worth in my children. Maybe that was my father's problem. He worked too hard all his life and never had time for teaching or communicating positively with his family. Most of the comments he could muster were belittling, critical, and bullying. Unsurprisingly, both my brother and sister have some confidence anxieties as well.

It's a difficult balance. I have a friend whose father was the complete opposite of mine. All his life, my friend was told that he was brilliant and could do what he wanted. He ended up a drug addict. His brother, a very likeable person, has hardly been out socially for years now. It's only one family, but it does make me wonder if somewhere there is an equilibrium between telling children they are great and being a proper disciplinarian.

4. Increased body confidence

Apparently UK schools are being urged to hold classes in body confidence, as research has shown that two-thirds of teachers say that pupils arrive at secondary school (aged 11) anxious and insecure about their shape and appearance (Griffiths, 2014). They potentially feel embarrassed to raise their hands in class or to take part in physical education activities. They don't measure up to the "ideal" bodies and fashionable clothes seen on western society TV and in magazines.

Spending time with stand-up comedians, I realised it wasn't the performer's looks or clothes that made an act funny. It was the material and persona on stage that counted. One of my favourite comedians is Daniel Kitson, who normally performs in a pair of old jeans, an unironed shirt, and a big beard. What I took away from Daniel and others was to believe in myself without worrying about what I am wearing or how my hair looks (when I had hair). I didn't learn to like my appearance so much as stop caring about it.

5.   Improved desensitization to and acceptance of stuttering

Stuttering was a subject that audiences seemed to find interesting. The more stand-up I did, the more I talked about stuttering and the more desensitized I became to it. It opened a road to acceptance. Rather than making out that I didn't have a stutter or simply ignoring it, my speech became an important part of me and my act. By confronting the problem head on week after week I improved it.

It's hard to add up the number of hours I spent on the London Comedy circuit writing, practicing, and performing material about my life and my stutter, but it must have run into the thousands. All that time and effort helped me to realize that stuttering wasn't shameful but actually a character trait that could be celebrated and applauded.

Before doing stand-up, I could not talk to strangers very easily. I would clam up in front of adults, particularly authority figures. One of my coping mechanisms was to deny the existence of the impediment, relieving myself from the pain by simply acting as though my stuttering didn't exist.   But although denial can offer protection, it also forces separation from the problem. At school I concentrated on what I did well, such as passing exams or writing coursework. In that way, I was able to diminish the effect that stuttering was having on my life. I should have practiced speaking more, but doing so would have forced me to admit that I had a real problem. Then as an adult, having to express myself well to pass an interview or handle a date, denial was no longer possible and, in fact, became a self-destructive act. Stuttering became a ghost that haunted me every time I faced a new day. Stand-up comedy forced me to bring that ghost into the open. For the first time, I could practice speaking with an end pay off. This endeavour by far had the biggest positive impact on my attitudes toward speech.

6. A view to helping my children

Children provide hope—that a little piece of us lives on after death. And even in the present, looking after one's self becomes a more serious responsibility with dependents who will be close by for at least the next two decades.

One of the problems with the mistreatment I received growing up is that I do not always realize when my behaviour is uncaring. If bullying is the norm, after all, it's accepted as part of life, even viewed as typical (which of course it's not).

I believe that childhood bullying is connected to challenges in handling emotions, a lack of self-discipline, and an inability to manage stress, which causes people to react to difficulty in snappy and impulsive ways. When parents use abuse as the means to converse, children grow up without proper communication skills. They, in turn, display frustration and poor communication with their children, and so on. I wanted to avoid the cycle.

Healthy relationships can also be difficult to establish coming from a home in which the father was sometimes abusive towards the mother. The message a child potentially receives—that women are weak and need to be controlled—could affect not only the partner, but their offspring as well.

Stand-up comedy allowed me to view life from a new perspective and become a more positive and functioning person. I feel my hundreds of gigs taught me better communication skills, eased my frustration, and hopefully made me a more tolerant person. I do admit that I am not as calm and patient as Jenn, who grew up in a more stable household. Her model has taught me much about love and understanding, vital lessons to learn. Children aren't too worried if parents are rich or poor, after all; what is essential to their wellbeing is the parents' unconditional love.

Because childhood is such a crucial time of life, I want my children to grow up in a more reassuring way than I did. If you want and expect less from life, it becomes simpler and smoother. With lofty hopes comes extra pressure and stress. I therefore hope my children don't have such high expectations of life as I did.

My father said to me recently that he didn't think spending time with young children was worth it as they won't remember it anyway. From my perspective, however, learning to trust a parent takes a long time. In some cases—speaking personally here—it never happens. I want to have a good relationship with my children and want them to always trust me. I don't need them growing up to write a book about my failures!

To be fair, most men I know are not particularly adept at looking after children. They see it as a difficult task and would rather watch rugby highlights. Our ancestors spent their days hunting and gathering, and I think modern day man is still programed to do this. He would rather work and gather money. I took my son to swimming classes and children centre groups, and for walks to the woods. I know how looking after young children requires a great deal of patience, understanding, and love, traits I could not inherit from my father.

I met a guy at work who said he's never been happier now that he's divorced. He can travel to where he wants and do the things he's always wanted to do (e.g., go down route 66 on a Harley Davidson). He said that when a friend rings him up to announce an impending child, rather than congratulating the friend, he commiserates with, "Well that's your life over for the next 20 years. Bad luck mate."

It is a testament to women that, given the pool of possibilities available to them, most are still shrewd enough to pick partners trainable enough to raise children.

7. Helped me understand the meaning of (my) life

Comedy gave a temporary meaning to my life, but certainly not a true understanding of why I exist. Stuttering may yet help with the latter. I think people who stutter can be quite spiritual and insightful, as we are perhaps more sensitive to our surroundings in comparison to the general population. That skill—maintaining harmony with the environment—is more or less how I define spirituality. I don't believe in an afterlife. There are, of course, many people who subscribe to the idea of an eternal self which lies in the soul or other karmic entity and lives on in some form, either in a heaven or new bodily incarnation. To me, existence is determined by the brain, and when its complex interaction of organised neurones and cells stops functioning, we surely go from lights on to lights out permanently. I think if religions could understand and appreciate the basis of science more, the world might have a chance of making it. Instead, we fight over that which we don't even understand.

As noted, the meaning of *my* life changed by finding a partner and having two children with her. I am a useful person to my children (at least until they stop speaking to me when they are teenagers!). Writing this book has also added meaning, as does seeing my family and good friends, and also the occasional holiday.

Life is a bit like a movie. It's made up of thousands and thousands of moments, with a beginning, middle, and an end. It is difficult to make sense of the whole film without understanding each of the scenes. To watch a movie while distracted keeps the viewer from appreciating the full meaning of what the director was trying to show. Maybe the meaning of life reveals itself the same way and we fill in the gaps as we age. Apparently, people are happiest after age 50 (Stone, 2013), so perhaps that is the time when the pieces begin to form an understandable whole. If we use our time in fulfilling ways, it seems less likely that we will be distracted from the true importance of each significant situation. If so, we can increase the chances that the meaning of our own stories will eventually become evident.

I hope comedy is a worthwhile chapter of my life. I have worked in some miserable jobs where the one sentence I heard the most was "Think of the money." In other words, people were working not for the love of the job, or the self-fulfilment it gave them. They were doing it purely to pay their bills. Comedy was certainly not a "think of the money" activity (especially considering the low amount the average gig actually paid).

On the contrary, it could be an incredibly enlightening and fulfilling experience.

Still, I have trouble listing what specific significance comedy has given my life. I suppose it provided an identity, and there is meaning in that. I can make a room full of strangers laugh (often at my expense). Too many times, however, I walked off the stage to problem drinking, hangovers, illness, and depression. It was a lifestyle dominated by a cycle of extreme highs and lows, which became spiritually exhausting and confusing. Did the alcohol provide any meaning? All I know is that if someone found true meaning in his life, he probably wouldn't then ruin it by being drunk all day!

According to Viktor E. Frankl (1946), we derive meaning in life by creating, accomplishing, experiencing, encountering, rising above a hopeless situation, and turning personal tragedy into triumph. By that definition, stand-up comedy clearly provided meaning. Creativity begat accomplishments, which led to unique experiences and encounters with interesting people. In the process, I rose above my miserable stutter, turning my predicament into a human achievement. If meaning requires such struggle, perhaps life isn't supposed to be rosy.

Alternatively, of course, it could be that life isn't meant to have any grand meaning at all. We are just mammals that have evolved as an intelligent species, who have learnt how to communicate very effectively with each other, some of us while stuttering.

8. Helped me utilize some (hidden) talents

The complexity of performing professionally requires many different skills, such as communication, timing, and the empathy required to read an audience. Even though the material will not change much from night to night, the delivery is altered according to the different dynamics of each audience. It is not just reciting jokes. It's expressing thoughts and checking in with the listeners now and then to see if they are following. As noted earlier, the best comedians have a relationship with the audience and are very attentive to them. A stutter taught me how to charm people more than the average person perhaps, as I had to fine-tune attributes besides speech. However it's done, persuading a crowd to listen, appreciate, and laugh for 20 minutes is a real skill. One must put to use pathos, charm, listening skills, empathy, patience, respect, calmness, command, control, body language, openness, and positivity, all difficult attributes to learn. Even when my material wasn't great, I felt I had the personality attributes to get me through.

9. Helped resolve some of my negativity/anger/frustration issues

I don't think I used laughter to defend myself against any psychological issues. I primarily wanted to become more comfortable in my own skin and reduce my stammer. Comedy saved me when all else around me failed, particularly my speech. It was a valve to release the pressure inside me, an escape which at the time I was very lucky to have. It also helped me to explore my feelings about life and relationships, emotions I had been repressing.

11. Taught me to be more positive and pushed my comfort zones

There is no doubt that having a stutter takes away positivity, but through stand-up comedy I learned how to laugh at myself and appreciate my own sense of humour and uniqueness. Not taking myself or my impediment too seriously definitely improved my outlook. When life was not going to plan, I began to look for solutions rather than dwelling on problems. So what if I can't get the job I want or go out with the girl of my dreams? Does it matter in the grand scheme of things? Brooding over failed job interviews or lost relationships is a waste of time as life is too short. Acceptance taught me that there are other ways of finding happiness.

Laughing at previous relationships, or just relationships in general, also took away the worries about never speaking to ex-girlfriends again. I went from "oh no" to "so what?" There was happiness to be found in freedom. I could basically do what I liked, and no one would tell me off or have any issues about it.

My life today is by no means sorted out. I'm still looking to open new comfort zones and put myself into quite extreme environments. Whatever the next challenge is, I will push through with it and face the consequences. From that perspective, performing stand-up comedy was really a stepping stone to becoming a happier and more fulfilled person.

12. Potential to be (slightly) famous

The American singer Lady Gaga once said, "I had a boyfriend who told me I'd never succeed, never be nominated for a Grammy, never have a hit song, and that he hoped I'd fail. I said to him, 'Someday, when we're not together, you won't be able to order a cup of coffee at the deli without hearing or seeing me'" (Spines, 2010). In my early thirties I would have liked to have been as well-known as Lady Gaga. I wanted to be so famous that when the name Jaik Campbell was mentioned, anyone in the world would have heard of me. I don't really know why I wanted that. Perhaps because of all the girls I could not speak to at school, university, or beyond; or all the failed job interviews; or the pointless negative remarks from my father. Who knows? One thing I learnt is that inward richness is much harder to achieve than material wealth.

400

The desire for fame has reduced with age thankfully, but it hasn't completely extinguished. I managed to be on TV and headline shows, and this sort of attention is intriguing. Being world famous would not only be exciting, but would solve some of my writing struggles. Let's face it, well-known comics get away with some really bad material because audiences no longer make them prove themselves. In addition, there have been times when I was chatting with top TV comics and thinking, "Yes, this is really cool." It must be fulfilling to be on the other side of that exchange.

13. Taught me entrepreneurship, business, selling skills

There are certainly healthier ways to learn business than hanging out in dingy, smoky comedy clubs in London, but the process of trying to be a comedian progressed and developed my entrepreneurship skills. As my career advanced, I was becoming more salesman than comic, always trying to get the next paid gig or seeking the approval of an agent or TV producer. As mentioned in Chapter 13, performing at the Edinburgh Fringe was a real exposure to what competition in the marketplace is like. It was find a niche or fail. I learnt about risk, pursuing opportunities without regard for resources.

A job can define a person. "I'm a doctor," "I'm a lawyer," and "I'm an accountant" all conjure work-related mental images. Stand-up comedy made me realise how restricted such imaginings can be. "I'm a comedian" didn't begin to tell the story of what I did. I told jokes, but I was foremost an entrepreneur. Be it stand-up, writing a movie, being an extra, or trying to be in a TV sitcom, something was always out there that had my name on it. Show business taught me that I had to cut loose from working for other people if I had any chance of making it, and gave me the confidence to work for myself.

For a long time I was living on small incomes, which gives me a higher appreciation of money when I earn it now. I also learnt when to delegate tasks and have people work for me, be it writing or negotiating with venue managers or photographers. I accept that stand-up comedy wasn't the ideal business mountain, but at least I climbed it.

14. Immortality

Let's face it, most of us would like to be remembered in some way after we die. Stand-up was perhaps my way to be recollected by future generations. Hopefully, some of my material and writings can contribute something to society.

15. Liberation

Being allowed to use words and discuss topics not commonly acceptable in ordinary life felt very liberating, provided the audience was laughing

16. Unique insight

Having a stutter provided me a different view of the world. Comedy gave me a platform to express that view.

17. Helpful when on a date

As noted throughout the book, my stutter and associated lack of eye contact definitely affected my confidence with women. Given that men are supposed to actually look at and speak to their dates, many of my get-togethers did not go well. Instead of calling, I sometimes tried in vain to attract women via text messages, so my dreadful speech wouldn't interfere.

Success with stand-up comedy gave me enough of a confidence boost to handle dates, a welcome change from the past. And on the rare occasions that I have actually been able to attract a woman, I was certainly not above using my comedic skills to my advantage. First dates go much better with laughter. In addition to learning how to deliver funny lines naturally, stand-up taught me the eye contact I had always avoided and how to be positive and pleasant instead of moody and brooding.

18. The art of management

Many of the happiest times of my life are spent alone, writing, jogging, sunbathing etc. Because of my stutter, I developed a love/hate relationship with communicating. Good management involves effective communication however, and thus speech is a necessary organizational skill. It can serve as a way to impress and lead. Unfortunately, it is also utilized to display vanity and disrespect. Some talk only to control and dominate conversations, or to show off their self-perceived intelligence. Due to insecurities and lack of empathy, they speak too much, in the apparent belief that communication is a competition and the highest word total wins. Comedy can likewise be an ego driven event dependent upon controlling a room, but hopefully not in a way that isolates others.

In school, I was taught some leadership skills, but it was comedy that stopped me from becoming an institutionalised droid. I'm a bit of a reluctant leader, but stand-up brought out the extrovert in me. I learnt to think outside the box, to problem solve, to adjust on the fly, deal with pressure, and be all that I could be as a person. The state school system in the UK is rather conformist, encouraging students to fit in and accept their academic and personal limitations, but stand-up comedy permitted me to explore my limits in ways that most jobs or educational establishments can't allow. Successful management is a heady mix of self-discipline, self-control, patience, understanding, likeability, charisma, charm, pathos, and self-belief to inspire co-workers. Like a stand-up comedian, if managers don't believe in what they are saying, neither will the listeners. Leaders need to have an appealing personality to keep their followers coming back. A comedian's success is no different.

Cons of Doing Stand-up

Of course, there were also drawbacks to the life I chose.

1. Increase in anxiety and stress levels

In chapter 3, I wrote that because of childhood stress, performing on stage was relatively easy and, for the most part, that's true. But there were also times that I found the pressure of performing even just once a week quite overwhelming. Perhaps I inherited an anxiety gene from my parents, or learnt to be anxious from watching and overreacting to my father (who could literally become stressed from making a cup of tea), but then gradually became accustomed to such anxiety. I learnt to manage it, even to adapt to it quickly, but it was still there.

Comedy is a competitive activity, as most comedians want to be the one who generates the most laughs. Writing original material was also very difficult. The process was like going to the darkest place of my mind and trying to return whole. My need for quiet time became much greater, perhaps triggering an associated upsurge in the more addictive side of my personality, most notably in terms of drinking. Addictions brought out the maverick in me which, although quite fun, wasn't conducive with responsibility in a proper and controlled everyday work environment.

In terms of making it as a comedian, a degree of obsessiveness is useful. Without it, gaining the stage time required to become any good would be impossible. Anxiety-related side effects are less needed though. Kate Copstick, a Scotsman newspaper critic, referred to me in 2003 as, "A nervous guy with a stutter," an indication of how my stage nerves were not thoroughly resolved. The more gigs I did the less anxious I became. Apparently making people enter and stay in their feared situations has become a standard and effective treatment technique. Repeated exposure to feared situations can result in the long term reduction of anxiety. Dreaded activities lose their power. It's like starting a new job—stressful at first but over the weeks it becomes easier to handle. In general, I become less reactive to situations as I get accustomed to them.

However, after a few months of not gigging, the anxiety can quite easily come back. It was a nerve wracking process, never knowing if all the jokes were going to work. The process of writing a good joke, learning my lines to a high standard, getting to the gig on time, not stuttering too much during the performance, and dealing confidently with the odd heckle, all helped to increase my anxiety levels. Unsuccessfully handling these stresses results in costs to a comedian's mental health that are unlikely to be outweighed by the benefits. Effectively, it amounts to making an audience feel good while slowly turning into a nervous wreck.

I once met someone who was in the Army and I asked him why he enlisted.

He said, "To see the world."

"Well you might have to kill people," I pointed out.

"Yes," he answered. "But there are pros and cons with any job."

In other words, costs don't have to be absent. They just need to be exceeded by the benefits. In comedy, such was not always the case. The comic is only as good as his or her last show, television series, or whatever other impression was made publically. Results require constant risk, which leads to anxiety. If comics could wait until they were 100% ready before doing anything, stress would be absent. But so would accomplishment.

2. Criticism was hard to handle

Often adding to the stress were the words of the critics. Perhaps because of the criticism I received growing up, I'm still not very good at recovering after being told off or put down. Human nature also plays a part however. Putting hundreds of hours of preparation into writing and practicing an Edinburgh show only to then be told it's terrible would be a fairly soul destroying experience for any-one. Still, I may have taken it to heart more than most. I once read a Fringe review that said I presented "consistently weak material" (Cox, 2005) and that took me weeks to get over.

3. Precious time potentially used up

People sometimes forget that time is finite. When I was in my twen-ties, time was a less precious commodity and always seemed avail-able. I knew that comedy success, like any worthwhile dream, was going to take a long time and I was prepared to pay that cost. But the thousands of hours I spent trying to acquire wealth and fame from comedy via performing 800 or so gigs cannot be reclaimed. It might have been used toward a more stable profession. Even bet-ter, I could have spent it with friends and family.

4. It's expensive

As written in Chapter 13, the Edinburgh Fringe was seriously expensive. The owners of the paid venues have a great laugh on holiday after the festival is over, whilst the performer languishes in financial regret at the sweet elixir of fame. The cost of living in London as well, without a well-paid or full time job, meant that most of the time I didn't have any money to actually enjoy my life. I had to be in the city though, as that's where the circuit exists, but working it often meant eating out in overpriced cafes and restaurants. And even if I met a nice woman, I couldn't afford to take her out to a fancy place or buy her a present! There was potentially a bit of funding available from places like the "UK Arts Council," but there was always a definite need to make more money. The challenge was finding ways to do so around the time and effort that stand-up required.

And if money is made, what if the work dries up? Comedians get no retirement funds, have no definitive career path, and their curriculum vitae demonstrate no obvious focus. My knowledge of the commercial "real world" is dreadful. I became a family man without a stable income or even a basic knowledge of how a mortgage works.

5. Too tiring and emotionally draining

In order for a gig to go well, I had to use up a great deal of positive energy, which was usually in short supply. Then I would get back late and have to be up early in the morning for work. The resulting tiredness diminished my on-the-job productivity and dedication, which of course had a negative effect on my job references. Sometimes the lack of sleep, hangovers, and overall fatigue would also make my stutter worse.

Add to that the isolation from friends and family and the sum is a process that in many respects was distressing.

6. My housemates hated me (understandably!)

If I was back late from a gig, I often woke my housemates up. This pattern was unacceptable, as they had proper 9 – 5 jobs. In addition, when we were all awake at the same time, the overall stress, tiredness, and need for solitude made me a relatively unpleasant person to be around.

7. Dangerous

Walking through the streets of London late at night or being on a twilight bus full of drunks on the way back from a gig could be perilous. There was no relaxing or daydreaming, as I needed my wits about me at all times.

8. Lack of relationships

Maybe it was just me, but as a male wannabe comic in London, it was difficult to attract a girlfriend. It seems females don't want to date someone who's out most evenings and weekends, has no money or car, and is often stressed out, anxious, and/or depressed. Many of my cohorts went out with female comedians or actresses, who understood the lifestyle involved. It's a shame because having a girlfriend in London seriously improves the quality of life.

I was actually a bit tired of relationships when I first entered stand-up. The unwritten rule of "break up with someone, then never speak to her again" was always quite difficult for me to understand. The one person who was held incredibly close has to become the one pushed furthest away.

It was not a situation I was anxious to repeat again quickly. The healing time took too long and used up too much energy.

9. Unhealthy lifestyle

A lifestyle of stress, late nights, alcohol, smoking, and fast food, was, obviously, less than ideal. The damage we were doing to ourselves was accentuated by the smoky venues prevalent until England's smoking ban in 2007. As previously discussed, my excessive alcohol use was because I was convinced I was only funny after having a drink, and we all know about the dangers of alcohol abuse. I experienced first-hand the devastation of a friend of mine, who died from cirrhosis of the liver at age 45.

Much of the drinking passages in this book are in chapter 13, the one about Edinburgh. In retrospect, I started performing Fringe shows too early and the alcohol was basically making up for a lack of material and polish. But once in the comedy system, it pays to keep the ball rolling. In addition, my parents were keen for me to flush the comedy bug out of my system and so pushed me to perform while I was young. So I continued telling jokes and engaging in bad habits.

The problem was not only the regularity with which I drank, but also the binges. According to the UK Daily Mail (Hope, 2015), research suggests that men should limit their drinking to one unit a day until they are 34 years old. Doctors warn against binge drinking, as this can, among other effects, slow brain function, leading to impairments of balance, breathing, and heartbeat. It probably also caused one or two extra fillings in my teeth.

To prepare for each Edinburgh show, I would consume a can of strong lager, followed by another during the show, a total of about

4-5 units. Such drinking can become a dangerous habit. Studies have shown that those who drink regularly in their teens and early twenties are up to twice as likely as light drinkers to be binge drinking 25 years later ("Cracking down…", 2014).

I know I never suffered from alcohol poisoning but a full Edinburgh run usually took at least a month to recover from and that was purely my body readjusting from the abuse. During the post Edinburgh month, I was typically anti-social, depressed, and withdrawn.

Now it is easy to see how my alcohol use was neither responsible nor particularly mature. It was binging to be funny, forgetting the many top UK comedians (e.g., Jimmy Carr, Daniel Kitson, Michael McIntyre) who do not need alcohol before they go on stage. All in all, it nearly ruined me. Now I hardly drink at all.

10. Difficult to spend time any quality time with my friends or family

The downside of choosing a solitary vocation is lost time with those I love. I could go great lengths of time without seeing my mother, whose company I like very much. Writing this book has been a wakeup call to the remainder of my life. I'm lucky to have met a very intelligent and capable woman, without whose help and energy my life would not be as enriched or interesting. Now that we have children, I can see even better the value of making time for those most important.

11. Using self-deprecating material has its drawbacks

My mother used to say to me, "Don't worry, your stutter gives you a special relationship with children and old people."

I said, "Really?"

She said, "Yes, they'll both hate you equally."

The audience seemed to laugh more when I made fun of myself. The material I used was generally self-deprecating, which made for a likeable and endearing persona but had a gradual and deleterious effect on my self-esteem. The more I criticized myself, the better the audience response and the more hooked I became into putting myself down. Ultimately, however, the least wanted and socially inept persona took away my confidence. Too much self-reflection and introspection to find that "killer" joke led to excessive self-loathing both on and off stage. For example, if I said, "Because of my stutter, I normally text the girl back after a date, which luckily works OK," the audience wouldn't have laughed. Whereas if I said, "Apparently it's best not to text too soon after a date. I waited two years. She texted back saying she would have preferred longer," it's well received. Such jokes became self-fulfilling prophecies. I believed what I was saying on stage to such an extent that I lived it off stage as well.

What I need to write is a more self-empowering routine that makes the audience laugh. The UK comedian Peter Kay, for example, uses a great deal of material that does not put him or others down. His act lacks cruelty and he hardly ever swears. It's normally clever observations about life in northern UK and he avoids jokes about sex and politics. Examples of two of his jokes are:

My dad used to say "always fight fire with fire," which is probably why he got thrown out of the fire brigade.

So I went down the local supermarket. I said, "I want to make a complaint. This vinegar's got lumps in it." He said, "Those are pickled onions."

12. Lose touch with reality

My brother Guy once said to me that, since becoming a comedian, I had lost touch with reality, that I'd become "too self-obsessed." If so, I was in the right occupation. Self-obsession is a real issue in comedy. It can become a showing off process, one in which the performer cares more about him- or herself than about making the audience laugh. Once a comedian's act becomes ego- and not audience-focused, it's not serving its purpose.

Self-absorption is not the only way in which comics distance themselves from reality, however. My old friend Jamie once listed all of the drawbacks of stand-up—such as lack of stability, relationships, and material possessions—in an attempt to get me to reduce the effort I was devoting to it. There is no denying that by his definition of reality, my existence was abnormal. Then again, what is normal? One person's dream is another's nightmare.

In general, the comedians I met were emotionally impaired in some way, with stories of bad relationships or tragic family events (then again, most people I've met in my time have some kind of emotional hang-up, so at least comedians are facing their demons head on). Although they typically got along fine, even rooted for one another, there were some who were prone to bitterness if peers passed them by (especially if high paid TV contracts were in the mix). But few presented really serious mental health issues. If they had, they couldn't have coped with being on stage. They were not all sad people either, although there were a few who seemed to have some kind of mild depressive disorder. Indeed, Claridge (2014), in one of the few academic papers on the psychology of comedians, found that stand-ups had high levels of psychotic traits with "a paradoxical high score on both depressive and impulsive, non-conformist traits… that's equivalent to manic depression or bipolar."

Conclusion… Moving on. What Next?

I've enjoyed telling my story via this book. I'm glad that I took the time to reassess and question life while there's time to do so. My goal was to visit the past without reliving it, so I can keep moving forward.

I feel that writing this textbook has been a more constructive use of my time than is life on the comedy circuit. In fact, a reduced schedule—the occasional Suffolk or London gig—seems to satisfy my need to be on stage and perform. And it helps pay the bills, which, as a responsible father, should be a priority now.

Between gigs, I do occasionally miss the buzz of stepping out onto that stage, but I guess it's time to be more practical with my life. I still believe that stand-up comedy is a powerful medium, however, and the ability to make people laugh and think at the same time is genuinely something special.

For me, stand-up cured many ills, but caused others. I enjoyed honing and improving my act, but the costs were greater than I expected. So was it worth it?

In a word: Yes. Because of comedy, my speech barrier is less of an issue than it could have been. It also allowed me to view the world positively. And, at the risk of sounding vain, I accomplished much in a field for which stuttering presented a significant obstacle. If nothing else, I can one day look back on my life and say "I did that."

In terms of *What next?*, the story isn't over yet. I'll still be learning lines and getting up on stage, as those tasks help my speech. Transferring a stuttering based script to TV or a movie is still an ambition of mine. I might finish off my stuttering action comedy film screenplay one day (with co-author Dale's help of course!). Beyond show business, simply seeking happiness is important to me, as is finding the balance between making money and enjoying life. Given that touching the hands of my son and daughter after they were born are among the happiest moments of my life, and not a single pound was exchanged in the transaction, perhaps the best things in life really are free. With that in mind, I mustn't forget my good fortune in having a soulmate and two beautiful children. With or without anything else, they keep my degree of happiness quite high.

I once wrote that the only problem with stuttering is that it tends to ruin absolutely every facet of life, including the meaning of it and the ability to hold down a proper job. Apart from that, absolutely no problem. I'm not sure whether that was a joke. I know that if stammering were less of an issue, I wouldn't have been so worried about trying to figure it out.

Questions for Discussion

Jaik claimed that he rarely stutters when talking to his partner because she handles stuttering "with intelligence, patience, and understanding." Do you believe listener reactions affect stuttering frequency? Why or why not?

What would your response be if a client said, "I realise children tend to duplicate how their parents speak and act and I certainly didn't want them to copy my stutter."

In chapter 3, we learned that Jaik's father hated being called "Daddy." However, Jaik's daughter apparently uses the term with him. Is there any significance to that disparity?

Do you see any merit in Jaik's speculation that more supportive behavior on the part of his father during Jaik's early childhood might have kept him from stuttering? Explain your answer.

When Jaik contemplates nature vs. nurture, one of his questions about his father—*What if I had been allowed to have a year off before going to university, or had some support for the jobs I wanted to do?*—has nothing to do with his early speech development. Why do you think he included it?

Respond to Jaik's statement that, "Genetically there is a high chance that one of my children will stutter."

There is a recurring theme of changing priorities with parenthood. How might these changes affect stuttering recovery, or even the progression of therapy?

On the list of comedy benefits, help with stuttering is only fourth.

What might that tell you about Jaik's recovery progress?

Jaik argues that laughing at stuttering is "a step in defeating it." How do you get clients to the point where they can laugh at such a sensitive topic?

What do you believe to be the relationship between the client's self-esteem and progress in therapy?

Jaik stated, "…the more I talked about stuttering…the more desensitized I became to it." What is the lesson for stuttering clients?

What is the most difficult stage of life to stutter? Explain your answer.

Jaik wrote that he didn't learn to like his appearance so much as stop caring about it. Is that a good explanation of acceptance? If so, how could it be applied to stuttering?

Do you believe, as Jaik does, that people who stutter are "perhaps more sensitive to (their) surroundings in comparison to the general population?" Why or why not?

Jaik's childhood stressors taught him to deal with pressure, yet sometimes the stress of getting on stage got to him. How do you explain this seeming contradiction?

The section on anxiety and stress as stand-up "cons" was generally devoted to stage fright, with stuttering only mentioned once. What do you feel is the significance of that discrepancy?

Jaik has a tendency to look back at some aspects of his life with regret.

How might such a tendency impact therapy?

Jaik learned that stand-up comedy requires "pathos, charm, listening skills, empathy, patience, respect, calmness, command, control, body language, openness, and positivity." How are these traits impacted by a lifetime of stuttering?

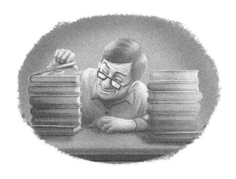

Chapter 16: Life

On New Year's Eve 1973, a child was born in Suffolk, England. He joined an older brother. A sister would soon follow. Their mother doted on the three children, making sure they were busy and well fed. Their father saw his parenting role much differently, preferring to focus on being a good provider. He worked long hours and gained a great many rewards, including the resources needed to send his children to private schools. But the hard work came at a cost: It was difficult to be patient with his children or feign interest in their activities. The rest of the family described the father's behavior as argumentative and demeaning. The children feared him. For a time, his wife fought back against the abuse, but eventually she too let him have his way. Stress was prevalent in the household and, in time, beyond. Family vacations were hell. Others in town—from business partners to the local vicar—also felt the father's wrath, leaving few spots in Suffolk where family members didn't hear whispers.

The father stuttered and family members wondered whether that added to his seemingly perpetual frustration. There was also a story about a rock band that never made it big, a lost dream that might also help explain the bitterness. Mostly, though, they figured it was the stress of paying the bills. To help cover the expenses, the mother started a business of her own. It was quite successful, but occupied enough of her time that protecting her children became more difficult.

The child and his older brother became close, spending their days playing games and riding bikes. Within the home, they barricaded themselves from the father with the help of television and movies. They especially liked comedies. They would record pretend shows together, among child's happiest boyhood memories.

The child also found refuge in school, performing well and fulfilling the parents' plan that he be well educated. A bit reserved, though with occasional lapses of disruptive behavior, he preferred the company of close friends, but did play rugby and join the school's drama club. Within the latter, he gained a few small roles, for which he learned his lines so well that he delivered them flawlessly. He didn't tell his family, but that was the hardest he studied anything during his school years.

At University, he continued to excel, graduating with honors. Socially, he was adequate, getting along with his roommates for as long as was required; generally, by the time they got on his nerves, another semester had finished and he could move out without confrontation. He gradually lost touch with all of the roommates, rarely thinking about them by the time he finished University. His plan then was to travel with a few close friends, but his father nixed the idea because he wanted his son to get started on a graduate science degree. So the child—now a young man—returned to school. Upon completion, he finally did travel, despite his father's objections. Work could wait, he decided; he'd earned some fun. He was not about to repeat the mistake of letting his father direct his adult plans. The subsequent holiday was one of his life's highlights, as he could relax and do as he pleased without worrying about studies or any other stressors. He also enjoyed seeing parts of Europe he had previously only heard about.

With schooling done, the family business awaited him, for good and for bad. The young man was glad he didn't have to deal with job interviews but, once his older brother moved to London, much of the company responsibility fell to him. Working closely with his father day in and day out, he found the older man behaviorally difficult, but, with time, somewhat easier to understand. Their arguments were frequent at first. With the son's recent education came innovations and modern ideas. The father, however, resisted anything new, fearing that lost income would result from following the unknown. The conflicts lessened as time went by. The young man better understood the pressures of running a business and the father came to rely on his son, although he never admitted it.

When he first joined the family business, the young man moved back in with his parents, as that seemed the easiest course of action. His social life suffered, however, as he felt that he lacked true independence. His parents always knew who he was going to see and when. Therefore, he found an apartment nearby. Although it cut into his savings, the new freedom was worth it.

The young man worked hard during the week. On weekends, he regularly met up with a group of old friends at one of several local pubs. Drinking seemed to cure his shyness and some nights he was the life of the party. It also helped with his fear of women, as he always was at least tipsy when approaching someone who caught his eye.

One Saturday night he saw a woman who looked familiar. When he finally placed the face, he realized that he knew her from primary school, many, many years before. Even though he had a reason to initiate a conversation, he still drank a can of lager before speaking to her. He need not have worried. They had much to talk about, as their experiences nearly mirrored one another's: She had gone away to school, earned two degrees, and decided to resettle in Suffolk as well. They made plans to meet for drinks the following evening. One night after that, they talked on the phone for an hour. For weeks thereafter, they were in contact nearly every day. They went to movies or out to eat, but always ended the evening in a familiar pub, with the young man's friends. Eventually his new girlfriend was accepted into the group. They became a couple within a larger collection.

The young man's social life had increased to 4-5 nights per week. He was somewhat concerned about the frequency of drinking, but he was having fun and didn't want to lose the thrill that came with a new relationship. Mornings became a challenge, however. He was too often tired and hungover. Sometimes he arrived to work late and, even when he didn't, his productivity suffered. Arguments with his father started up again. These were so difficult to endure through the headaches and fatigue that he often conceded just to end the discussion. At one point, the father threatened to fire his son, but the young man figured that was just a ploy to keep him from asking for a raise.

He began to wonder whether settling down would cure his ills. Two people in his drinking group were recently engaged and talked about entering the next phase of life. For the young man, this phase seemed to have arrived. He and his girlfriend had dated long enough that the familiarity of their usual places and activities was growing stale.

He also knew that his prospects in Suffolk consisted of the girlfriend and no one else. The decision was easy.

After a short engagement, they had a rather large wedding that was marred by the two fathers getting into an argument in which punches were nearly exchanged. Their honeymoon in Mallorca was a whirlwind of beaches, flamenco music, and Galilea Ale. I need to travel more, he vowed to himself. When he suggested this aloud, however, his new wife pointed out how difficult that would be, given their differing schedules, which would only intensify after they had children.

The newlyweds bought a house and quickly started a family of their own. With the first pregnancy came the end of their participation in the drinking group, or what was left of it. Each looked for new ways to fill the gap, he with work, she with learning about raising children. The birth of the child was a joyous occasion, followed by the disjointed schedule that comes with any new baby. Occasionally, the young man's mother or one of his wife's parents would babysit so they could go out. When they did, they rarely saw anyone from the old gang anymore, so they mostly talked about the baby.

It wasn't long before the second pregnancy. The young man again became motivated to work hard, much to the delight of his father. But the birth of the new child increased parenting demands exponentially and he and his wife soon felt perpetually exhausted. They talked some, always about child-related responsibilities. At times, the young man missed the pub conversations of a lifetime ago, so free and full of humor. The children were now the highlight of his life, but were sustainable as a conversation topic for only so long.

He and his wife retreated into their respective worlds, as the young man's parents had done a generation before. When they tried to communicate, things got worse, as both resented the same old topics. They struggled and clashed until neither could stand it any longer. The couple divorced when the children were 6 and 4 years of age. Although the young man's father rarely spoke to his wife or children, he was nevertheless furious about the split, viewing it as a moral failing on the part of his son. Thus, not even the workplace provided any sort of respite from the young man's trials.

He never stopped adoring his children and saw them regularly. The only awkward part of those visits was seeing his ex-wife, especially after she remarried. The young man did travel more for a time, visiting both North and South America. He tired of journeying alone, however, and coordinating plans with friends who were married and working became quite difficult.

The family business had its ups and downs, but the young man proudly stuck it out. Still, he vowed never to coerce his own children into becoming involved. This declaration originated in part because he saw so much potential in them that he felt they should be free to follow their own dreams and talents. In addition, he wondered how his former wife would take to the idea of the children working for him. That was a discussion he wished to avoid. Also, in his most honest moments, he wondered if keeping the business afloat was worth devoting one's life.

The young man has not remarried yet. He would like to find his soulmate, but feels he'd have to leave Suffolk to do so and that's where his kids and job are. He's considering joining the local theatre group. He might meet some new people and besides, learning to act could help with marketing the family business. Thinking about theatre reminds him of those childhood cassette recorded shows he performed with his brother. He figures any activity that brings back those happy memories can't be all bad. And who knows—maybe he'd turn out to have some talent. Wouldn't that be something? He smiles at the thought of his father and ex-wife one day watching him on TV.

Sometimes he wonders whether he should have pursued drama back in the day. Oh well, he figures, so few make it in show business that even if he had tried, he would probably have ended up right where he is today anyway.

Is that how Jaik's life would have unfolded without a stutter? Of course not. Is it close? I cannot say. I did not consult Jaik before I wrote it. I have no idea if he would have returned to Suffolk after graduate school, if old friends would have been waiting, or if any girls from primary school returned home single. I have no insight into his father's opinions about divorce. I do not know if Jaik would have considered the pursuit of acting or, for that matter, if Suffolk has a theatre troupe. I've never even been there.

(I did send it to him after it was finished. He said that some parts "hopefully won't happen," but did take away that "life without a stutter is potentially more disastrous than my actual life, so maybe having a stutter is a good thing and has expanded my horizons.")

The point is not to present exactly what would have happened (as if I could), but simply to illustrate that there would have been differences. Too many, in fact, to reasonably identify. Some would be large and some too small to see, but all would have had a ripple effect of further change. Thus, the story above is one of billions of possibilities for a fluent Jaik Campbell. One cannot specify the influence of stuttering on life any more than a cook can describe exactly where a seasoning mixes with a sauce.

Aspects of stuttering—the breakdowns, reactions, emotions, and attempts to hide it, among all of the others—form a whole that cannot easily be subtracted from life. Furthermore, each one exerts an influence all its own. Is a child embarrassed to speak less apt to become an adult leader? Not always, but it is not inappropriate to wonder whether a stuttering person had difficulty developing leadership skills simply because he or she was never given the opportunity to lead. Does the embarrassment of stuttering with a coworker mean that he or she will never be the speaker's friend? Again, sometimes no, sometimes yes, and sometimes yes but in a very different way.

It is not often clear how stuttering impacts key features of life (or, for that matter, how *any* of life's aspects interact). Take, for example, the confidence issues so prevalent in Jaik's story. Did they stem from stuttering? It does seem possible that his speech affected confidence with women, but only in combination with other factors. After all, not every male who stutters is afraid of females.

He admits that growing up without paternal support sucked away some confidence, even noting that his siblings suffer from the same deficiency. On the other hand, once his self-assurance was reduced, the negative listener reactions that come with stuttering surely did not help. One thing is certain: the indecision experienced during speech situations in some way mirrors (or at least reminds Jaik of) feelings of generalized indecisiveness. But in answer to the question of whether confidence would have been higher without stuttering, all we can really speculate is that speech-associated confidence may well have been better.

Similarly, Jaik's relationship with his father, rocky at best, might not have been affected by his stuttering in a general sense (that is, his childhood memories may well have been what they are now, even without the stutter), but problems speaking certainly could have added to the stress within specific situations. And given that stuttering was the trait for which Jaik was most self-conscious, angry reactions to it would have been devastating for a young child.

In school, Jaik wanted to prove that he was as smart as anyone else, despite his difficulty talking, so one could easily argue that stuttering affected that aspect of his life. Without question, participation in activities in and out of the classroom suffered to some extent. Jaik noted that time he might have spent socializing (if he did not stutter, but also if his father was more agreeable to friends coming over) was available for studying. It is worth noting that Jaik *did* excel at school, however, which does not happen solely through time and effort. So while there is no denying that his school years would have been different with fluency, I would argue that he still would have performed well.

On the topic of isolation, it is important to differentiate that from his preference for spending time alone. If the former led to the latter—that is, if forced seclusion led him to discover advantages to being alone—it seems likely that he would have eventually realized such advantages anyway. As an adult, Jaik enjoyed solitary pursuits such as writing and researching more, it seems, because he accomplished worthwhile goals without interference rather than for any reasons having to do with communicative fears. Could such times have still been valued but perhaps shortened if talking to people were easier? It seems like a reasonable assumption, given that traits such as social anxiety and social phobia occur relatively often with adults who stutter (in comparison to the general population) (Blumgart, Tran, & Craig, 2010). Again, however, there is no way to know with any certainty.

Another common theme throughout Jaik's story was a desire to travel. In chapter 3 he noted that traveling involves communicating with people, which makes the process less than relaxing for him. Later, he laments not doing it enough because of the time he devoted to stand-up, an activity that requires far more in terms of communicative skills than does visiting someplace new. So was it stuttering or life events that kept him from traveling? Perhaps that is a false dichotomy, given the impact one had on the other.

Jaik's drinking is another example of a life choice not totally divorced from stuttering, but not directly related either. He drank to lower inhibitions, which allowed him to feel more comfortable before audiences. How much of the inhibition was due to stuttering? Surely some was. On the other hand, there are few non-stutterers who could perform stand-up without some signs of overt reticence, an observation supported by Jaik's account of the amount of alcohol consumed by comedians in general. And given the large number of people who enjoy the lowered inhibitions they experience with drinking, it seems more likely than not that Jaik would have discovered this particular "benefit" of alcohol even had he never stuttered.

Another wrinkle to the stuttering-drinking association is Jaik's claim that, if not for his speech, he would never have become a comedian (rendering his reason for alcohol abuse non-existent). This declaration seems to stem from the idea that he entered stand-up as a way to improve speech-related confidence that had been eroded by a lifetime of stuttering. On this matter, I take him at his word—I even based this chapter's introductory story on the idea that normal fluency would have led him in another direction. However, from boyhood on he watched comedians perform not because he stuttered, but because he enjoyed them. It seems likely that he would have at least become a fan of comedy, if for no other reason than his brother and other childhood influences. More importantly, he came away from some acts convinced that he could do better. And that was *with* a stutter. If anything, that conviction would have been even stronger without one. Would it have been enough to push him to Michael Knighton's class? Again, Jaik appears to think not.

Taking a different perspective on the matter of why Jaik entered comedy, success in show business could be viewed as an effective way to outshine his father, the wannabe rock star. Notably, the dismissive behavior of his father toward Jaik's comedy career is consistent with his (the father's) regrets and the resentment he displayed toward anyone who achieved even a modicum of fame. It is likely that nobody (not even Jaik) can be sure whether paternal competitiveness was part of the motivation to pursue comedy, but it is not unreasonable to wonder whether Jaik inherited the desire and talent to perform from his father, then used them to jab back at the man who made his childhood so difficult.

Of course, any forays into comedy would have changed drastically without his stutter. Perspective and preparation, to name just two examples, would have both been very different. He might have become one of those comics talking about relationships, airport security, and all the other topics he noted were common on the circuits. And although there would have been no need to continually rewrite scripts to avoid feared words, his writing struggles would have been intensified without having the one unique perspective he brought to the stage.

In chapter 15, Jaik wrote of changing priorities with the birth of his children. In short, his focus has shifted to them. Certainly this is a normal reaction to parenting, but even this sort of near-universal emotion is not free from the influence of stuttering, as Jaik made the case that a stutter-free life would have resulted in less apprehension when it came to raising children. He wrote: "I realise children tend to copy how their parents speak and act and I certainly didn't want them to copy my stutter." Again, stuttering is too complex a disorder to be caused by simple imitation. Moreover, it appears that children do not "copy how their parents speak" so much as absorb the language features of their culture. Were that not the case, I would speak with a German accent. In actuality, I can't even imitate one.

So what has Jaik's story taught us? Here is another incomplete list, one that does not really capture a life lived.

- Stuttering is complex. So are people. Combining them is like multiplying two multiline equations. The potential effects on an individual seem endless. Stuttering's reputation as an individualized disorder did not occur by accident, after all. Jaik's story did include some familiar stuttering disabilities—for example, situational fears, shame, and embarrassment—but others that are decidedly uncommon, namely, the use of stand-up comedy as a desensitizer. A father who does not laud his children is also atypical. Significantly, Jaik addresses his relationship with his father right from the start of his summary chapter.

- And speaking of complexity, stuttering humor is also a complicated endeavor. And it is not for everyone.

- Stuttering is not easy. Neither is life. The difference is that the latter seems to go by quickly.

- There is no cure for stuttering. However, acceptance can go a long way toward putting the handicapping effects of stuttering in the rear view mirror. Unfortunately, acceptance is a long, but I would argue necessary, road. Stuttering individuals need to understand their strengths, but also their limitations. That way, they can set realistic personal goals and use their skills and personality assets to their advantage. Life is not a linear process. We are all too aware of its ups and downs. With that in mind, there is no reason to assume that acceptance would be easy or straightforward. As a stuttering comedian (not Jaik) once told me, "Every time you think you've accepted stuttering, you find new things that challenge that" (G, N., personal correspondence, 2015).

- On the topic of challenges, good things come from proactively confronting one's demons. Stuttering solutions are not easy to come by, in part because new problems emerge as we stumble through life. Avoiding challenges means avoiding life. Hoping for miraculous answers is less efficient than persistence.

- For many, stuttering can be better controlled once the speaker has given him- or herself permission to stutter, even if it is in front of a large audience or bank of television cameras. Talking without worrying about when the next disfluency is going to occur can be an effective way to counteract all those environmental reminders of past stuttering.

- People should do what they want to do and say what they have to say, even if they sometimes stutter.

Jaik wanted to tell jokes. He wanted to utilize humor to educate. He accomplished both. Yes, he has some doubts about the extent to which comedy will play a part in his future, but he never has to wonder, "What if...?"

One of his possible future projects is to "finish off (his) stuttering action comedy film screenplay…with…Dale's help of course…" To be honest, that was the first I had heard of the idea, but it fits perfectly into this discussion. What the world needs is a hero for whom stuttering is his or her super power. When mere mortals hear the disfluencies, they realize immediately that they are in the presence of greatness. That would be the ultimate in turning an impairment into a strength.

Questions for Discussion

How do you think Jaik's life plays out if he did not stutter?

More specifically, different aspects of life could have been different without the element of stuttering. Many are listed in this chapter. Can you think of others?

Jaik stated that if not for stuttering, he would not have become a comedian. Do you agree? Why or why not?

What did Jaik's story teach you about stuttering?

References

Abdalla, F. A., & Louis, K. O. S. (2012). Arab school teachers' knowledge, beliefs and reactions regarding stuttering. *Journal of Fluency Disorders, 37*(1), 54-69.

Alberge, D. (2002). Review [Review of comedian *Jaik Campbell*]. *The Fringe.*

Allard, E. R., & Williams, D. F. (2008). Listeners' perceptions of speech and language disorders. *Journal of Communication Disorders*, 41(2), 108-123.

Alm, P. A. (2014). Stuttering in relation to anxiety, temperament, and personality: review and analysis with focus on causality. *Journal of Fluency Disorders, 40*, 5-21.

Alm, P. A., & Risberg, J. (2007). Stuttering in adults: The acoustic startle response, temperamental traits, and biological factors. *Journal of Communication Disorders*, 40(1), 1-41.

Alpert, M., Kotsaftis, A., & Pouget, E. R. (1997). At issue: speech fluency and schizophrenic negative signs. *Schizophrenia Bulletin, 23*(2), 171.

Ambrose, N. G., & Yairi, E. (1999). Normative disfluency data for early childhood stuttering. *Journal of Speech, Language, and Hearing Research, 42*(4), 895-909.

American Speech-Language-Hearing Association. (2007). *Scope of practice in speech-language pathology* [Scope of practice]. Available at: www.asha.org/policy.

Anderson, J. D. (2007). Phonological neighborhood and word frequency effects in the stuttered disfluencies of children who stutter. *Journal of Speech, Language, and Hearing Research, 50*, 229–247.

Anderson, J. D., Pellowski, M. W., Conture, E. G., & Kelly, E. M. (2003). Temperamental Characteristics of Young Children Who Stutter. *Journal of Speech, Language, and Hearing Research, 46*(5), 1221-1233.

Anderson, T. K., & Felsenfeld, S. (2003). A thematic analysis of late recovery from stuttering. *American Journal of Speech-Language Pathology,* 12 (2), 243-253.

Andrews, C., O'Brian, S., Harrison, E., Onslow, M., Packman, A., & Menzies, R. (2012). Syllable-timed speech treatment for school-age children who stutter: A phase I trial. *Language, Speech, and Hearing Services in Schools, 43*(3), 359-369.

Andrews, G., & Cutler, J. (1974). Stuttering therapy: The relation between changes in symptom level and attitudes. *Journal of Speech and Hearing Disorders, 39*(3), 312-319.

Andrews, G., Guitar, B., & Howie, P. (1980). Meta-analysis of stuttering treatment. *Journal of Speech and Hearing Disorders, 45,* 287-307.

Andrews, G., & Harris, M. (1964). The Syndrome of Stuttering: Clinics in Developmental Medicine 17.

Andrews, G., Howie, P. M., Dozsa, M., & Guitar, B. E. (1982). Stuttering Speech Pattern Characteristics Under Fluency-Inducing Conditions. *Journal of Speech, Language, and Hearing Research, 25*(2), 208-216.

Andrews G, Morris-Yates A, Howie P, Martin NG. (1991). Genetic factors in stuttering confirmed. *Archives of General Psychiatry, 48,* 1034–1035.

Arnold, H. S., Li, J., & Goltl, K. (2015). Beliefs of teachers versus non-teachers about people who stutter. *Journal of Fluency Disorders, 43,* 28-39.

Arthur, D. (2012). *Recruiting, interviewing, selecting & orienting new employees.* AMACOM Div American Mgmt Assn.

Azevedo, J. C., Lopes, R., Curral, R., Esteves, M. F., Coelho, R., & Roma Torres, A. (2012). Clozapine induced palilalia? *Acta Neuropsychiatrica*, 24(2), 122-124.

Baken, R. J., McManus, D. A., & Cavallo, S. A. (1983). Prephonatory chest wall posturing in stutterers. *Journal of Speech, Language, and Hearing Research*, 26(3), 444-450.

Bakker, K., & Brutten, G. J. (1987). Labial and laryngeal reaction times of stutterers and nonstutterers. In Peters, H. F. M. & Hulstijn, W., *Speech Motor Dynamics in Stuttering* (pp. 177-183). Vienna: Springer.

Bakker, K., & Brutten, G. J. (1989). A comparative investigation of the laryngeal premotor, adjustment, and reaction times of stutterers and nonstutterers. *Journal of Speech, Language, and Hearing Research*, 32(2), 239-244.

Barlow, D. H. (2000). Unraveling the mysteries of anxiety and its disorders from the perspective of emotion theory. *American Psychologist*, 55(11), 1247.

Battle, D. E. (2011). *Communication disorders in multicultural populations* (4th Ed.). Elsevier Health Sciences.

Bauman, J., Hall, N. E., Wagovich, S. A., Weber-Fox, C. M., & Ratner, N. B. (2012). Past tense marking in the spontaneous speech of preschool children who do and do not stutter. *Journal of Fluency Disorders*, 37(4), 314-324.

BBC News (2006, Feb 2). New research to help stammering. *BBC News*. Retrieved from http://news.bbc.co.uk/2/hi/uk_news/england/suffolk/4674080.stm

Beilby, J. M., Byrnes, M. L., & Yaruss, J. S. (2012). Acceptance and commitment therapy for adults who stutter: Psychosocial adjustment and speech fluency. *Journal of Fluency Disorders*, 37(4), 289-299.

Beilby, J. M., Byrnes, M. L., & Young, K. N. (2012). The experiences of living with a sibling who stutters: a preliminary study. *Journal of Fluency Disorders, 37*(2), 135-148.

Bennett, S. (2001). Review [Review of comedian *Jaik Campbell*]. *Chortle*. Available at: http://www.chortle.co.uk/comics/j/323/jaik_campbell

Berkowitz, G. (2005). Review [Review of the comedy show *I've Stuttered So I'll F-F-Finish*]. *The Stage*. Available at: http://www.thestage.co.uk/reviews/2005/jaik-campbell-i-ve-stuttered-so-i-ll-f-f-finish-review-at-co2/

Bernardini, S., Vanryckeghem, M., Brutten, G. J., Cocco, L., & Zmarich, C. (2009). Communication attitude of Italian children who do and do not stutter. *Journal of Communication Disorders, 42*(2), 155-161.

Berry, M. F. (1938). A study of the medical history of stuttering children. *Communications Monographs, 5*(1), 97-114.

Bleek, B., Montag, C., Faber, J., & Reuter, M. (2011). Investigating personality in stuttering: Results of a case control study using the NEO-FFI. *Journal of Communication Disorders, 44*(2), 218-222.

Bleek, B., Reuter, M., Yaruss, J. S., Cook, S., Faber, J., & Montag, C. (2012). Relationships between personality characteristics of people who stutter and the impact of stuttering on everyday life. *Journal of Fluency Disorders, 37*(4), 325-333.

Block, S., Ingham, R. J., & Bench, R. J. (1996). The effects of the Edinburgh Masker on stuttering. *Australian Journal of Human Communication Disorders, 24*(1), 11-18.

Blomgren, M. (2010). Stuttering treatment for adults: An update on contemporary approaches. *Seminars in Speech and Language, 31*, 272-282.

Blood, G. (2014). Bullying Be Gone. *The ASHA Leader* (May), 36-43.

Blood, G. W., & Blood, I. M. (2004). Bullying in adolescents who stutter: Communicative competence and self-esteem. *Contemporary Issues in Communication Science and Disorders*, *31*, 69-79.

Blood, G. W., Blood, I. M., Dorward, S., Boyle, M. P., & Tramontana, G. M. (2011). Coping strategies and adolescents: Learning to take care of self and stuttering during treatment. *SIG 4 Perspectives on Fluency and Fluency Disorders*, *21*(3), 68-77.

Blood, G. W., Blood, I. M., Maloney, K., Meyer, C., & Qualls, C. D. (2007). Anxiety levels in adolescents who stutter. *Journal of Communication Disorders*, *40*, 452-469.

Blood, G. W., Blood, I. M., Tellis, G. M., & Gabel, R. M. (2003). A preliminary study of self-esteem, stigma, and disclosure in adolescents who stutter. *Journal of Fluency Disorders*, *28*(2), 143-159.

Blood, G.W., Blood, I.M., Tramontana, G.M., Sylvia, A.J., Boyle, M.P., & Motzko, G.R. (2011). Self-reported experience of bullying of students who stutter: Relations with life satisfaction, life orientation, and self-esteem 1. *Perceptual and Motor Skills*, *113*(2), 353-364.

Blood, G. W., Boyle, M. P., Blood, I. M., & Nalesnik, G. R. (2010). Bullying in children who stutter: Speech-language pathologists' perceptions and intervention strategies. *Journal of Fluency Disorders*, *35*(2), 92-109.

Bloodstein, O. (1950). A rating scale study of conditions under which stuttering is reduced or absent. *Journal of Speech and Hearing Disorders, 15*, 29-36.

Bloodstein, O. (1958). Stuttering as an anticipatory struggle reaction. In J. Eisenson, (Ed.), *Stuttering: A Symposium* (pp. 3–69). New York: Harper & Row.

Bloodstein, O. (1960). The development of stuttering: I. Changes in nine basic features. *Journal of Speech and Hearing Disorders, 25*, 219-237.

Bloodstein, O. (1981). *A Handbook on Stuttering* (3rd ed.). Chicago, IL: National Easter Seal Society.

Bloodstein, O. (1993). *Stuttering: The Search for a Cause and Cure.* Needham Heights: Pearson College Division.

Bloodstein, O. (1995). *A Handbook on Stuttering* (5th ed.). Chicago, IL: National Easter Seal Society.

Bloodstein, O., & Bernstein Ratner, N. (2008). *A Handbook on Stuttering* (6th ed.). New York: Thomson Delmar Learning.

Blumgart, E., Tran, Y., & Craig, A. (2010). Social anxiety disorder in adults who stutter. *Depression and Anxiety, 27*(7), 687-692.

Boberg, J. (1997). Spouses of people who stutter. In M. Hughes (Ed.), *Good people: The best of speaking out.* St. John, Canada: Speak Easy Inc.

Boberg, J. M., & Boberg, E. (1990). The other side of the block: The stutterer's spouse. *Journal of Fluency Disorders, 15*(1), 61-75.

Boller, F., Boller, M., Denes, G., Timberlake, W. H., Zieper, I., & Albert, M. (1973). Familial palilalia. *Neurology 23, 1117-25.*

Bonfanti, B. H., & Culatta, R. (1977). An analysis of the fluency patterns of institutionalized retarded adults. *Journal of Fluency Disorders, 2*(2), 117-128.

Borden, G. J. (1983). Initiation versus execution time during manual and oral counting by stutterers. *Journal of Speech, Language, and Hearing Research, 26*(3), 389-396.

Borden, G. J. (1990). Subtyping adult stutterers for research purposes. *In J.A. Cooper (Ed.), Research needs in stuttering: Roadblocks and future directions (pp. 58-62).*

Borden, G. J., Baer, T., & Kenney, M. K. (1985). Onset of voicing in stuttered and fluent utterances. *Journal of Speech, Language, and Hearing Research, 28*(3), 363-372.

Boström, P. K., Broberg, M., & Hwang, P. (2010). Parents' descriptions and experiences of young children recently diagnosed with intellectual disability. *Child: Care, Health and Development, 36*(1), 93-100.

Bothe, A., Davidow, J., Bramlett, R., & Ingham, R. (2006). Stuttering treatment research 1970-2005: I. Systematic review incorporating trial quality assessment of behavioral, cognitive, and related approaches. *American Journal of Speech-Language Pathology, 15*, 321-341.

Boucand, V. A., Millard, S., Packman, A. (2014). Early intervention for stuttering: Similarities and differences between two programs. *SIG Perspectives on Fluency and Fluency Disorders, 24*(1), 8-19.

Boyd, A., Dworzynski, K., & Howell, P. (2011). Pharmacological agents for developmental stuttering in children and adolescents: A systematic review. *Journal of Clinical Psychopharmacology, 31*(6), 740-744.

Boyle, M. P. (2013). Psychological characteristics and perceptions of stuttering of adults who stutter with and without support group experience. *Journal of Fluency Disorders, 38*(4), 368-381.

Boyle, M. P. (2015). Identifying correlates of self-stigma in adults who stutter: Further establishing the construct validity of the Self-Stigma of Stuttering Scale (4S). *Journal of Fluency Disorders, 43*, 17-27.

Brady, J. P. (1991). The pharmacology of stuttering: A critical review. *American Journal of Psychiatry, 148*(1), 1309-1316.

Bricker-Katz, G., Lincoln, M., & Cumming, S. (2013). Stuttering and work life: An interpretative phenomenological analysis. *Journal of Fluency Disorders, 38*(4), 342-355.

Brocklehurst, P. H., Drake, E., & Corley, M. (2015). Perfectionism and stuttering: Findings of an online survey. *Journal of Fluency Disorders, 44,* 46-62.

Brosch, S., Häge, A., & Johannsen, H. S. (2002). Prognostic indicators for stuttering: The value of computer-based speech analysis. *Brain and Language, 82*(1), 75-86.

Brown, S. F., & Moren, A. (1942). The Frequency of Stuttering in Relation to Word Length During Oral Reading. *Journal of Speech Disorders, 7*(2), 153-159.

Brown, S., Ingham, R. J., Ingham, J. C., Laird, A. R., & Fox, P. T. (2005). Stuttered and fluent speech production: An ALE meta-analysis of functional neuroimaging studies. *Human Brain Mapping, 25*(1), 105-117.

Bruder, C. E., Piotrowski, A., Gijsbers, A. A., Andersson, R., Erickson, S., De Ståhl, T. D., & Dumanski, J. P. (2008). Phenotypically concordant and discordant monozygotic twins display different DNA copy-number-variation profiles. *The American Journal of Human Genetics, 82*(3), 763-771.

Brundage, S. B., & Hancock, A. B. (2015). Real enough: Using virtual public speaking environments to evoke feelings and behaviors targeted in stuttering assessment and treatment. *American Journal of Speech-Language Pathology, 24,* 139-149.

Brutten, E. J., & Shoemaker, D. J. (1967). *The Modification of Stuttering*. Englewood Cliffs, N.J: Prentice-Hall.

Brutten, G.J. & Vanryckeghem, M. (2003). BAB Behavior Assessment Battery, A multi-dimensional and evidence-based approach to diagnostic and therapeutic decision making for adults who stutter. Destelbergen: SIG.

Brutten, G., & Vanryckeghem, M. (2006). Behavior Assessment Battery for children who stutter. San Diego, CA: Plural Publishing.

Brutten, G. & Vanryckeghem, M. (2010). BigCAT: Communication Attitude Test for Adults. San Diego, CA: Plural Publishing

Buscaglia, L. (1975). *The Disabled & Their Parents: A Counseling Challenge*. Thorofare, N. J.: C. B. Slack.

Cavenagh, P., Costelloe, S., Davis, S., & Howell, P. (2015). Characteristics of young children close to the onset of stuttering. *Communication Disorders Quarterly*, *36*(3), 162-171.

Centers for Disease Control and Prevention (2010). Youth risk behavior surveillance – United States, 2009. Surveillance summaries. *Morbidity and Mortality Weekly Report*, 59(SS-5).

Chang, S. E. (2011). Using brain images to unravel the mysteries of stuttering. *The Stuttering Foundation.* Retrieved from: http://www.stutteringhelp.org/using-brain-imaging-unravel-mysteries-stuttering

Chang, S. E., Kenney, M. K., Loucks, T. M., & Ludlow, C. L. (2009). Brain activation abnormalities during speech and non-speech in stuttering speakers. *Neuroimage*, *46*(1), 201-212.

Chang, S. E., Horwitz, B., Ostuni, J., Reynolds, R., & Ludlow, C. L. (2011). Evidence of left inferior frontal–premotor structural and functional connectivity deficits in adults who stutter. *Cerebral Cortex*, *21*(11), 2507-2518.

Chapman, A. H., & Cooper, E. B. (1973). Nature of stuttering in a mentally retarded population. *American Journal of Mental Deficiency. 78(2), 153-157*.

Cheasman, C. & Everard, R. (2015). Stuttering: Acceptance and Commitment. *Advance Healthcare Network for Speech & Hearing.* Available at: http://speech-language-pathology-audiology.advanceweb.com/Features/Articles/Acceptance-and-Commitment.aspx.

Cheng, L. & Williams, D. F. (2012) Multicultural issues in CSD. In Williams, D. F. *Communication Sciences and Disorders: An Introduction to the Professions.* New York: Taylor & Francis.

Claridge, G. Ando, V., & Clark, K. (2014). Psychotic traits in comedians. *British Journal of Psychiatry, 204,* 341-345.

Clark, C. E., Conture, E. G., Frankel, C. B., & Walden, T. A. (2012). Communicative and psychological dimensions of the Kiddy-CAT. *Journal of Communication Disorders, 45*(3), 223-234.

Coleman, C. (2013). SIGnatures: Widening the Treatment Circle Involving parents enhances treatment for children who stutter. So why not include the child's siblings, friends, teachers and other communication partners? *The ASHA Leader, 18*(2), 54-56.

Collins, C. R., & Blood, G. W. (1990). Acknowledgment and severity of stuttering as factors influencing nonstutterers' perceptions of stutterers. *Journal of Speech and Hearing Disorders, 55*(1), 75-81.

Conture, E.G. (1996). Treatment Efficacy: Stuttering. *Journal of Speech and Hearing Research, 39,* S18-S26.

Conture, E. G. (2001). *Stuttering: An Integrated Approach to its Nature and Treatment* (3rd ed.). Needham Heights, MA: Allyn & Bacon.

Conture, E. G., & Guitar, B. E. (1993). Evaluating efficacy treatments of stuttering: School age children. *Journal of Fluency Disorders, 18*(2-3), 253-287.

Conture, E. G., & Kelly, E. M. (1991). Young stutterers' nonspeech behaviors during stuttering. *Journal of Speech, Language, and Hearing Research, 34*(5), 1041-1056.

Cooper, E. B. (1972). Recovery from stuttering in a junior and senior high school population. *Journal of Speech, Language, and Hearing Research, 15*(3), 632-638.

Cooper, E. B. (1986). The mentally retarded stutterer. *In K. O. St. Louis (Ed.), The Atypical Stutterer: Principles and practices of rehabilitation (pp. 123-154). Florida: Atlantic Press.*

Cooper, E.B. (1987). The chronic preservative stuttering syndrome: Incurable stuttering. *Journal of Fluency Disorders, 12,* 381-388.

Cooper, E. B. (2003). Understanding the process. In J. Fraiser (Ed.) *Effective counseling in stuttering therapy.* Memphis, TN: Stuttering Foundation of America.

Cooper, E. B., & Cooper, C. S. (1985). Clinician attitudes toward stuttering: A decade of change (1973–1983). *Journal of Fluency Disorders, 10*(1), 19-33.

Cooper, E. B., Parris, R., & Wells, M. T. (1974). Prevalence of and recovery from speech disorders in a group of freshmen at the University of Alabama. *ASHA, 16*(7), 359.

Coppens-Hofman, M. C., Terband, H. R., Maassen, B. A. M., van Schrojenstein Lantman-De Valk,Henny M J., van Zaalen-op't Hof, Y., & Snik, A. F. M. (2013). Dysfluencies in the speech of adults with intellectual disabilities and reported speech difficulties. *Journal of Communication Disorders, 46*(5-6), 484.

Copstick, K. (2003). [Review of the comedy show *BIRDS*]. *The Scotsman.*

Corcoran, J. A., & Stewart, M. (1998). Stories of stuttering: A qualitative analysis of interview narratives. *Journal of Fluency Disorders, 23*(4), 247-264.

Cordes, A. K. (2000). Individual and consensus judgments of disfluency types in the speech of persons who stutter. *Journal of Speech, Language, and Hearing Research, 43*(4), 951-964.

Coriat, I. (1928). Stammering: A psychoanalytic interpretation. *Nervous & Mental Disorders Monographs, 47,* 1-68.

Cox, N. J., Seider, R. A., & Kidd, K. K. (1984). Some environmental factors and hypotheses for stuttering in families with several stutterers. *Journal of Speech, Language, and Hearing Research, 27*(4), 543-548.

Cox, R. (2005, August 22). I've Stuttered So I'll F-F-Finish [Review of the comedy show *I've Stuttered So I'll F-F-Finish*]. *The Scotsman*. Retrieved from: http://www.scotsman.com/news/ i-ve-stuttered-so-i-ll-f-f-finish-1-730282

Cracking down on binge drinking (2014). Retrieved from: http:// marca.wikia.com/wiki/Research.

Craig, A. R. (1998). Relapse following treatment for stuttering: A critical review and correlative data. *Journal of Fluency Disorders, 23*, 1-30.

Craig A. (2010). The importance of conducting controlled clinical trials in the fluency disorders with emphasis on cluttering. In: K. Bakker, L.J. Raphael, F.L. Myers (Eds.). *Proceedings of the First World Conference on Cluttering. International Cluttering Association* (pp. 220-219).

Craig, A. (2014). Major controversies in fluency disorders: Clarifying the relationship between anxiety and stuttering. *Journal of Fluency Disorders, 40*, 1-3.

Craig, A., Blumgart, E., & Tran, Y. (2011). Resilience and stuttering: Factors that protect people from the adversity of chronic stuttering. *Journal of Speech, Language, and Hearing Research, 54*(6), 1485-1496.

Craig, A., Hancock, K., Tran, Y., Craig, M., & Peters, K. (2002). Epidemiology of stuttering in the community across the entire life span. *Journal of Speech, Language, and Hearing Research, 45*(6), 1097-1105.

Craig, A., Hancock, K., Tran, Y., Craig, M., & Peters, K. (2003). Stereotypes towards stuttering for those who have never had direct contact with people who stutter: A randomized and stratified study. *Perceptual and Motor Skills, 97*, 235-245.

Cross, D. E., & Olson, P. (1987). Interaction between jaw kinematics and voice onset for stutterers and nonstutterers in a VRT task. *Journal of Fluency Disorders, 12*(5), 367-380.

Crowe, T. (1997). *Applications of Counseling in Speech-Language Pathology and Audiology*. Baltimore: Williams & Wilkins.

Crowe Hall, B.J. (1991). Attitudes of fourth and sixth graders toward peers with mild articulation disorders. *Language, Speech, and Hearing Services in Schools, 22*, 334-340.

Culatta, R., & Goldberg, S. A. (1995). *Stuttering Therapy: An integrated approach to theory and practice*. Needham Heights, MA: Allyn & Bacon.

Cullinan, W. L., & Springer, M. T. (1980). Voice initiation and termination times in stuttering and nonstuttering children. *Journal of Speech, Language, and Hearing Research, 23*(2), 344-360.

Cummins, F. (2012) Gaze and blinking in dyadic conversation: A study in coordinated behaviour among individuals. *Language and Cognitive Processes, 27:10*, 1525-1549.

Cykowski, M. D., Fox, P. T., Ingham, R. J., Ingham, J. C., & Robin, D. A. (2010). A study of the reproducibility and etiology of diffusion anisotropy differences in developmental stuttering: a potential role for impaired myelination. *Neuroimage, 52*(4), 1495-1504.

Dahm, B. (2015). Barbara Dahm thoughts on dynamic stuttering therapy. Available at http://www.isastutter.org/alternative-therapies/barbara-dahm-thoughts-on-dynamic-stuttering-therapy.

Dake, J. A., Price, J. H., & Telljohann, S. K. (2003). The nature and extent of bullying at school. *Journal of School Health, 73*(5), 173-180.

Daly, D. & Burnett, M. (1996) Cluttering: Assessment, treatment planning, and case study illustration. *Journal of Fluency Disorders, 21,* 239-244.

Daniels, D. E., Gabel, R. M., & Hughes, S. (2012). Recounting the K-12 school experiences of adults who stutter: A qualitative analysis. *Journal of Fluency Disorders, 37*(2), 71-82.

Daniels, D. E., Hagstrom, F., & Gabel, R. M. (2006). A qualitative study of how African American men who stutter attribute meaning to identity and life choices. *Journal of Fluency Disorders, 31*(3), 200-215.

Davidow, J. H., Crowe, B.T., & Bothe, A. K. (2004). Gradual increase in length and complexity of utterance and extended length of utterance treatment programs for stuttering: Assessing the implications of strong but limited evidence. In A.K. Bothe (Ed.), *Evidence-based treatment of stuttering: Empirical bases and clinical applications* (pp. 201-229). Mahwah, NJ: Lawrence Erlbaum.

Defloor, T., Van Borsel, J., & Curfs, L. (2000). Speech fluency in Prader-Willi syndrome. *Journal of Fluency Disorders, 25*(2), 85-98.

DeNil, L. F. (1998). Some thoughts on the multidimensional nature of stuttering from a neurophysiological perspective. *In 1st International Stuttering Awareness Day Online Conference (ISAD1).* Available at: http://www.mnsu.edu/comdis/isad/papers/denil.html

DeNil, L. F., & Brutten, G. J. (1987). Communication attitudes of stuttering, speech disordered and normal speak children. Paper presented at the American Speech-Language-Hearing Association Convention, New Orleans, LA.

DeNil, L. F., Kroll, R. M., Lafaille, S. J., & Houle, S. (2004). A positron emission tomography study of short-and long-term treatment effects on functional brain activation in adults who stutter. *Journal of Fluency Disorders, 28*(4), 357-380.

DePaulo, B. (2009). Children of single mothers: How do they really fare? *Psychology Today*. Available at: https://www.psychologytoday.com/blog/living-single/200901/children-single-mothers-how-do-they-really-fare.

de Sonneville-Koedoot, C., Stolk, E., Rietveld, T., & Franken, M-C (2015). Direct versus Indirect Treatment for Preschool Children who Stutter: The RESTART Randomized Trial. *PLoS ONE 10(7)*:e0133758.

Devices are not a cure, Foundation reports (2004). *Advance for Speech-Language Pathologists and Audiologists, 14 (19)*, 14.

Dietrich, S. (2000). Tension control therapy: A model of integrated approaches to treatment. *Journal of Fluency Disorders, 25*(3), 170.

Disability Now. (2004, August). [Review of the comedy show *D-D-D-Don't Mention the Disability...I did once and it took 15 minutes*]. *Disability Now Magazine.* Retrieved from: http://www.disabilitynow.org.uk/living/arts/feature_fringe.htm

Dominques, C. E. F., Olivera, C. M. C., Oliveira, B. V., Juste, F. S., Andrade, C. R. F., Giacheti, C. M., Moretti - Ferreria, D. & Drayna, D. (2014). A genetic linkage study in Brazil identifies a new locus for persistent developmental stuttering on chromosome 10. *Genetics and molecular research: GMR, 13*(1), 2094.

Donaher, J. (2003). Intervention strategies for the school-aged child who stutters. Workshop presented at the National Stuttering Association Convention, Nashville.

Donaher, J. & Scott, L. (2014, May). Be prepared to help at-risk clients. *The ASHA Leader,*19, 45-50.

Doody, I., Kalinowski, J., Armson, J., & Stuart, A. (1993). Stereotypes of stutterers and nonstutterers in three rural communities in Newfoundland. *Journal of Fluency Disorders, 18*(4), 363-373.

Dorsey, M., & Guenther, R. K. (2000). Attitudes of professors and students toward college students who stutter. *Journal of Fluency Disorders*, 25(1), 77-83.

Douglass, E. & Quarrington, B. (1952). The differentiation of interiorized and exteriorized secondary stuttering. *Journal of Speech and Hearing Disorders, 17*, 377-385.

Dowell, B. (2003). [Review of the comedy show *BIRDS*]. *The Stage.*

Duffy, J. R. (1995). *Motor Speech Disorders*. Toronto: Mosby.

Dugan, C. (1998, April/May). Book review/Case review. *Reaching Out.*

Dunn, L. M., & Dunn, D. M. (2007). Picture Peabody Vocabulary Test (4th ed.). Pearson Clinical.

EdFringe, (2004). Review [Review of the comedy show *D-D-D-Don't Mention Disability. I Did Once and it Took me 15 Minutes*]. Available at: http://edfringereview.com/

Eggers, K., DeNil, L. F., & Van den Bergh, B. R. (2010). Temperament dimensions in stuttering and typically developing children. *Journal of Fluency Disorders, 35*(4), 355-372.

Einarsdóttir, J., & Ingham, R. J. (2005). Have disfluency-type measures contributed to the understanding and treatment of developmental stuttering? *American Journal of Speech-Language Pathology, 14*(4), 260-273.

Eldridge, K. (1997). A Conversation With My Stutter. Available on the Stuttering Home Page at http://www.mnsu.edu/comdis/kuster/casestudy/eldridge.html

Erickson, R. L. (1969). Assessing communication attitudes among stutterers. *Journal of Speech, Language, and Hearing Research, 12*(4), 711-724.

Evans, D., Healey, E. C., Kawai, N., & Rowland, S. (2008). Middle school students' perceptions of a peer who stutters. *Journal of Fluency Disorders*, *33*(3), 203-219.

Feinberg, A. (1990, July, 14). Stuttering protest and TV censorship. *Chicago Tribune.* Retrieved from: http://articles.chicagotribune.com/1990-07-14/news/9002270431_1_national-stuttering-project-trim-tv-notes

Felsenfeld, S., Kirk, K. M., Zhu, G., Statham, D. J., Neale, M. C., & Martin, N. G. (2000). A study of the genetic and environmental etiology of stuttering in a selected twin sample. *Behavior Genetics*, *30*(5), 359-366.

Fenichel, O. (1945). *The Psychoanalytic Theory of Neurosis.* New York: W. W. Norton & Company.

Finn, P. (1996). Establishing the validity of recovery from stuttering without formal treatment. *Journal of Speech, Language, and Hearing Research*, *39*(6), 1171-1181.

Finn, P. (1997). Adults Recovered From Stuttering Without Formal Treatment: Perceptual Assessment of Speech Normalcy. *Journal of Speech, Language, and Hearing Research*, *40*(4), 821-831.

Finn, P. (2004). Self-change from stuttering during adolescence and adulthood. In A.K. Bothe (Ed.), *Evidence-based treatment of stuttering: Empirical bases and clinical applications* (pp. 117-136).

Finn, P. (2005). The epigenisis of stuttering. *Journal of Fluency Disorders, 30,* 163-188.

Fluharty, N. B. (2000). *Fluharty Preschool speech and language screening test* (2nd ed.). Austin, Pro-Ed.

Foundas, A. L., Bollich, A. M., Corey, D. M., Hurley, M., & Heilman, K. M. (2001). Anomalous anatomy of speech–language areas in adults with persistent developmental stuttering. *Neurology*, *57*(2), 207-215.

Foundas, A. L., Cindass Jr, R., Mock, J. R., & Corey, D. M. (2013). Atypical caudate anatomy in children who stutter 1, 2. *Perceptual & Motor Skills*, *116*(2), 528-543.

Foundas, A. L., Corey, D. M., Angeles, V., Bollich, A. M., Crabtree–Hartman, E., & Heilman, K. M. (2003). Atypical cerebral laterality in adults with persistent developmental stuttering. *Neurology*, *61*(10), 1378-1385.

Fox, P. T., Ingham, R. J., Ingham, J. C., Hirsch, T. B., Downs, J. H., Martin, C., Jerabek, P., Glass, T. & Lancaster, J. L. (1996). A PET study of the neural systems of stuttering. *Nature, 382,* 158-162.

Franken, MC. J., Kielstra-Van der Schlak, C. J., Boelens, H. (2005). Experimental treatment of early stuttering: A preliminary study. *Journal of Fluency Disorders, 30*(3), 189-199.

Frankl, V. (1946). *Man's search for meaning: The Classic Tribute to Hope from the Holocaust.* Boston: Beacon Press.

Fringe, The. (2014). The Edinburgh fringe society annual review 2014. Available at: https://www.edfringe.com/uploads/docs/About_Us/Fringe%20Annual%20Review%202014.pdf

Fry, J. (2009). Introduction to Cognitive Therapy. *The Stuttering Foundation.* Retrieved from: http://www.stutteringhelp.org/introduction-cognitive-therapy.

Fry, J., Botterill, W., & Pring, T (2009). *The effect of an intensive group therapy programme for young adults who stutter: A single subject study. International Journal of Speech-Language Pathology*, 11 (1): 12-19.

Frymark, T., Venediktov, R., & Wang, B. (2010). Effectiveness of interventions for preschool children with fluency disorders: A comparison of direct versus indirect treatments. Rockville, MD: American Speech-Language-Hearing Association. Retrieved from www.asha.org/members/ebp/EBSRs/.

G, N. & D, G. (2012, January 22). Shit fluent people say to people who stutter [YouTube video]. Retrieved from: https://www.youtube.com/watch?v=stCCXC4KYPc

Gabel, R. M., Blood, G. W., Tellis, G. M., & Althouse, M. T. (2004). Measuring role entrapment of people who stutter. *Journal of Fluency Disorders, 29*(1), 27-49.

Gabel, R. M., Hughes, S., & Daniels, D. (2008). Effects of stuttering severity and therapy involvement on role entrapment of people who stutter. *Journal of Communication Disorders, 41*(2), 146-158.

Gallop, R. F., & Runyan, C. M. (2012). Long-term effectiveness of the SpeechEasy fluency-enhancement device. *Journal of Fluency Disorders, 37*(4), 334-343.

Goldiamond, I. (1965). Stuttering and fluency as manipulatable operant response classes. In L. Krasner & L. Ullman (Eds.), *Research in behavior modification* (pp. 106-156). New York: Holt, Rinehart & Winston.

Goodhue, R., Onslow, M., Quine, S., O'Brian, S., & Hearne, A. (2010). The Lidcombe program of early stuttering intervention: mothers' experiences. *Journal of Fluency Disorders, 35*(1), 70-84.

Gregory, H. (1991). Therapy for elementary school-age children. *Seminars in Speech and Language, 12,* 323-335.

Gregory, H. H. (2003). *Stuttering Therapy: Rationale and Procedures.* Boston: Allyn & Bacon.

Griener, J. R., Fitzgerald, H. E., Cooke, P. A., & Djurdjlc, S. D. (1985). Assessment of sensitivity to interpersonal stress in stutterers and nonstutterers. *Journal of Communication Disorders, 18,* 215-225.

Griffiths, S. (2014, Oct 12). Body confidence lessons for pupils. *The Sunday Times.* Available at: http://www.thesundaytimes.co.uk/sto/news/uk_news/Education/article1470349.ece.

Guitar, B. (1998). *Stuttering: An Integrated Approach to its Nature and Treatment.* Baltimore: Williams & Wilkins.

Guitar, B. (2013). *Stuttering: An Integrated Approach to its Nature and Treatment* (4th ed). Baltimore, MD: Lippincott, Williams, & Wilkins.

Guitar, B., & Conture, E. G. (2005). *The Child who Stutters: To the Pediatrician* (4th ed.). Memphis, TN: Stuttering Foundation of America.

Guitar, B., Kazenski, D., Howard, A., Cousins, S. F., Fader, E., & Haskell, P. (2015). Predicting treatment time and long term outcome of the Lidcombe program: A replication and reanalysis. *American-Journal of Speech-Language Pathology, 24,* 533-544.

Guitar, B. & Tozier, N. (2002). A different kind of electronic device for stuttering therapy for children. *In 5th International Stuttering Awareness Day Online Conference (ISAD5).* Available at: https://www.mnsu.edu/comdis/isad5/papers/guitar.html

Gunthert, K. C., Cohen, L. H., & Armeli, S. (1999). The role of neuroticism in daily stress and coping. *Journal of Personality and Social Psychology, 77*(5), 1087.

Hancock, K., & Craig, A. (1998). Predictors of stuttering relapse one year following treatment for children aged 9 to 14 years. *Journal of Fluency Disorders, 23*(1), 31-48.

Hand, C. R., & Haynes, W. O. (1983). Linguistic processing and reaction time differences in stutterers and nonstutterers. *Journal of Speech, Language, and Hearing Research, 26*(2), 181-185.

Hanson, D. M., Jackson, A. W., Hagerman, R. J., Opitz, J. M., & Reynolds, J. F. (1986). Speech disturbances (cluttering) in mildly impaired males with the Martin-Bell/fragile X syndrome. *American Journal of Medical Genetics, 23*(1-2), 195-206.

Harasym, J., Langevin, M., & Kully, D. (2015). Video self-modeling as a post-treatment fluency recovery strategy for adults. *Journal of Fluency Disorders, 44,* 32-45.

Harris, P. (2014, Jan 7). *Only 2% of applicants actually get interviews: Here's how to be one of them.* Available at http://www.workopolis.com/content/advice/article/only-2-of-applicants-actually-get-interviews-heres-how-to-be-one-of-them/

Harrison, K. (2013). *Self confidence and self efficacy* [PowerPoint slides]. Available at: http://www.slideshare.net/klharrison/self-confidence-and-selfefficacy-2013?related=1

Hay, M. (2007, February 5). The state of London's comedy circuit. *Timeout London.* Retrieved from: http://www.timeout.com/london/comedy/the-state-of-londons-comedy-circuit

Healey, E. C. (2010). What the literature tells us about listeners' reactions to stuttering: Implications for the clinical management of stuttering. *Seminars in Speech and Language, 31(4),* 227-235.

Healy, S. (2004, August 5). The List [Review of the comedy show *The 3 Monkeys*]. *Glasgow and Edinburgh Events Guide.*

Hearne, A., Packman, A., Onslow, M., & Quine, S. (2008). Stuttering and its treatment in adolescence: The perceptions of people who stutter. *Journal of Fluency Disorders, 33(2),* 81-98.

Hegde, M. N., & Davis, D. (1999). *Clinical methods and practicum in speech-language pathology* (3rd ed.). San Diego, CA: Singular Publishing Group.

Hegde, M. N., & Hartman, D. E. (1979). Factors affecting judgments of fluency: I. Interjections. *Journal of Fluency Disorders, 4(1),* 1-11.

Helgadottir, F. D., Menzies, R. G., Onslow, M., Packman, A., & O'Brian, S. (2014). Safety Behaviors and Speech Treatment for Adults Who Stutter. *Journal of Speech, Language, and Hearing Research, 57*(4), 1308-1313.

Hicks, B. (2005). Love All the People: Letters, Lyrics, Routines. London: Constable.

Hicks, R. (1997). In On the Lighter Side, Stuttering Home Page, at: http://www.mnsu.edu/comdis/kuster/humor.html#hicks

Hood, S. (2003). Desirable Outcomes From Stuttering Therapy. *In 6th International Stuttering Awareness Day Online Conference (ISAD6).* Available at: http://www.mnsu.edu/comdisi-sad6/papers/hood6.html

Hood, S. & Roach, C. (2001). "I've Got a Secret – And It's Scaring Me to Death! (The Story of a Covert Stutterer)." In 4th International Stuttering Awareness Day Online Conference (ISAD4). Available at: http://www.mankato.msus.edu/dept/comdis/4/papers/hood.html

Hope, J. (2015). Why drinking is bad for you until your mid-30s. *Daily Mail.* Retrieved from: http://www.dailymail.co.uk/health/article-130020/Why-drinking-bad-mid-30s.html

Howell, P., Au-Yeung, J., & Sackin, S. (1999). Exchange of stuttering from function words to content words with age. *Journal of Speech, Language, and Hearing Research, 42*(2), 345-354.

Howell, P. & Davis, S. (2011). The epidemiology of cluttering with stuttering. In D. Ward & K. Scaler-Scott, *Cluttering: A Handbook of Research, Intervention and Education.* Hove: Psychology Press.

Howell, P., El-Yaniv, N., and Powell, D. J. (1987). Factors affecting fluency in stutterers when speaking under altered auditory feedback. In Peters, H., and Hulstijn, W. (Eds.), *Speech motor dynamics in stuttering* (pp. 361-369). New York: Springer.

Howie, P. M. (1981). Intrapair similarity in frequency of disfluency in monozygotic and dizygotic twin pairs containing stutterers. *Behavior Genetics, 11*(3), 227-238.

Hugh-Jones, S., & Smith, P. K. (1999). Self-reports of short-and long-term effects of bullying on children who stammer. *British Journal of Educational Psychology, 69,* 141-158.

Hulit, L. M. (2006). *Straight talk on stuttering: Information, encouragement and counsel for stutterers, caregivers, and speech-language clinicians* (2nd ed.). Springfield, IL: Charles C. Thomas Publisher Ltd.

Hulstijn, W., Van Lieshout, P. H. H. M., & Peters, H. F. M. (1991). On the measurement of coordination. In H. F. M. Peters, W. Hulstijn, & C. W. Starkweather (Eds.), *Speech motor control and stuttering* (pp. 211-231). Amsterdam: Elsevier Science Publishers.

Hunt, B. (1987). Self-help for stutterers – Experience in Britain. In L. Rustin, H. Purser, & D. Rowley (Eds.), *Progress in the treatment of fluency disorders.* London: Whurr.

Hurst, M. A, & Cooper, E. B. (1983a). Employer attitudes toward stuttering. *Journal of Fluency Disorders, 8*(1), 1-12.

Hurst, M. A., & Cooper, E. B. (1983b). Vocational rehabilitation counselors' attitudes toward stuttering. *Journal of Fluency Disorders, 8*(1), 13-27.

Ingham, R. J., Bothe, A. K., Wang, Y., Purkhiser, K., & New, A. (2012). Phonation interval modification and speech performance quality during fluency-inducing conditions by adults who stutter. *Journal of Communication Disorders, 45*(3), 198-211.

Ingham, R. J., Gow, M., & Costello, J. M. (1985). Stuttering and Speech Naturalness Some Additional Data. *Journal of Speech and Hearing Disorders, 50*(2), 217-219.

Ingham, R. J., & Packman, A. C. (1978). Perceptual assessment of normalcy of speech following stuttering therapy. *Journal of Speech, Language, and Hearing Research, 21*(1), 63-73.

Iverach, L., O'Brian, S., Jones, M., Block, S., Lincoln, M., Harrison, E., Hewat, S., Menzies, R. G., Packman, A., & Onslow, M. (2010). The five factor model of personality applied to adults who stutter. *Journal of communication disorders, 43*(2), 120-132.

Janssen, P., Kraaimaat, F., & Brutten, G. (1990). Relationship between stutterers' genetic history and speech-associated variables. *Journal of Fluency Disorders, 15*(1), 39-48.

Janssen, P., Wieneke, G., & Vaane, E. (1983). Variability in the initiation of articulatory movements in the speech of stutterers and normal speakers. *Journal of Fluency Disorders, 8*(4), 341-358.

Jayaram, M. (2014). Some perceptual and acoustical correlates of stuttering: a pre-post therapy comparison. Available at: http://hdl.handle.net/10603/15937

Johnson, W. (1942). A Study of the Onset and Development of Stuttering1.*Journal of Speech Disorders, 7*(3), 251-257.

Johnson, W. (1950). Teaching children with speech handicaps. *National Society for the Study of Education, 49*, 177-193.

Johnson, W., Brown, S., Curtis, J., Edney, C, & Keaster, J. (1967). *Speech handicapped school children*. New York: Harper & Row.

Johnson, W., & Knott, J. R. (1937). Studies in the psychology of stuttering: I. The distribution of moments of stuttering in successive readings of the same materials. *Journal of Speech Disorders, 2*, 17-19.

Johnson-Root, B. A. (2015). *Oral-Facial Evaluation for Speech-Language Pathologists.* Plural Publishing.

Jokel, R., DeNil, L., & Sharpe, K. (2007). Speech disfluencies in adults with neurogenic stuttering associated with stroke and traumatic brain injury. *Journal of Medical Speech-Language Pathology*, 12(3), 243-261.

Jones, T. J. (2004). Toni's research findings. Available at the Canadian Association of People Who Stutter Web site: http://www.stutter.ca/research.html.

Jones, R. M., Conture, E. G., & Walden, T. A. (2014). Emotional reactivity and regulation associated with fluent and stuttered utterances of preschool-age children who stutter. *Journal of Communication Disorders, 48*, 38-51.

Jones, M., Onslow, M., Harrison, E., Packman, A. (2000). Treating stuttering in young children. *Journal of Speech, Language, and Hearing Research, 43*, 1440-1450.

Jones, M., Onslow, M., Packman, A., O'Brian, S., Hearne, A., Williams, S., Ormond, T., & Schwarz, I. (2008). Extended follow up of a randomized controlled trial of the Lidcombe Program of Early Stuttering Intervention. *International Journal of Language & Communication Disorders, 43*(6), 649-661.

JS (2003, August 11). [Review of the comedy show *BIRDS*]. *Three Weeks (an Edinburgh Fringe Free Newspaper).*

Kahneman, D. (2011). *Thinking, fast and slow.* New York, NY: Farrar, Straus and Giroux

Kale, K., & Williams, D. F. (2014). MyLynel: Customizable Therapy Platform for Clinical Therapy Outside of a Clinic, ASHA Convention, Orlando.

Kalinowski, J., Noble, S., Armson, J., & Stuart, A. (1994). Pretreatment and posttreatment speech naturalness ratings of adults with mild and severe stuttering. *American Journal of Speech-Language Pathology*, 3(2), 61-66.

Kay, A. (2004, August 26). [Review of the comedy show *BIRDS*]. Retrieved from: www.EdinburghGuide.com

Kefalianos, E., Onslow, M., Ukoumunne, O., Block, S., & Reilly, S. (2014). Stuttering, temperament, and anxiety: Data from a community cohort ages 2–4 years. *Journal of Speech, Language, and Hearing Research, 57*(4), 1314-1322.

Kendall, D.L., (2000). Counseling in communication disorders. *Contemporary Issues in Communication Science and Disorders, 27*, 96-103.

Kent, R. D. (1983). Facts about stuttering: Neuropsychologic perspectives. *Journal of Speech and Hearing Disorders, 48*(3). 249-255.

Kidd, K. K. (1980). Genetic models of stuttering. *Journal of Fluency Disorders, 5*(3), 187-201.

Kidd, K. K. (1984). Stuttering as a genetic disorder. In R. F. Curlee & W. H. Perkins (Eds.). *Nature and treatment of stuttering: New directions* (pp. 149-169). Baltimore: Lippincott, Williams & Wilkins.

Kiser, A.M., Lass, N.J., Lockhart, P., Mussa, A.M., Pannbacker, M., Ruscello, D.M., & Schmidt, J.F. (1994). School administrator' perceptions of people who stutter. *Language, Speech, and Hearing Services in Schools*, 25, 90-93.

Klein, J. F., & Hood, S. B. (2004). The impact of stuttering on employment opportunities and job performance. *Journal of Fluency Disorders, 29*(4), 255-273.

Kleppe, S. A., Katayama, K. M., Shipley, K. G., & Foushee, D. R. (1990). The speech and language characteristics of children with Prader-Willi syndrome. *Journal of Speech and Hearing Disorders, 55*(2), 300-309.

Krauss-Lehrman, T., & Reeves, L. (1989). Attitudes toward speech-language pathology and support groups: Results of a survey of members of the National Stuttering Project. *Texas Journal of Audiology and Speech Pathology, 15*(1), 22-25.

Krishnan, G., & Tiwari, S. (2013). Differential diagnosis in developmental and acquired neurogenic stuttering: Do fluency-enhancing conditions dissociate the two? *Journal of Neurolinguistics*, 26(2), 252.

Kuster, J. (2004). Electronic Devices and Stuttering Treatment. Available on the Stuttering Home Page at: http://www.mnsu.edu/comdis/kuster/TherapyWWW/dafjanus.html.

Langevin, M. & Boberg, E. (1996) Results of intensive stuttering therapy with adults who clutter and stutter. *Journal of Fluency Disorders, 21,* 315-328.

Lankford, S. D., & Cooper, E. B. (1974). Recovery from stuttering as viewed by parents of self-diagnosed recovered stutterers. *Journal of Communication Disorders*, 7(2), 171-180.

LaSalle L. R. (2014) Slow Speech Rate Effects on Stuttering Preschoolers with Disordered Phonology. *Communication Disorders, Deaf Studies and Hearing Aids, 2*, 105-113.

LaSalle, L. R., & Conture, E. G. (1995). Disfluency Clusters of Children Who StutterRelation of Stutterings to Self-Repairs. *Journal of Speech, Language, and Hearing Research*, *38*(5), 965-977.

Lass, N. J., Ruscello, D. M., Bradshaw, K. H., & Blankenship, B. L. (1991). Adolescents' perceptions of normal and voice-disordered children. *Journal of Communication Disorders*, 24(4), 267-274.

Lass, N. J., Ruscello, D. M., Pannbacker, M., Schmitt, J. F., Kiser, A. M., Mussa, A. M., & Lockhart, P. (1994). School administrators' perceptions of people who stutter. *Language, Speech, and Hearing Services in Schools, 25*(2), 90-93.

Latulas, M., Tetnowski, J., & Bathel, J. (2003). Getting ready for therapy: Self-esteem and "coachability." Paper presented at the National Stuttering Association Convention, Nashville.

Lebrun, Y, & Van Borsel, J. (1990). Final sound repetitions. *Journal of Fluency Disorders 15*, 107- 113.

Lee, G. (2003) Bully pulpit: Forum takes on schools toughs. *Illionoistimes Online*, May 3rd. Available at http://illionoistimes.com/gbase/Gyrosite/Content?oid=oid%3A1975.

Leith, W. R. (1993). *Clinical methods in communication disorders.* Austin: Pro-Ed.

Lew, G.W., (2000). What parents can do for your child when he is being teased for stuttering. *In 3rd International Stuttering Awareness Day Conference (ISAD3).* Available at: http://www.parentcomdis/ISAD3/papers/lew.html.

Lincoln, M., Packman, A., Onslow, M., & Jones, M. (2010). An experimental investigation of the effect of altered auditory feedback on the conversational speech of adults who stutter. *Journal of Speech, Language, and Hearing Research, 53*(5), 1122-1131.

Logan, K. J. (2014). *Fluency Disorders.* San Diego: Plural Publishing.

Logan, K. J., & Haj-Tas, M. A. (2007). Effect of sample size on the measurement of stutter-like disfluencies. *SIG 4 Perspectives on Fluency and Fluency Disorders, 17*(3), 3-6.

Logan, K. J., & LaSalle, L. R. (1999). Grammatical characteristics of children's conversational utterances that contain disfluency clusters. *Journal of Speech, Language, and Hearing Research, 42*(1), 80-91.

Logan, K.J. & LaSalle, L.R. (2003). Developing intervention programs for children with stuttering and concomitant impairments. *Seminars in Speech and Language, 24(1)*, 13-19.

Logan, K. J., & O'Connor, E. M. (2012). Factors affecting occupational advice for speakers who do and do not stutter. *Journal of Fluency Disorders, 37*(1), 25-41.

Ludlow, C. L., Hoit, J., Kent, R., Ramig, L. O., Shrivastav, R., Strand, E., Yorkston, K., & Sapienza, C. (2008). Translating principles of neural plasticity into research on speech motor control recovery and rehabilitation. *Journal of Speech, Language, and Hearing Research, 51*(1), S240-S258.

Lyttle, J. (2002, March 27). "Heaps of laughter: Toward a philosophy of humor." Presentation as part of the Richard L. Connolly Faculty Forum at Long Island University, Brooklyn, NY.

Mackie, D.M., Hamiliton, D.L., Susskind, J., & Rosselli, F. (1996). Social psyschological foundations of stereotype formation. In C.N. Macrae, C. Stagnor, & M. Hewstone (Eds.), *Stereotypes and stereotyping*. New York: Guilford.

MacKinnon, S. P., Hall, S., & MacIntyre, P. D. (2007). Origins of the stuttering stereotype: Stereotype formation through anchoring–adjustment. *Journal of Fluency Disorders, 32*(4), 297-309.

Maguire, G. A., Yeh, C. Y., & Ito, B. S. (2012). Overview of the diagnosis and treatment of stuttering. *Journal of Experimental & Clinical Medicine, 4*(2), 92-97.

Maguire, G. A., Franklin, D. L., & Kirsten, J. (2011). Asenapine for the treatment of stuttering: an analysis of three cases. *The American Journal of Psychiatry, 168*(6), 651-652.

Manning, W. H. (1999). Progress under the surface and over time. In N. Bernstein Ratner & E. C. Healey (Eds.), *Stuttering Research and Practice: Bridging the Gap* (123-129). Mahwah, NJ: Lawrence Erlbaum Associates, Inc.

Manning, W. H. (2001). The demands and capacities model. *Journal of Fluency Disorders, 25*(4), 317-319.

Manning, W., & Beck, J. G. (2013). Personality dysfunction in adults who stutter: Another look. *Journal of Fluency Disorders, 38*(2), 184-192.

Manning, W. H., Dailey, D., & Wallace, S. (1984). Attitude and personality characteristics of older stutterers. *Journal of Fluency Disorders, 9*(3), 207-215.

Mansson H. (2007). Complexity and diversity in early childhood stuttering. In J. Au-Yeung & M. Leahy (Eds.), *Proceedings of the Fifth World Congress on Fluency Disorders* (pp. 98-101). Dublin, Ireland: The International Fluency Association.

Market, K. E., Montague, J. C., Buffalo, M. D., Drummond, S. S. (1990). Acquired stuttering. Descriptive data and treatment outcome. *Journal of Fluency Disorders, 15*, 21-33.

Marland, D. (2013, June 11). Healing the Stuttering Self. Retrieved December 8, 2014, from http://blog.asha.org/2013/06/11/healing-the-stuttering-self/

Martin, N. A. (2010). *Expressive One Word Picture Vocabulary Test* (4th ed.). San Antonio: Pearson Clinical.

Martin, N. A., & Brownwell, R. (2010). *Receptive One Word Picture Vocabulary Test* (4th ed.). San Antonio: Pearson Clinical.

Martin, R. R., & Lindamood, L. P. (1986). Stuttering and spontaneous recovery: Implications for the speech-language pathologist. *Language, Speech, and Hearing Services in Schools, 17*(3), 207-218.

Martineau, W. H. (1972). A model of the social functions of humor. *The psychology of humor: Theoretical perspectives and empirical issues*, 101-125.

Mass, E., Robin, D. A., Austermann Hula, S. A., Freedman, S. E., Wulf, G., Ballard, K. J., & Schmidt, R. A. (2008). Principles of motor learning in treatment of motor speech disorders. *American Journal of Speech-Language Pathology, 17*, 277-298.

Max, L., & Baldwin, C. J. (2010). The role of motor learning in stuttering adaptation: Repeated versus novel utterances in a practice–retention paradigm. *Journal of Fluency Disorders*, *35*(1), 33-43.

Max, L., Guenther, F. H., Gracco, V. L., Ghosh, S. S., & Wallace, M. E. (2004). Unstable or insufficiently activated internal models and feedback-biased motor control as sources of dysfluency: A theoretical model of stuttering. *Contemporary Issues in Communication Science and Disorders*, *31*,105-122.

Mayo, R., Mayo, C. M., Jenkins, K. C., & Graves, L. R. (2004). Public knowledge of stuttering: Cross-cultural perspectives. *SpeechPathology.com*, *1*.

McAllister, J., Collier, J., & Shepstone, L. (2012). The impact of adolescent stuttering on educational and employment outcomes: Evidence from a birth cohort study. *Journal of Fluency Disorders*, *37*(2), 106-121.

McClean, M. D., Kroll, R. M., & Loftus, N. S. (1990). Kinematic analysis of lip closure in stutterers' fluent speech. *Journal of Speech, Language, and Hearing Research*, *33*(4), 755-760.

McClean, M. D., & Runyan, C. M. (2000). Variations in the relative speeds of orofacial structures with stuttering severity. *Journal of Speech, Language, and Hearing Research*, *43*(6), 1524-1531.

McClure, J. A., & Yaruss, S. (2003). Stuttering survey suggests success of attitude changing treatment. *ASHA Leader, 8*(9), 3, 19.

McCroskey, J. C., Daly, J. A., Richmond, V. P., & Falcione, R. L. (1977). Studies of the relationship between communication apprehension and self-esteem. *Human Communication Research, 3(3)*, 269-277.

McKeehan, A. & Child, D. R. (1991). *Parents as partners: Treatment of childhood stuttering.* Logan, UT: Utah State University Dept. of Communicative Disorders.

McKenna, P. (2006). *Instant confidence.* United Kingdom: Bantam Press.

McLellan, D. (1989, March, 29). Stutter group pickets over 'Wanda' role. *Los Angeles Times.* Retrieved from: http://articles.latimes.com/1989-03-29/entertainment/ca-716_1_wanda-insults-people.

McNamee, K. (2014, June 26). Laughing your way to health. *Urbino Now.* Available at: http://2014.inurbino.net/laughing-your-way-to-health/

Meduna, L. J. (1948). Alteration of neurotic pattern by use of CO_2 inhalations. *Journal of Nervous and Mental Diseases, 108*, 373-374.

Menzies, R. G., O'Brian, S., Onslow, M., Packman, A., St Clare, T., & Block, S. (2008). An experimental clinical trial of a cognitive-behavior therapy package for chronic stuttering. *Journal of Speech, Language, and Hearing Research, 51*(6), 1451-1464.

Mewherter, M. (2012). Cincinnati Children's Hospital Medical Center: Best evidence statement: Evidence based practice for stuttering home programs in speech-language pathology. Retrieved from www.cincinnatichildrens.org/svc/alpha/h/health-policy/best.htm

Meyers, S. C., & Freeman, F. J. (1985). Interruptions as a variable in stuttering and disfluency. *Journal of Speech, Language, and Hearing Research, 28*(3), 428-435.

Miles, S., & Bernstein-Ratner, N. (2001). Parental language input to children at stuttering onset. *Journal of Speech, Language, and Hearing Research, 44*(5), 1116-1130.

Miles, T. (2014). No greater foe? Rethinking emotion and humour, with particular attention to the relationship between audience members and stand-up comedians. *Comedy Studies, 5* (1)

Millard, S. K., Edwards, S., & Cook, F. M. (2009). Parent-child interaction therapy: Adding to the evidence. *International Journal of Speech-Language Pathology, 11*(1), 61-76.

Millard, S. K., Nicholas, A., & Cook, F. M. (2008). Is parent-child interaction therapy effective in reducing stuttering? *Journal of Speech, Language, and Hearing Research, 51*(3), 636-650.

Miller, N. B., & Sammons, C. C. (1999). *Everybody's Different: Understanding and Changing Our Reactions to Disabilities.* Baltimore: Paul H. Brookes Publishing Co.

Molt, L. (1998). A Perspective On Neuropharmacological Agents And Stuttering: Are There Implications For A Cause As Well As A Cure?. *In 1st International Stuttering Awareness Day Online Conference (ISAD1).* Available at: http://www.mnsu.edu/comdis/isad/papers/molt.html

Molt, L. (2002). Fluency master/Speakeasy devices. In S. Hood, J. Kuster, D. Mallard, W Manning, L. Molt, R. W. Quesal, N. E. B. Ratner, P. Ramig, K. O. St. Louis, L. Shields, J. A. Tetnowski, D. F. Williams, & J. S. Yaruss. (2002). Office hours: The professor is in. *Interactive discussion on the 5th International Stuttering Awareness Day On-Line Conference (ISAD5).*

Montgomery, A. A., & Cooke, P. A. (1976). Perceptual and acoustic analysis of repetitions in stuttered speech. *Journal of Communication Disorders, 9*(4), 317-330.

Montgomery, B. M., & Fitch, J. L. (1988). The prevalence of stuttering in the hearing-impaired school age population. *Journal of Speech and Hearing Disorders, 53*(2), 131-135.

Moore, W. H. (1976). Bilateral tachistoscopic word perception of stutterers and normal subjects. *Brain and Language, 3*(3), 434-442.

Moore, W. H. (1984). Hemispheric alpha asymmetries during an electromyographic biofeedback procedure for stuttering: A single-subject experimental design. *Journal of Fluency Disorders, 9*(2), 143-162.

Moore, W. H. (1990). Pathophysiology of stuttering: Cerebral activation differences in stutterers vs. nonstutterers. *ASHA Reports Series (American Speech-Language-Hearing Association), 18.* 72-80.

Morreall, J. (1982). A new theory of laughter. *Philosophical Studies, 42*(2), 243-254.

Mundkur, N. (2005). Neuroplasticity in children. *Indian Journal of Pediatrics, 72*(10), 855-857.

Murphy, B. (2000). Speech pathologists can help children who are teased because they stutter. *In 3rd International Stuttering Awareness Day Online Conference (ISAD3).* Available at: http://www.mnsu.edu/dept/ comids/ISAD3/papers/murphy. html.

Murphy, W. P., & Quesal, R. W. (2002, August). Strategies for addressing bullying with the school-age child who stutters. *Seminars in Speech and Language, 23*(3), 205-212.

Murphy, W. P., Yaruss, J. S., & Quesal, R. W. (2007). Enhancing treatment for school-age children who stutter: I. Reducing negative reactions through desensitization and cognitive restructuring. *Journal of Fluency Disorders, 32*(2), 121-138.

Murray, F. P. & Edwards, S. G. (1994) *A Stutterer's Story* (Third printing). Memphis: Stuttering Foundation of America.

Myers, F. L., Bakker, K., St Louis, K. O., & Raphael, L. J. (2012). Disfluencies in cluttered speech. *Journal of Fluency Disorders, 37*(1), 9-19.

National Alliance on Mental Illness (2012). Available at: http://www.nami.org.

Neelley, J. N., & Timmons, R. J. (1967). Adaptation and consistency in the disfluent speech behavior of young stutterers and nonstutterers. *Journal of Speech, Language, and Hearing Research, 10*(2), 250-256.

Neilson, M. D., & Neilson, P. D. (1987). Speech motor control and stuttering: A computational model of adaptive sensory-motor processing. *Speech Communication, 6*(4), 325-333.

Newcomer, P. & Hammill, D. (2008). Test of Language Development-Primary (4th ed.). Austin: Pro-Ed.

Nsabimana, D. (2011). Report of the study of therapy for stuttering in Africa. *In 15th International Stuttering Awareness Day Online Conference (ISAD15)*. Available at: https://www.mnsu.edu/comdis/isad15/papers/rwanda15/nsabimana15.html

Ntourou, K., Conture, E. G., & Lipsey, M. W. (2011). Language abilities of children who stutter: A meta-analytical review. *American Journal of Speech-Language Pathology, 20*(3), 163-179.

Okasha, A., Bishry, Z., Kamel, M., & Hassan, A. H. (1974). Psychosocial study of stammering in Egyptian children. *The British Journal of Psychiatry, 124*(583), 531-533.

Onslow, M., Adams, R., & Ingham, R. (1992). Reliability of speech naturalness ratings of stuttered speech during treatment. *Journal of Speech, Language, and Hearing Research, 35*(5), 994-1001.

Onslow, M. & O'Brian, S. (2013). Management of childhood stuttering. *Journal of Paediatrics and Child Health, 49*(2).

Onslow, M., Packman, A., & Harrison, E. (2003). *The Lidcombe Program of early stuttering intervention: A clinician's guide.* Austin: Pro-Ed.

Orben, R. (2001). Some thoughts on humor. *The Gilner Center for Humor Studies.* Available at: http://www.amst.umd.edu/humorcenter/essays/orben1.htm

Otto, F. M., & Yairi, E. (1974). An analysis of speech disfluencies in Down's syndrome and in normally intelligent subjects. *Journal of Fluency Disorders, 1*(4), 26-32.

Özdemir, R. S., Louis, K. O. S., & Topbaş, S. (2011). Stuttering attitudes among Turkish family generations and neighbors from representative samples. *Journal of Fluency Disorders, 36*(4), 318-333.

Paden, E. P., Ambrose, N. G., & Yairi, E. (2002). Phonological progress during the first 2 years of stuttering. *Journal of Speech, Language, and Hearing Research, 45*(2), 256-267.

Palasik, S. (2013). Stuttering Suicide: Our experiences responsibilities. *Department of Speech-Language Pathology and Audiology.* Available at: http://works.bepress.com/scott_palasik/15.

Palasik, S., Gabel, R., Hughes, C., & Rusnak, E. (2012). Perceptions about occupational experiences by people who stutter. *SIG 4 Perspectives on Fluency and Fluency Disorders, 22*(1), 22-33.

Parry, W. (2009). Fighting employment discrimination for people who stutter – under the amended Americans with disabilities act. Available at: http://www.stutterlaw.com/adaaa.htm

Perkins, W., Rudas, J., Johnson, L., & Bell, J. (1976). Stuttering: Discoordination of phonation with articulation and respiration. *Journal of Speech, Language, and Hearing Research, 19*(3), 509-522

Perkins, W. H., Kent, R. D., & Curlee, R. F. (1991). A theory of neuropsycholinguistic function in stuttering. *Journal of Speech, Language, and Hearing Research, 34*(4), 734-752.

Plexico, L. W., & Burrus, E. (2012). Coping with a child who stutters: A phenomenological analysis. *Journal of Fluency Disorders, 37*(4), 275-288.

Plexico, L., Manning, W. H., & DiLollo, A. (2005). A phenomenological understanding of successful stuttering management. *Journal of Fluency Disorders, 30*(1), 1-22.

Pollard, R., Ellis, J. B., Finan, D., & Ramig, P. R. (2009). Effects of the SpeechEasy on objective and perceived aspects of stuttering: a 6-month, phase I clinical trial in naturalistic environments. *Journal of Speech, Language, and Hearing Research, 52*(2), 516-533.

Poulos, M. G., & Webster, W. G. (1991). Family history as a basis for subgrouping people who stutter. *Journal of Speech, Language, and Hearing Research, 34*(1), 5-10.

Prasse, J. E., & Kikano, G. E. (2008). Stuttering: An overview. *American Family Physician, 77*(9), 1271.

Preuss, J.B., Fewell, R.R., and Bennet, F.C. (1989). Vitamin therapy and children with Down syndrome: a review of research. *Exceptional Children, 55*, 336-341.

Quarrington, B. (1977). How do the various theories of stuttering facilitate our therapeutic approach? *Journal of Communication Disorders, 10*(1), 77-83.

Ramig, L. O., Fox, C., & Sapir, S. (2007). Speech disorders in Parkinson's disease and the effects of pharmacological, surgical and speech treatment with emphasis on Lee Silverman voice treatment (LSVT®). *Handbook of Clinical Neurology, 83*, 385-399.

Ramig, P. R. (1993). High reported spontaneous stuttering recovery rates fact or fiction? *Language, Speech, and Hearing Services in Schools, 24*(3), 156-160.

Ramig, P. R. (2003). Don't ever give up! In: *Advice to those who stutter* (3rd ed) (46-51). Memphis: Stuttering Foundation of America.

Ramig, P. R., Dodge, D. M. (2005). *The child and adolescent stuttering treatment and activity resource guide.* Clifton Park: Thomson Delmar Learning.

Ramig, P. R., Ellis, J. B., Pollard, R., & Finan, D. (2010). Application of the SpeechEasy to stuttering treatment: Introduction, background, and preliminary observations. *Treatment of stuttering: Conventional and emerging interventions.* Baltimore: Lippincott, Williams & Wilkins.

Ratyńska, J., Szkiełkowska, A., Markowska, R., Kurkowski, M., Mularzuk, M., & Skarżyński, H. (2012). Immediate speech fluency improvement after application of the Digital Speech Aid in stuttering patients. *Medical science monitor: international medical journal of experimental and clinical research, 18*(1), CR9.

Rautakoski, P., Hannus, T., Simberg, S., Sandnabba, N. K., & Santtila, P. (2012). Genetic and environmental effects on stuttering: a twin study from Finland. *Journal of Fluency Disorders, 37*(3), 202-210.

Raza, M. H., Gertz, E. M., Mundorff, J., Lukong, J., Kuster, J., Schäffer, A., Drayna, D. (2013). Linkage analysis of a large African family segregating stuttering suggests polygenic inheritance and assortative mating. *Human Genetics 132*, 385-396.

Records, M. A., Kidd, K. K., & Kidd, J. K. (1976). *Stuttering among relatives of stutters.* Address to the annual meeting of the American Speech and Hearing Association, Houston.

Reilly, S., Onslow, M., Packman, A., Cini, E., Conway, L., Ukoumunne, C. O., Bavin, E. L., Prior, M., Eadie, P., Block, S., & Wake, M. (2013). Natural history of stuttering to 4 years of age: A prospective community-based study. *Pediatrics, 132*(3), 460-467.

Resch, J. A., Elliott, T. R., & Benz, M. R. (2012). Depression among parents of children with disabilities. *Families, Systems, & Health, 30*(4), 291.

Results of survey on electronic devices (2004). *Stuttering Foundation of America* (newsletter), Winter.

Rice, M., & Kroll, R. (1994). A survey of stutterers' perceptions of challenges and discrimination in the workplace. *Journal of Fluency Disorders, 19*(3), 203.

Richels, C., Buhr, A., Conture, E., & Ntourou, K. (2010). Utterance complexity and stuttering on function words in preschool-age children who stutter. *Journal of Fluency Disorders, 35*(3), 314-331.

Riley, G. (2009). *The Stuttering Severity Instrument for Adults and Children* (SSI-4) (4th ed.). Austin: Pro-Ed.

Robb, M.P. (2012) *Invited Presentation: Application of motor learning principles in speech and nonspeech tasks.* Sun City, South Africa: South African Speech-Language-Hearing Association Congress (SASLHA), 3-6 Nov 2012.

Robles, M. M. (2012). Executive perceptions of the top 10 soft skills needed in today's workplace. *Business Communication Quarterly, 75*(4), 453-465.

Robinson, T., & Crowe, T. (2002). Fluency disorders. In E. Battle (Ed.), *Communication Disorders in Multicultural Populations*. Boston: Butterworth-Heinemann.

Rollin, W. J. (1987). *The psychology of communication disorders in individuals and their families*. Englewood Cliffs, NJ: Prentice-Hall.

Roth, F. P., Worthington, C. K. (2001). *Treatment resource manual for speech-language pathology* (2nd ed.). San Diego: Singular/Thompson Learning.

Roth, I., & Beal, D. (1999). Teasing and bullying of children who stutter. Retrieved from: http://www.stutteringhomepage.com

Rustin, L., & Cook, F. (1995). Parental involvement in the treatment of stuttering. *Language, Speech, and Hearing Services in Schools, 26*(2), 127-137.

Ryan, B. P. (2003). Treatment efficacy research and clinical treatment. *Perspectives on Fluency and Fluency Disorders, 13*(1), 31-33.

Sacco, P. (1992). The treatment of fluency disorders: From grandchild to grandparent. Workshop presented in Fort Pierce, FL, November 7.

Saxon, K. G., & Ludlow, C. L. (2007). A critical review of the effect of drugs on stuttering. In E. Conture & R. F. Curlee (Eds.), Stuttering and related disorders of fluency (3rd ed., pp. 277-293). New York: Thieme.

Schlagheck, A., Gabel, R., & Hughes, S. (2009). A mixed methods study of stereotypes of people who stutter. *Contemporary Issues in Communication Science and Disorders, 36*, 108-117.

Schlanger, B. B., & Gottsleben, R. H. (1957). Analysis of speech defects among the institutionalized mentally retarded. *The Journal of Speech and Hearing Disorders, 22*(1), 98-103.

Schloss, P. J., Freeman, C. A., Smith, M. A., & Espin, C. A. (1987). Influence of assertiveness training on the stuttering rates exhibited by three young adults. *Journal of Fluency Disorders, 12*(5), 333-353.

Schwartz, H. D. (1999). *A Primer of Stuttering Therapy*. Needham Heights, MA: Allyn and Bacon.

Schwartz, H. D., & Conture, E. G. (1988). Subgrouping Young Stutterers: Preliminary Behavioral Observations. *Journal of Speech, Language, and Hearing Research, 31*(1), 62-71.

Schwenk, K. A., Conture, E. G., & Walden, T. A. (2007). Reaction to background stimulation of preschool children who do and do not stutter. *Journal of Communication Disorders, 40*(2), 129-141.

Scotsman, The. (2002, June 12). Unusually funny. *The Scotsman.* Retrieved from: http://www.scotsman.com/news/unusually-funny-1-1374107

Sen, E., & Yurtsever, S. (2007). Difficulties experienced by families with disabled children. *Journal for Specialists in Pediatric Nursing, 12*(4), 238-252.

Shames, G., & Florence, C. (1980). *Stutter-free Speech: A Goal for Therapy.* Columbus: Charles Merrill.

Shapiro, D. A. (2011). *Stuttering intervention: A collaborative journey to fluency freedom* (2nd ed.). Austin: Pro-Ed.

Shearer, W. M., & Williams, J. D. (1965). Self-recovery from stuttering. *Journal of Speech and Hearing Disorders, 30*(3), 288-290.

Sheehan, J. (1958). Conflict theory of stuttering. In *Stuttering: A Symposium* (pp. 121-166). New York: Harper.

Sheehan, J. G. (1997). Message to a Stutterer. Available on the Stuttering Home Page at: http: https://www.mnsu.edu/comdis/kuster/Infostuttering/sheehanmessage.html

Sheehan, J. G. (2003). Message to a Stutterer. In: *Advice to Those who Stutter* (3rd ed.) (31-35). Memphis: Stuttering Foundation of America.

Sheehan, J. G., & Martyn, M. M. (1970). Stuttering and its Disappearance. *Journal of Speech, Language, and Hearing Research, 13*(2), 279-289.

Sheehan, V., Williams, D. F., & Dugan, P. (2001). Stuttering therapy: Treating the whole dis-order. *American Academy of Private Practice in Speech Pathology and Audiology Spring Conference*

Shenker, R. C., Kully, D., & Meltzer, A. (1998). Letter to the Editor Concerning the Leadership Conference. *American Speech-Language-Hearing Association Special Interest Division 4, Fluency & Fluency Disorders newsletter, 8(3)*, 9-10.

Sidavi, A., & Fabus, R. (2010). A review of stuttering intervention approaches for preschool-age elementary school-age children. *Contemporary Issues in Communication Science and Disorders, 37*, 14-26.

Siegel, G. M., & Gold, C. (1999). Principles and practices of current stuttering therapy. In R. F. Curlee (Ed.), *Stuttering and related disorders of fluency* (297-325). New York: Thieme.

Silverman, F. H., & Bongey, T. A. (1997). Nurses' attitudes toward physicians who stutter. *Journal of Fluency Disorders, 22(1)*, 61-62.

Silverman, F. H., & Paynter, K. K. (1990). Impact of stuttering on perception of occupational competence. *Journal of Fluency Disorders, 15(2)*, 87-91.

Silverman L. K. (2003). Gifted children with learning disabilities. In Colangelo N. & Davis G. A. (Eds.), *Handbook of gifted education* (3rd ed., pp. 533-543). Boston: Allyn & Bacon.

Smith, A., & Kelly, E. (1997). Stuttering: A dynamic, multifactorial model. *Nature and treatment of stuttering: New directions, 2*, 204-217.

Soderberg, G. A. (1967). Linguistic factors in stuttering. *Journal of Speech, Language, and Hearing Research, 10(4)*, 801-810.

Sommer, M., Koch, M. A., Paulus, W., Weiller, C., & Büchel, C. (2002). Disconnection of speech-relevant brain areas in persistent developmental stuttering. *The Lancet, 360*(9330), 380-383.

Sommers, R. K., Brady, W. A., & Moore Jr, W. H. (1975). Dichotic ear preferences of stuttering children and adults. *Perceptual and Motor Skills, 41*(3), 931-938.

Spines, C. (2010, April). Lady Gaga wants you. *Cosmopolitan, 34.*

St. Louis, K. O. & Myers, F. (1995). Clinical management of cluttering. *Language, Speech, and Hearing Services in the Schools, 26,* 187-194

St. Louis, K. O. S., Przepiorka, A. M., Beste-Guldborg, A., Williams, M. J., Blachnio, A., Guendouzi, J., Reichel, I. K., & Ware, M. B. (2014). Stuttering attitudes of students: Professional, intracultural, and international comparisons. *Journal of Fluency Disorders, 39,* 34-50.

St. Louis, K. O. S., Raphael, L. J., Myers, F. L., & Bakker, K. (2003). Cluttering updated. *ASHA Leader, 8*(4–5), 20-22.

St. Louis, K. O. S., & Westbrook, J. B. (1987). The effectiveness of treatment for stuttering. In L. Rustin, H. Purser, & D. Rowley (Eds.), *Progress in the treatment of fluency disorders.* London: Whurr.

Stager, S. V., & Ludlow, C. L. (1993). Speech production changes under fluency-evoking conditions in nonstuttering speakers. *Journal of Speech, Language, and Hearing Research, 36*(2), 245-253.

Stansfield, J., Collier, R., & King, R. (2012). Adults with intellectual impairment who stammer: A clinical case study. *British Journal of Learning Disabilities, 40*(1), 23-30.

Starkes, J. L., & Allard, F. (1993). *Cognitive issues in motor expertise.* Amsterdam: Elsevier.

Starkweather, C. W. (1987). *Fluency and stuttering.* Englewood Cliffs, NJ: Prentice-Hall.

Starkweather, C. W. (1990). Current trends in therapy for stuttering children and suggestions for future research. *ASHA Reports Series (American Speech-Language-Hearing Association), 18,* 82-90.

Starkweather, C.W. (2000). Talking to Parents about Stuttering. *In 3rd International Stuttering Awareness Day Online Conference (ISAD3).* Available at: https://www.mnsu.edu/comdis/ISAD3/papers/starkweather3.html.

Starkweather, C. W., & Givens-Ackerman, J. (1997). *Stuttering.* Austin: Pro-Ed.

Steele, C. M., & Southwick, L. (1985). Alcohol and social behavior: I. The psychology of drunken excess. *Journal of Personality and Social Psychology, 48*(1), 18.

Stein, J. (1993). Vocal alterations in schizophrenic speech. *Journal of Nervous and Mental Disease, 181*(1), 59-61.

Stocker, B., Goldfarb, R. (1995). The Stocker Probe for Fluency and Language. Vero Beach: Speech Bin, Inc.

Stone, A. (2010). Proceedings of the National Academy of Sciences. Available at http://www.webmd.com/balance/news/20100518/people-happier-less-stressed-after-middle-age.

Stuttering Foundation of America (2006). *Effective Counseling in Stuttering Therapy (2nd ed.).* Memphis: Stuttering Foundation of America.

Stromswold, K. (2006). Why aren't identical twins linguistically identical? Genetic, prenatal and postnatal factors. *Cognition, 101*(2), 333-384.

Styxx (2003, August 9). [Review of the comedy show *BIRDS*]. *The Edinburgh Festival Fringe*. Retrieved from: http://www.jaik-campbell.com/index.php/review-quotes?font-size=larger

Suicide Prevention Resource Center, & Rodgers, P. (2011). Understanding risk and protective factors for suicide: A primer for preventing suicide. Newton, MA: Education Development Center, Inc.

Sultanoff, S. (1995). Levity Defies Gravity; Using Humor in Crisis Situations. *Therapeutic Humor, 9*(3), 1-2.

Susca, M. (1997). Normalization of speech patterns in people who stutter. *Journal of Fluency Disorders, 22*(2), 123.

Takahama, V. (1991, February 11). When he talks about stuttering, filmmakers listen. *Orlando Sentinel*. Retrieved from: http://articles.orlandosentinel.com/1991-02-11/lifestyle/9102091161_1_stuttering-zimmerman-wanda.

Thatchell, R. H., Van den Berg, S., & Lerman, J. W. (1983). Fluency and eye contact as factors influencing observers' perceptions of stutterers. *Journal of Fluency Disorders, 8*(3), 221-231.

Theys, C., van Wieringen, A., & DeNil, L. F. (2008). A clinician survey of speech and non-speech characteristics of neurogenic stuttering. *Journal of Fluency Disorders, 33*(1), 1-23.

Throneburg, R. N., & Yairi, E. (1994). Temporal Dynamics of Repetitions During the Early Stage of Childhood Stuttering: An Acoustic Study. *Journal of Speech, Language, and Hearing Research, 37*(5), 1067-1075.

Throneburg, R. N., & Yairi, E. (2001). Durational, Proportionate, and Absolute Frequency Characteristics of Disfluencies: A Longitudinal Study Regarding Persistence and Recovery. *Journal of Speech, Language, and Hearing Research, 44*(1), 38-51.

Trajkovski, N., Andrews, C., Onslow, M., O'Brian, S., Packman, A., Menzies, R. (2009). Using syllable timed speech to treat preschool children who stutter: A multiple baseline experiment. *Journal of Fluency Disorders, 34*(1), 1-10.

Trajkovski, N., Andrews, C., Onslow, M., O'Brian, S., Packman, A., Menzies, R. (2011). A phase II trial of the Westmead program: Syllable-timed speech treatment for pre-school children who stutter. *International Journal of Speech-Language Pathology, 13*(6), 500-509.

Travis, L. E. (1978). The cerebral dominance theory of stuttering: 1931–1978. *Journal of Speech and Hearing Disorders, 43*(3), 278-281.

Travis, L. E. (1957). *Handbook of speech pathology and audiology.* New York: Appleton-Century-Crofts and Fleschner Publishing Company.

Trichon, M., & Tetnowski, J. (2011). Self-help conferences for people who stutter: A qualitative investigation. *Journal of Fluency Disorders, 36*(4), 290-295.

Tsiamtsiouris, J., & Cairns, H. S. (2013). Effects of sentence-structure complexity on speech initiation time and disfluency. *Journal of Fluency Disorders, 38*(1), 30-44.

Tudor, M. (1939). *An experimental study of the effect of evaluative labeling of speech fluency.* Unpublished master's thesis, University of Iowa.

Tuong, T. J., Traystman, R. J., & Hurn, P. D. (1998). Estrogen-mediated neuroprotection after experimental stroke in male rats. *Stroke, 29*, 1666-1670.

Turnbaugh, K. R., Guitar, B. E., & Hoffman, P. R. (1979). Speech clinicians' attribution of personality traits as a function of stuttering severity. *Journal of Speech, Language, and Hearing Research, 22*(1), 37-45.

Utterly Global (2015). Available at: http://antibullyingprograms.org.

Van Borsel, J., Brepoels, M., & De Coene, J. (2011). Stuttering, attractiveness and romantic relationships: The perception of adolescents and young adults. *Journal of Fluency Disorders*, *36*(1), 41-50.

Van Borsel, J.V, Drummond, D., & de Britto Pereira, M. M. (2010). Delayed auditory feedback and acquired neurogenic stuttering. *Journal of Neurolinguistics*, 23(5), 479-487.

Van Riper, C. (1973). *The Treatment of Stuttering*. Englewood Cliffs, NJ: Prentice-Hall.

Van Riper, C. (1982). *The Nature of Stuttering*, Second Edition, Englewood Cliffs, N.J.: Prentice-Hall.

Vanryckeghem, M., & Brutten, G., J. (2006) Communication Attitude Test for Preschool and Kindergarten Children Who Stutter (KiddyCAT). San Diego, CA: Plural Publishing.

Vanryckeghem, M., Brutten, G. J., & Hernandez, L. M. (2005). A comparative investigation of the speech-associated attitude of preschool and kindergarten children who do and do not stutter. *Journal of Fluency Disorders*, *30*(4), 307-318.

van Zaalen-Op 't Hof, Y., Wijnen, F., & De Jonckere, P. H. (2009). Differential diagnostic characteristics between cluttering and stuttering--part one. *Journal of Fluency Disorders*, 34(3), 137-154.

Wall, M. J., & Myers, F. L. (1995). *Clinical management of childhood stuttering*. Austin: Pro-ed.

Walton, P. (2008). A Multidimensional approach for Preschool Stuttering. SID-4 Leadership / Clinical Conference, Phoenix, AZ.

Walton, P., & Wallace, M. (1998). *Fun with fluency: Direct therapy with the young child*. Austin: Pro-Ed.

Ward, D. (2010). Sudden onset stuttering in an adult: Neurogenic and psychogenic perspectives. *Journal of Neurolinguistics*, 23(5), 511-517.

Ward, D., Connally, E., Pliatsikas, C., & Watkins, K. E. (2015). The neurological underpinnings of cluttering: Some initial findings. *Journal of Fluency Disorders*, 43, 1-16.

Ward, D., & Scaler-Scott, K. S. (2011). Treatment of cluttering: a cognitive-behavioral approach centered on rate control. *Cluttering: A handbook of research, intervention, and education*. Hove: Psychology Press.

Watkins, K. E., Smith, S. M., Davis, S., & Howell, P. (2008). Structural and functional abnormalities of the motor system in developmental stuttering. *Brain*, *131*(1), 50-59.

Watkins, R. V., & Yairi, E. (1997). Language production abilities of children whose stuttering persisted or recovered. *Journal of Speech, Language, and Hearing Research*, *40*(2), 385-399.

Watson, B. C., &: Alfonso, P. J. (1987). Physiological bases of acoustic LRT in nonstutterers, mild stutterers, and severe stutterers. *Journal of Speech and Hearing Research*, 30, 434-447.

Weber-Fox, C., Wray, A. H., & Arnold, H. (2013). Early childhood stuttering and electrophysiological indices of language processing. *Journal of Fluency Disorders*, *38*(2), 206-221.

Webster, D. (1999). *Neuroscience of Communication*. San Diego: Singular.

Webster, E. J. & Ward, L. M. (1993). *Working with Parents of Young Children with Disabilities* (Early Childhood Intervention Series). San Diego: Singular.

White, P. A., & Collins, S. R. (1984). Stereotype Formation by Inference: A Possible Explanation for the Stutterer Stereotype. *Journal of Speech, Language, and Hearing Research*, *27*(4), 567-570.

Wilder, L. (2013, Oct 19). *Stuttering and marriage.* Available at: http://www.stutter.ca/articles/research/121-stutter-ing-and-marriage.html

Williams, D. (1992, May 4). Remembering Wendell Johnson. Daily Iowan.

Williams, D. E., & Kent, L. R. (1958). Listener evaluations of speech interruptions. *Journal of Speech, Language, and Hearing Research, 1*(2), 124-131.

Williams, D. F. (2006). *Stuttering recovery: Personal and empirical perspectives.* Mahwah, N.J: Lawrence Erlbaum Associates.

Williams, D. F. (2008). Treating the gifted client. *Perspectives on Fluency and Fluency Disorders, 18,* 60-63, August.

Williams, D. F. (2012). *Communication Sciences and Disorders: An Introduction to the Professions.* New York: Taylor & Francis.

Williams, D. F., & Brutten, G. J. (1994). Physiologic and aerody-namic events prior to the speech of stutterers and nonstut-terers. *Journal of Fluency Disorders,19*(2), 83-111.

Williams, D. F. & Diaz, C. F. (2006). The stereotyping of people who stutter. In D. F. Williams, *Stuttering recovery: Personal and empirical perspectives* (75-82). Mahwah, NJ: Lawrence Er-lbaum Associates.

Williams, D. F. & Dugan, P. M. (2002). Administering stuttering mod-ification therapy in school settings. *Seminars in Speech and Language, 23*(3), 187-194.

Williams, D. F., G. N., & Campbell, J. (2015). Stuttering Comedians: What Can They Teach Us? *In 19th International Stuttering Awareness Day Online Conference (ISAD19).* Available at: http://isad.isastutter.org/isad-2015/papers-present-ed-by-2015/research-therapy-and-support/stuttering-come-dians-what-can-they-teach-us/

Williams, D. F., & Wener, D. L. (1996). Cluttering and stuttering exhibited in a young professional. *Journal of Fluency Disorders, 21*(3), 261-269.

Williams, D. F. & Williams, M. L. (2000). Helping the child who stutters: Guidelines for parents. *Parenting Plus*, March.

Wilson, C. (2007, August 10). [Review of the comedy show *L-L-Lost For Words: My life with a Stutter*]. *The Stage*.

Wilson, M. E. (2013). Stroke: Understanding the Differences between Males and Females. *Pflügers Archiv: European Journal of Physiology, 465*(5), 595–600.

Wingate, M. E. (1964). A standard definition of stuttering. *Journal of Speech and Hearing Disorders, 29*(4), 484-489.

Wingate, M. E. (1967). Stuttering and word length. *Journal of Speech, Language, and Hearing Research, 10*(1), 146-152.

Wingate, M. E. (1988). *The structure of stuttering: A psycholinguistic approach.* New York: Springer-Verlag.

Wolk, L., Edwards, M. L., & Conture, E. G. (1993). Coexistance of stuttering and disordered phonology in young children. *Journal of Speech, Language, and Hearing Research, 36*(5), 906-917.

Wolpe. J. (1982). *The practice of behavior therapy* (3rd ed.). New York: Pergamon Press.

Wong, C. T., Cheng, Y. Y., & Chen, L. M. (2013). Multiple perspectives on the targets and causes of school bullying. *Educational Psychology in Practice, 29*(3), 278-292.

Woods, C. L., & Williams, D. E. (1976). Traits attributed to stuttering and normally fluent males. *Journal of Speech, Language, and Hearing Research, 19*(2), 267-278.

Worchel, S. & Rothgerber, H. (1997). Changing the stereotype of the stereotype. In Spears, R., Oakes, P. J., Ellemers, N., & Haslam, S. A. *The Social Psychology of stereotyping and group life: Emphasizing the side of group perceptions* (pp. 72-93). London: Sage.

World Health Organization (2010). ICD-10 F95.8 - Stuttering. Retrieved from: http://apps.who.int/classifications/icd10/browse/2010/en#/F98.5

Worrell, P. R., Dreber, A., Rand, D. G., Wernerfelt, N., Zeckhauser, R. J. (2013). The decisions of entrepreneurs and their agents: Revealed levels of risk aversion and betrayal version. *Available at SSRN 2263282.*

Wright, P. (2002). From emotions to advocacy: The parents' journey. *Apraxia –Kids.* Available at http://www.wrightslaw.com/advoc/articles/Emotions.html

Wu, J. C., Maguire, G., Riley, G., Lee, A., Keator, D., Tang, C., James, F. & Najafi, A. (1997). Increased dopamine activity associated with stuttering. *Neuroreport, 8*(3), 767-770.

Yairi, E. (1981). Disfluencies of normally speaking two-year-old children. *Journal of Speech, Language, and Hearing Research, 24*(4), 490-495.

Yairi, E. (1990). Subtyping child stutterers for research purposes. *ASHA Reports, 18,* 50-57.

Yairi, E. (1997). Speech characteristics of early childhood stuttering. In R. Curlee and G. Siegel (Eds.), *Nature and treatment of stuttering.* Needham Heights, MA: Allyn and Bacon.

Yairi, E., & Ambrose, N. (1992). Onset of Stuttering in Preschool Children: Selected Factors. *Journal of Speech, Language, and Hearing Research, 35*(4), 782-788.

Yairi, E., & Ambrose, N. G. (2005). *Early childhood stuttering for clinicians by clinicians.* Austin: Pro Ed.

Yairi, E., Ambrose, N. G., Paden, E. P., & Throneburg, R. N. (1996). Predictive factors of persistence and recovery: Pathways of childhood stuttering. *Journal of Communication Disorders, 29*(1), 51-77.

Yairi, E., & Carrico, D. M. (1992). Early Childhood Stuttering Pediatricians' Attitudes and Practices. *American Journal of Speech-Language Pathology, 1*(3), 54-62.

Yairi, E., & Curlee, R. (November, 1995). *Early intervention in childhood stuttering: Myths and facts.* Paper presented at the annual convention of the American Speech-Language-Hearing Association, Orlando, FL.

Yairi, E., & Williams, D. E. (1970). Speech clinician's stereotypes of elementary-school boys who stutter. *Journal of Communication Disorders, 3*(3), 161-170.

Yaruss, J. S. (2010). Assessing quality of life in stuttering treatment outcomes research. *Journal of Fluency Disorders, 35*(3), 190-202.

Yaruss, J. S., & Quesal, R. W. (2001). The many faces of stuttering: Identifying appropriate treatment goals. *The ASHA Leader, 14*, 4-5.

Yaruss, J. S., & Quesal, R. W. (2006). Overall Assessment of the Speaker's Experience of Stuttering (OASES): Documenting multiple outcomes in stuttering treatment. *Journal of Fluency Disorders, 31*(2), 90-115.

Yaruss, J. S., & Quesal, R. W. (2010). *Overall Assessment of the Speaker's Experience of Stuttering.* Bloomington, MN: Pearson Assessments.

Yeakle, M. K., & Cooper, E. B. (1986). Teacher perceptions of stuttering. *Journal of Fluency Disorders, 11*(4), 345-359.

Zackheim, C. T., & Conture, E. (2003). Childhood stuttering and speech disfluencies in relation to children's mean length of utterance: A preliminary study. *Journal of Fluency Disorders, 28*, 115-142.

Zebrowski, P. M., & Conture, E. G. (1989). Judgments of disfluency by mothers of stuttering and normally fluent children. *Journal of Speech, Language, and Hearing Research, 32*(3), 625-634.

Zhang, Y., & Tan, A. (2011). Impact of mass media during the 2008 US presidential election: A cross-cultural study of stereotype change in China and the United States. *Communication Studies, 62*(4), 353-371.

Zimmerman, I. L., Steiner, V. G., & Pond, R. E. (2011). Preschool Language Scales (5th ed.). San Antonio: Pearson Clinical.

Zocchi, W., Estenne, M., Johnston, S., Del Ferro, L., Ward, M. E., & Macklem, P. T. (1990). Respiratory Muscle Incoordination in Stuttering Speech1-3. *American Review of Respiratory Disease, 141*, 1510-1515.

Index

A

B

H

I

J

K

L

CPSIA information can be obtained
at www.ICGtesting.com
Printed in the USA
LVHW051312250420
654387LV00013B/109

9 780987 347626